Voice and Communication Therapy for the Transgender/Gender Diverse Client

A Comprehensive Clinical Guide

Third Edition

Voice and Communication Therapy for the Transgender/Gender Diverse Client

A Comprehensive Clinical Guide

Third Edition

Edited by

Richard K. Adler, PhD, CCC-SLP
Sandy Hirsch, MS, CCC-SLP
Jack Pickering, PhD, CCC-SLP

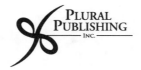

PLURAL
PUBLISHING
INC.

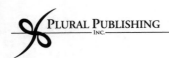

5521 Ruffin Road
San Diego, CA 92123

e-mail: information@pluralpublishing.com
Web site: http://www.pluralpublishing.com

FSC
www.fsc.org
MIX
Paper from
responsible sources
FSC® C011935

Typeset in 10.5/13 Garamond Book by Achorn International
Printed in the United States of America by McNaughton & Gunn, Inc.

Library of Congress Cataloging-in-Publication Data:

Names: Adler, Richard Kenneth, editor. | Hirsch, Sandy, editor. | Pickering, Jack, editor.
Title: Voice and communication therapy for the transgender/gender diverse client : a comprehensive clinical guide / [edited by] Richard K. Adler, Sandy Hirsch, Jack Pickering.
Other titles: Voice and communication therapy for the transgender/transsexual client
Description: Third edition. | San Diego, CA : Plural Publishing, [2019] | Preceded by Voice and communication therapy for the transgender/transsexual client / edited by Richard K. Adler, Sandy Hirsch, Michelle Mordaunt. 2nd ed. c2012. | Includes bibliographical references and index.
Identifiers: LCCN 2018028887| ISBN 9781944883300 (alk. paper) | ISBN 1944883304 (alk. paper)
Subjects: | MESH: Voice Training | Nonverbal Communication | Voice Quality |Transsexualism
Classification: LCC RF511.T73 | NLM WV 500 | DDC 616.85/500866—dc23
LC record available at https://lccn.loc.gov/2018028887

Contents

Preface

We are proud and humbled that 12 years on from our first edition in 2006, this text remains the only comprehensive clinical guide to voice and communication therapy for the transgender/gender diverse client. The number of voice clinicians, coaches, and trainers serving the needs of transgender/gender diverse people has continued to grow rapidly. The pressing need for such a text, as well as comprehensive graduate school planning around this topic, appears only to be increasing.

It was our hope at the writing of the second edition in 2012 that evidence-based practice would increase even further. This hope has been met by an exponential growth in research that touches on all aspects of working with transgender and gender diverse people. Since 2012, ASHA's special interest groups Voice and Voice Disorders, SIG 3, and Higher Education, SIG 10, have dedicated two online *Perspectives* publications to transgender work, the *International Journal of Transgenderism* has published a standards of care version 7 voice and communication companion document, and there has been a host of research articles published in the US and internationally that raise, and seek to answer, a multitude of critical questions.

In this third edition we have continued to blend research, clinically based guidelines, and art. Many of the same, and several new, contributing experts in the area of transgender voice and communication have consulted with one another and compared notes, and have further refined the crucible of the first and second editions. We have presented here the most up-to-date research and proven approaches to this challenging and endlessly satisfying specialty of voice. We are particularly honoured to have had Aaron Devor, PhD, from the University of Victoria, Canada, who holds the only chair in Transgender Studies, write our foreword. We are also pleased to have included the voice of the transgender actress Delia Kropp, whose perspective on voice sheds a personal and unique light for voice coaches, trainers, and speech-language pathologists.

In this edition, the transmasculine chapter is almost a text unto itself, with current research, and a comprehensive approach to assessment and therapy. Case studies are included, making the chapter excellent food for therapists embarking on working with trans men. We are also particularly pleased to have included a final chapter focusing on trans youth, entitled "A Call to Action." The increase in the number of young people transitioning has quite rightly gained the attention of clinicians and researchers across all disciplines. In our final chapter of this edition, we have provided a starting point for further discussion; a discussion that will hopefully lead to fluent and comprehensive services for young people in the school setting, and the integration of all necessary services in adolescent gender clinics.

Unique to this edition is a PluralPlus companion website with access to numerous resources, paired with each chapter, that enhance the already extensive in-text references. These include study questions as food for thought, which we hope will help graduate program planners and students to formalize their learning in this area of their voice training and clinical practica.

Working with transgender clients remains a humbling experience. It requires openness to the occasional intensely emotional session, and the ability to recognize the apparently fine line between voice clinician and psychotherapist. To this end, the psychotherapy and counseling chapters in this edition have been updated and extended to increase specific programmatic approaches, such as Adler's "Windows to the Voice." The Singing Chapter, also deeply grounded in the "soul" of our work, now includes a section on choral work.

The editors and contributing authors continue to assume that the reader has a moderate degree of voice as well as clinical expertise. As in the previous editions, we stress the importance of gaining voice experience before working with this population. Approaches that have been presented should still be interpreted as guidelines. Specific explanations and suggestions have been limited to allow for clinical individualism and creativity. We do not presume to know all of the answers.

We noted in the preface of the second edition that transgender women and men are transitioning with greater confidence. Support from employers and peers allows them to express who they are with openness and honesty. This continues to be the case, though we must never become complacent about educating the general population about transgender issues. We must continue to guide our clients as they navigate social and professional transitions across a landscape where consistent acceptance is not necessarily a given.

We remain deeply grateful to the many transgender and gender diverse clients who teach us to constantly question the meaning of "normal," and who entrust us with helping them to finally give an honest, genuine voice to personal truths that they may have heretofore kept silent. We continue to feel confident that any clinician, coach, or trainer embarking on a new journey in this area of expertise will feel honoured and equally grateful.

Sandy Hirsch, MS, CCC-SLP

Foreword

More than 30 years ago, when gender was still very binary and I was still in graduate school, I had my first practical lesson in voice therapy. I had made friends with a doctoral student named Alan. Although as a graduate student he was less athletic than he had once been, Alan had been an elite gymnast who had competed at the highest levels of sport. His background in sport showed in his broad shoulders, and in his heavily muscled upper body and arms. Alan was short in stature, but other than that, everything about his physical appearance was resolutely masculine and cisgender. However, Alan had an unusually high-pitched voice for a man and one day he complained to me that he was routinely mistaken for "Ellen" on the phone. I had no training as a voice therapist, but I had been studying gender for some years already, so I ventured to make a suggestion. "Alan," I said. "You're just too nice. Try being more rude on the phone." Sure enough, a couple of weeks later he came back to me to tell me that it had worked like a charm. When he stopped being so nice, the gender binary and sexism still being extremely strong, people on the phone recognized him as Alan, and the plague of being mistaken for "Ellen" was gone from his life.

Alan's story gave me just a very small glimpse into how much more goes into making a correct auditory gender impression. Most members of the general public, trans as well as cis, seem to assume that the most important, indeed the only, element that truly conveys gender is the pitch of one's voice. Although this is certainly important, as Alan's story and those of countless "whiskey-voiced" women illustrate, pitch alone may not be the deciding factor

tipping the scales toward, or away from, an individual being correctly gendered. As noted throughout this volume, voice generally remains a larger challenge for adult trans women than for trans men due to the powerful effects of testosterone on voice. As also noted throughout this book, such challenges for both transfeminine and transmasculine people are far from insurmountable with good training, much hard work, and patience.

In the decades since graduate school, I have devoted most of my career to working in trans and, more recently, non-binary communities, and with people who research and provide services to trans and non-binary folks. Despite the fact that voice is such a significant factor in attaining gender congruence, remarkably little professional attention had been given to voice until the inclusion of a section on voice and communication in the 2011 7th Version of the World Professional Association's *Standards of Care for the Health of Transsexual, Transgender, and Gender-nonconforming People*. Prior to 2011, other than speech and communications specialists, most professionals working in the field were heavily focused on hormone therapy and surgery as the requisite treatments for trans people. Speech and voice weren't considered core to a successful transition. As a member of the World Professional Association for Transgender Health (WPATH) *Standards of Care* committee for the 6th and 7th Versions, I witnessed the efforts of Richard Adler and his colleagues as they argued hard to convince the *Standards of Care* committee that we needed to include a small section on Voice and Communication Therapy in version 7. Thankfully, this is now an established part of the *Standards of Care,* which I have been assisting in having translated from English into an additional 17 languages. Voice and communications therapy are now recognized as essential to offer to people transitioning around the world.

I also know from numerous private one-to-one conversations with a great many trans and non-binary people that many people feel insecure about the sound of their voice. Despite this, there is relatively little public conversation among trans and non-binary folks about voice and speech training, especially among trans masculine people. I suspect that this is, in part, due to a certain degree of self-consciousness and reluctance to call attention to one's voice when one feels that it may be less persuasive than they wish it to be. I also suspect that some of the relative silence on this issue is born of the mistaken belief that there is little that can be done other than to live with the effects of testosterone—mostly happily for those on the transmasculine spectrum, not so for those on the transfeminine spectrum, and in complex ways for non-binary people. Certainly, the authors and consumers of this edited collection know that this is far from true, and one especially welcome addition in this third edition of *Voice and Communication Therapy for the Transgender/Gender Diverse Client* is a significant chapter addressing the previously underserved voice and communication needs of transmasculine individuals.

My positions as the world's only Chair in Transgender Studies and as the Founder and Academic Director of the world's largest Transgender Archives (part of the University of Victoria Libraries in Victoria, British Columbia, Canada) provide me with a unique perspective on the historical position of voice and communication therapy for the transgender/gender diverse client. There is simply nothing else like these books, now or in the past. The first two editions filled a void and have already made huge contributions to improving the lives of transgender people around the globe.

This third volume has the potential to make an even more valuable contribution to "training the trainers" by building on the work of the first two editions and by so doing, providing a larger and better informed cadre of speech language professionals with specialized skills of benefit to trans and non-binary people. It is my hope that the knowledge transmitted by this volume will encourage more trans and non-binary people to feel confident that, should they seek out professional help to reach their voice goals, they will be met with effective and compassionate assistance.

It has been an honour to be a part of this important project.

Aaron H. Devor, PhD, FSSS, FSTLHE
Chair in Transgender Studies
Founder and Academic Director
The Transgender Archives
Professor, Sociology Department
University of Victoria
Victoria, Canada

Acknowledgments

Dr. Adler would like to acknowledge the hundreds of transmasculine and transfeminine clients he has worked with over the past 35 years. Their enthusiasm, determination and bravery inspired Dr. Adler to advocate for equality and acceptance of Transgender Communities and to mentor other SLPs to do the same. Some special thanks go to his husband Dave Purcell for his support and encouragement. Dr. Adler would also like to thank his many undergraduate and graduate students over the many years of University teaching, supervision and research who have been excellent students, clinicians, researchers and learners. Their respect, acceptance and enthusiasm for training/therapy with Transmasculine and Transfeminine clients was very inspiring and helped him move forward each time an obstacle seemed to try and get in his way. Dr. Adler wants to thank his co-authors/ co-editors Sandy Hirsch and Jack Pickering for their encouragement, love, patience, and enthusiasm with this edition and for being able to be there to talk when he needed extra encouragement. Finally, he would also like to thank the ASHA staff who were helpful as he pursued his research, teaching, and clinical work with Transgender clients. Finally, he would like to thank the many ASHA members (professors, clinicians, and researchers) who he contacted and who had become mentors who encouraged him to continue his work throughout his career.

Sandy Hirsch would like to acknowledge her husband, Jim West, for his editing ears, eagle eye, and ever-loving patience; also her sons Finn and Johnny West, for their pride, love and encouragement; to her siblings, Nicky and Peter Hirsch for their listening and humour; and to innumerable friends who have buoyed her throughout this project. Thanks to her brilliant, passionate colleagues all over the world, tirelessly doing research and clinical work in the area of gender diverse voice and communication training. She expresses deep gratitude to her co-editors Richard Adler and Jack Pickering; their gracious, egoless intelligence and commitment is second-to-none. Sandy is humbled by her clients who teach her as much, and often more, than she teaches them. Finally, thanks to, and in loving memory of her parents, John and Becky Hirsch, who encouraged Sandy to turn a thing on its side so as to develop a unique perspective.

Jack Pickering would like to acknowledge all of the transgender and gender nonconforming people who have been involved in the Saint Rose program, as well as those he has met along the way because of his experience in transgender voice and communication. Thanks to Dan Kayajian, an incredible co-director, and the multitude of graduate students who have made the program work and grow for over 10 years. He wishes to thank Arlene Lev for that initial phone contact, asking if he knew anyone who worked on voice with people who are transgender. Jack is grateful for his colleagues at The College of Saint Rose who encourage, support, and provide an exceptional place to work. Jack thanks his wife, Kelly, and the boys, Matthew and Benjamin, for their love and support. Special thanks to Richard and Sandy for asking him to be part of this incredible project! Finally, Jack acknowledges John Pettit, his first mentor and the individual who got him interested in voice almost 40 years ago. Dr. Pettit encouraged him to do a thesis at the University of Maine, a study that focused on gender and voice.

Editors and Contributors

Editors

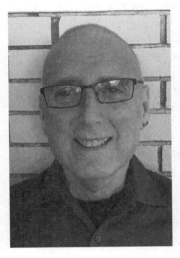

Richard K. Adler, PhD, CCC-SLP, ASHA Fellow, is now retired and a Professor Emeritus from Minnesota State University Moorhead, Moorhead, MN. He has a BA in speech correction from Long Island University, Brooklyn, an MA in Speech/Linguistics from New York University, an MA in Speech-Language Pathology from the University of Akron, Ohio, and a PhD in Psycholinguistics and Communication from the Ohio University, Athens, Ohio. Dr. Adler's career has spanned nearly 50 years as an SLP in public schools, hospitals, private practice, university teaching, clinical supervision, research, mentoring, consulting, and writing. He has published many articles on such subjects as Teaching, Voice and Communication for Transgender individuals, Voice Disorders, Counseling, and TBI.

Dr. Adler has also presented nearly 90 workshops and seminars at local, and several state and national conferences including the ASHA convention, The World Professional Association for Transgender Health (WPATH) symposia, and several State Speech and Hearing Association Conventions. He has provided voice and communication training/therapy for Transgender clients for the past 35 years and is currently mentoring students, faculty, and clinical SLPs in this area. Dr. Adler has also been an invited keynote speaker throughout the US, Europe, and Asia in the area of Transgender Voice and Communication. He was the first SLP to be appointed to the writing committee for the WPATH Standards of Care, VII and he was a founding member and the first chair of the standing committee on Voice and Communication issues for WPATH. Dr. Adler lives in Ann Arbor, Michigan with his husband Dave.

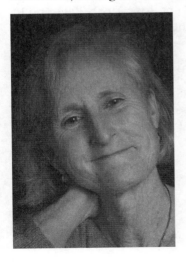

Sandy Hirsch, MS, CCC-SLP, is a private practitioner with Give Voice in Seattle, WA. She received her BA in French and Classics with a minor in music (singing) in 1981 from Lancaster University, UK. Following, she pursued a career in theatre and moved to the United States from London in 1982. Ms. Hirsch received her MS in Speech and Hearing Sciences from the University of Washington in 1989. She has been an ASHA-certified SLP since 1990, focusing on voice and neurological disorders. She has practiced in hospital and school settings. For over 25 years, Ms. Hirsch has made voice and communication modification with gender diverse people the focus of her private practice. She is a member of the Ingersoll Transgender Professional Consult

Group in Seattle, WA, WPATH, CPATH, the Voice Foundation, the Northwest Chapter of the Voice Foundation, VASTA and WSHLA.

Since 2007, Ms. Hirsch has been teaching workshops nationally and internationally to clinicians, voice coaches and trainers who are committed to improving the quality of life of gender diverse people. She has presented extensively on gender diverse voice and communication modification at the Esprit Gala in Port Angeles, WA, ASHA, the Voice Foundation Symposium, the Art and Science of Performance Voice in Seattle, WA, Gender Odyssey and CPATH. Ms. Hirsch has been a guest lecturer at the University of Washington and Western Washington University as well as for medical residents in Seattle. In addition to this text, she has contributed to ASHA's SIG 10 Higher Education *Perspectives* publication, and her work has been featured extensively in newsprint, as well as on national radio and television media. Privately, Ms. Hirsch continues to pursue her passion for languages as well as classical and jazz singing.

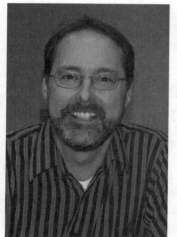

Jack Pickering, PhD, CCC-SLP, is a Professor of Communication Sciences and Disorders at The College of Saint Rose in Albany, New York and speech-language pathologist for Capital Region ENT. For over 10 years, he has directed the college's Voice and Communication Program for People in the Transgender Community with Dan Kayajian, MS, CCC-SLP. Jack has been an ASHA-certified SLP since 1984, focusing on the assessment and treatment of voice disorders. He received his BA and MA from the University of Maine, and his doctoral degree in Speech and Hearing Sciences at Ohio University in 1990. His teaching interests include voice disorders, transgender voice and communication, motor speech disorders, and counseling for communication disorders.

Jack has given over 160 presentations and has published in the areas of voice disorders, transgender voice and communication, issues in higher education, and computer applications. He was the Chair of the Department of Communication Sciences and Disorders at The College of Saint Rose, 1999–2004; and Interim Dean of the Saint Rose School of Education during the 2005–2006 academic year. Jack also served as the President of the New York State Speech-Language-Hearing Association in 2006. In 2010, he was presented with the Distinguished Clinician Award from the New York State Speech-Language-Hearing Association, and was the 2011 and 2012 American Speech-Language-Hearing Foundation's Clinical Achievement Award winner for the state of New York. This recognition was based on his work in transgender voice and communication. Jack is a member of the World Professional Association for Transgender Health (WPATH).

Contributors

Christine Adaire, MFA
Head of Voice
American Conservatory Theatre
San Francisco, California
Chapter 15

Christella Antoni, BA Hons, MSc, MRCSLT, HCPC
National Advisor, Royal College of Speech and Language Therapists
Independent Practice
ENT Department, Charing Cross Hospital
RCSLT Representative, British Laryngological Association
London, United Kingdom
Chapter 8

Christie Block, MA, MS, CCC-SLP
Clinical Speech-Language Pathologist
Owner, New York Speech and Voice Lab
BlueSleep Snoring and Sleep Apnea Center
ENT and Allergy Associates
New York, New York
Chapter 9

Joan Boonin, MS, CCC-SLP
Speech-Language Pathologist, Retired
University of Michigan Health System
Med Rehab
Ann Arbor, Michigan
Chapters 11 and 12

Darren Cosgrove, LMSW
Choices Counseling and Consulting
Albany, NY
Chapter 2

Timothy S. Crumley, LMHC
Clinical Director
Hospitality House TC Inc.
Psychotherapist

Choices Counseling
Albany, New York
Chapter 2

Georgia Dacakis, PhD, BAppSc (SpPath), MEd
Adjunct Lecturer
Discipline of Speech Pathology
School of Allied Health
La Trobe University
Melbourne, Australia
Chapter 7

Aaron H. Devor, PhD, FSSS, FSTLHE
Chair in Transgender Studies
Founder and Academic Director
The Transgender Archives
Professor, Sociology Department
University of Victoria
Victoria, Canada
Foreword

Cecilia Dhejne, MD
Centre for Psychiatry Research
Department of Clinical Neuroscience
Karolinska Institutet
ANOVA, Center of Expertise in Andrology, Sexual Medicine and Transgender Medicine
Karolinska University Hospital
Stockholm, Sweden
Chapter 1

Marylou Pausewang Gelfer, PhD, CCC-SLP
Professor and Graduate Program Coordinator
Department of Communication Sciences and Disorders
University of Wisconsin–Milwaukee
Milwaukee, Wisconsin
Chapters 10 and 11

McKenzee Greene, B.S.
College of Saint Rose
Albany, NY
Chapter 5

Linda Gromko, MD
Medical Director
Queen Anne Medical Associates, PLLC
Seattle, Washington
Chapter 4

Sandra C. Hammond, BA
Founder, Butterfly Music Transgender
    Chorus
Founder and President, Butterfly Partners,
    LLC
Boston, Massachusetts
Chapter 14

Kevin Hatfield, MD
The Polyclinic
Seattle, WA
Chapter 4

Leah B. Helou, PhD, CCC-SLP
Voice Pathologist
Director of Transgender Voice
    and Communication Training
    Program
UPMC Voice Center
Department of Otolaryngology
University of Pittsburgh Medical
    Center
Pittsburgh, Pennsylvania
Chapter 16

Stellan Hertegård, MD, PhD
Karolinska University Hospital
Department of Otorhinolaryngology
Karolinska Institutet
Department of Clinical Sciences and
    Intervention
Stockholm, Sweden
Chapter 1

Daniel M. Kayajian, MS, CCC-SLP
Speech Language Pathologist
Associate Director, Voice, Swallowing,
    and Airway Program
Albany Medical Center Hospital
Division of Otolaryngology
Adjunct Professor
Co-Director, Voice Modification Program
    for Transgender Individuals
The College of St. Rose
Albany, New York
Chapter 13

Anita L. Kozan, PhD, CCC-SLP
Director
Kozan Clinic for Voice, Speech and Spirit,
    LLC
Co-Producer and Co-Host
BI CITIES cable television show
St. Paul Neighborhood Network
Minneapolis, Minnesota
Chapter 14

Delia Kropp
Company Member
Pride Films and Plays
Chicago, Illinois
Chapter 15

Arlene Lev, LCSW-R, CASAC
University at Albany
School of Social Welfare
Clinical Director
Choices Counseling and Consulting
    Director
Director, The Institute for Gender,
    Relationships, Identity, and Sexuality
Albany, New York
Chapter 2

Michelle Mordaunt, MS, CCC-SLP
Speech Language Pathologist
Seattle, Washington
Chapters 10 and 13

Ulrika Nygren, PhD, SLP
Karolinska Institutet
Department of Clinical Science,
    Intervention and Technology
Division of Speech and Language
    Pathology
Karolinska University Hospital
Functional Area Speech and Language
    Pathology
Stockholm, Sweden
Chapter 1

Jennifer M. Oates, PhD
Associate Professor
Discipline of Speech Pathology
School of Allied Health
La Trobe University
Melbourne, Australia
Chapter 6

Viktória G. Papp, PhD, MSc, MA
Lecturer in Linguistics
University of Canterbury

New Zealand Institute of Language, Brain,
    and Behaviour Christchurch, New
    Zealand
Chapter 9

Rebecca Root, MA
Voice Studies
Voice Teacher and Actor
London, United Kingdom
Chapter 15

Maria Södersten, PhD, SLP
Associate Professor
Karolinska Institutet
Department of Clinical Science,
    Intervention and Technology
Division of Speech and Language
    Pathology
Karolinska University Hospital
Functional Area Speech and Language
    Pathology
Stockholm, Sweden
Chapter 1

To our families; with love and thanks for their undying patience, yet again

To our clients who trust us to help them with their courageous journey

In memory of those who lost hope

1

A Multidisciplinary Approach to Transgender Health

Maria Södersten, Ulrika Nygren, Stellan Hertegård, and Cecilia Dhejne

Introduction

Transgender health care varies around the world. In many countries, transgender people live on the margin of the society with insecure conditions to support themselves, with risks to become victims of hate crimes, including murder, or laws that make gender non-confirming expressions illegal (Winter et al., 2016). To support transgender health care around the world, the World Professional Association for Transgender Health (WPATH) issues Standards of Care (SOC). A multidisciplinary approach is recommended by WPATH in SOC number 7 (Coleman et al., 2012), since several specialized professionals are needed for assessments and different interventions to establish the best care for a transgender individual.

This chapter aims to introduce the reader to a multidisciplinary approach to transgender health from the standpoint of the field of voice and communication within the context of a multidisciplinary model established and implemented in Sweden. The chapter contains information about definitions and diagnoses; legislation and statistics of the large increase of transgender individuals seeking medical help; the organization of our multidisciplinary team; routines for voice assessment, voice and communication therapy, and pitch-raising surgery; and examples of educational and quality enhancement activities.

Definitions and Diagnoses

Gender identity refers to an innate and deeply felt psychological identification as a female, male, or a non-binary gender. Gender identity may be congruent or incongruent with the sex assigned at birth. Gender dysphoria refers to the discomfort or distress that gender incongruence may cause. The clinical presentation for a person with gender dysphoria generally includes discomfort with the sex characteristics of the assigned sex at birth and an urge for medical help to alter the phenotypic expression of the body. Requests may include treatment with sex hormones, surgery to change primary and secondary sex characteristics, voice modification, saving germ cells for later parenthood, pitch-raising surgery and hair removal in individuals who were assigned male at birth, psychiatric support or psychotherapy during the transition, and a new legal gender.

If gender incongruence causes distress, the individual could meet the criteria for a formal diagnosis. According to the American Psychiatric Association's (APA) current diagnostic system, the *Diagnostic and Statistical Manual for Mental Disorders, Fifth Edition* (DSM-5) from 2013, the diagnosis is labeled Gender Dysphoria. According to the World Health Organization's (WHO, 2010) *International Classification of Diseases and Related Health Problems, 10th Revision* (ICD-10), Gender Identity Disorders (F64) are Transsexualism (F64.0), Other Gender Identity Disorders (F64.8), or Gender Identity Disorder Not Otherwise Specified (F64.9).

For many years there has been a discussion questioning that a formal diagnosis of gender dysphoria is classified as a psychiatric diagnosis according to both DSM-5 and ICD-10. A revision of the diagnostic systems has been needed to meet the new research knowledge, policies and laws, human rights, as well as changed norms and attitudes in society. There has been a lot of effort made to move the gender dysphoria diagnosis from DSM-5 to reduce stigma (Pfäfflin, 2011), but to secure access to health care the diagnosis is still included in the DSM-5. In the revision of ICD-10 to ICD-11 it is proposed that gender identity disorders will be re-conceptualized to Gender Incongruence and moved from the Chapter "Mental and Behavioural Disorders" to a new chapter named "Conditions Related to Sexual Health" (Reed et al., 2016). The proposed changes in the ICD-11 are considered, according to the authors, "to be (a) more reflective of current scientific evidence and

best practices; (b) more responsive to the needs, experience, and human rights of vulnerable populations; and (c) more supportive of the provision of accessible and high-quality health care services" (Reed et al., 2016, p. 218). The ICD-11 is expected to be launched in 2018. The proposed move of the diagnoses from the psychiatric chapter to a chapter for conditions related to sexual health in ICD-11 will certainly affect transgender health care, but how is difficult to say.

The terminology and concepts within the area of gender incongruence and gender dysphoria have changed over the years. Previously it was common that experts talked about "sex change" from male-to-female (MtF) or from female-to-male (FtM) transsexuals, and later the word "sex correction" was used. Today the words "gender-affirming" or "gender-confirming" treatment are more and more used, which better reflect what the transition is about. Trans* (with an asterisk) is an umbrella term used if one wants to include all different trans identities, not only transgender women or men, within the gender identity spectrum. Transmasculine is a broad term used to describe a person assigned female sex at birth having a gender expression leaning toward the masculine, whereas transfeminine describes a person assigned male at birth having a gender expression leaning toward the feminine (Zeluf et al., 2016). Persons with gender identity in congruency with the sex assigned at birth are named cisgender persons or cispersons. WPATH recommends the use of "transgender woman" for someone with a female gender identity who was assigned male at birth and "transgender man" for someone with a male gender identity who was assigned female at birth. We will in this chapter use the terms "transgender women" and "transgender men," since they are so far in the majority among those who seek gender-affirming voice and communication therapy. All transgender individuals do not need medical health care, but some do. In this chapter, we will use the word "patient" when we describe the clinical work with transgender individuals who need assessments and interventions within medical health care.

Legislation and Statistics

The transgender health care organizations for transgender people differ around the world. In many countries, there are no medical services available at all, while multidisciplinary teams exist in some countries, although waiting time and costs for treatment differ.

Sweden was the first country in the world to enact a law regulating a person's legal right to change her or his sex assigned at birth. The law was created in 1972 and revised in 2013 by omitting a former sterilization prerequisite (Dhejne, 2017). The current law states that: (a) if the person has for a long time had a feeling of not belonging to the gender assigned at birth; (b) has lived in accordance with that experienced gender identity during a time; and (c) is anticipated to continue to live in this gender identity in the future, he or she can obtain permission for legal gender recognition and gender-affirming genital surgery. Requirements are that the person is over 18 years and has a residence permit in Sweden. Currently, there is a suggestion to legally allow change of assigned sex at birth at the age of 12 years with permission from parents or guardians, and at the age of 15 years without. The Legal Board of the National Board of Health and Welfare handles applications from all persons who re-

quest a legal sex change and permission for gender-affirming genital surgery. This procedure puts Sweden in a unique situation to assess trends and changes in number of applications and decisions about sex change over the years.

Statistics since 1960 are available regarding the number of applications, permissions, genital surgeries, new legal status, as well as withdrawals and regrets reported by Wålinder (1971), Landén, Wålinder, and Lundström (1996), and more recently Dhejne, Öberg, Arver, and Landén (2014). From 1972 to 2010 the incidence of applications increased significantly for both transgender men and transgender women. For transgender men, the increase was 0.16 to 0.42/100,000/year, and for transgender women from 0.23 to 0.73/100,000/year. The point prevalence in 2010 for transgender men was 1:13,120 and for transgender women 1:7,750. The average ratio during the period 1972 to 2010 was 1:1.66 (transgender men:transgender women) and the number of approved applications was 89%. A large increase of applications was found after 2000 as shown in Figure 1–1, especially after the 2013 law revision, when the request for sterilization was removed, along with the implicit requirement for gender-affirming genital surgery. A substantial increase of persons seeking medical help because of gender dysphoria or gender incongruence has been reported from many other countries as well, also including children, adolescents, and non-binary people (for an overview, see Dhejne, 2017).

The average regret rate, defined as applications to the National Board of Health and Welfare for reversal to the sex assigned at birth, was 2.2 percent for both sexes during the 50 years 1960 to 2010. From 2001 to 2010, the regret rate decreased significantly to 0.3 percent over the 10-year period (Dhejne

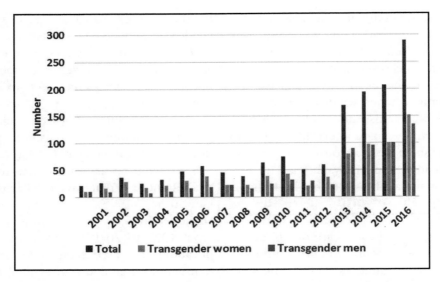

Figure 1–1. Number of applications for legal sex change and gender-affirming genital surgery to the National Board of Health and Welfare in Sweden from 2000 to 2016, presented as total number, and for transgender women and transgender men separated.

et al., 2014). During 2016, approximately 910 individuals >18 years of age and 410 youths <18 years of age were referred to the gender teams in all of Sweden to start assessment because of gender incongruence (Statistics from the Swedish Association for Transsexual Health).

There is a growing interest regarding a potential link between gender dysphoria and Autism Spectrum Disorder (ASD), and clinicians report seeing more gender dysphoric individuals with ASD (de Vries, Noens, Cohen-Kettenis, Berckelaer-Onnes, & Doreleijers, 2010; Jacobs, Rachlin, Erickson-Schroth, & Janssen 2014). A recent systematic review showed higher prevalence of ASD in children and adolescents with gender dysphoria, compared with the general population, whereas studies on adults showed conflicting results. Firm conclusions regarding adults were also hampered by a limited amount of studies (Glidden, Bouman, Jones, & Arcelius, 2016).

Organization of Specialized Multidisciplinary Gender Teams

Multidisciplinary gender teams are recommended by WPATH in the SOC 7 (Coleman et al. 2012), and in some countries, such teams have been developed. In Sweden, multidisciplinary teams have been developed since 2007, when the Swedish Association for Transsexual Health was launched. Today there are six specialized psychiatric gender teams, all at university hospitals. Those teams are responsible for the diagnostic assessments and coordination of gender-affirming medical interventions. One to four speech-language pathologists (SLPs) are for the moment associated with each gender team. Through the Swedish national health insurance system, the costs for medical care, such as diagnostic assessment, hormone treatment, voice and communication therapy, most surgeries including pitch-raising surgery, and hair removal, are covered. Because of the increasing number of patients seeking medical help, the waiting time for assessment and treatments are, for many patients, unacceptably long.

The psychiatric gender teams consist of psychiatrists, psychologists, and social workers and follow a consensus program for evaluating gender dysphoria. The program was updated in 2015 by the National Board of Health and Welfare to make it more congruent with WPATH's SOC 7 (Coleman et al., 2012). The main changes were: (a) a more flexible and individualized evaluation process; (b) that gender-affirming medical treatment should not be reserved for transgender persons who fulfill the criteria of Transsexualism, but could also be offered to those with "other gender identity disorders" and "unspecified gender identity disorder"; (c) fertility preservation should be offered to patients prior to gender-affirming medical

treatment; and (d) facial feminization surgery and hip liposuction could be offered in some cases. The guidelines also emphasize the importance of working in multidisciplinary teams. The diagnostic evaluation procedure is adjusted to the person's needs and varies between 6 and 12 months in Sweden (National Board of Health and Welfare, 2015), as seen in Figure 1–2.

A recent review of 38 cross-sectional studies showed that psychiatric disorders, such as depression and anxiety, are significantly more common among transgender people in the beginning and after the transition, compared with a cisgender population, but also that psychiatric well-being improves during gender-affirming medical interventions (Dhejne et al., 2011; Dhejne, Van Vlerken, Heylens, & Arcelus, 2016).

After the psychiatric assessment resulting in a confirmed diagnosis, the patients are referred to endocrinologists for hormonal treatment, speech-language pathologists for

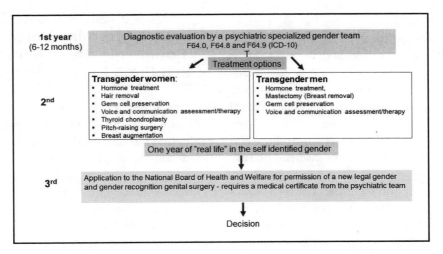

Figure 1–2. Flow chart showing the procedure for diagnostics and treatment options for transgender women and transgender men. The treatment starts after a diagnosis has been confirmed and can vary for different patients. Voice and communication therapy often continues later than during the second year. Pitch-raising surgery may be performed after voice therapy, often later than during the second year, and followed by post-surgery voice therapy. Hormone treatment will continue lifelong.

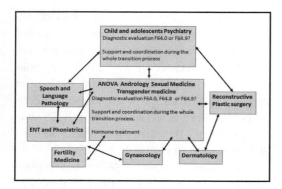

Figure 1–3. Flow chart showing the complex referral ways and interactions between the different specialists in the extended gender team at Karolinska University Hospital. Courtesy of Karolinska University Hospital.

voice assessment and if needed voice and communication therapy, ENT-physicians specialized in phoniatrics for laryngeal assessment, gynecologists for germ cell preservation, dermatologists for hair removal (for transgender women), and reconstructive plastic surgeons for gender-affirming surgical interventions. Individuals requesting a new legal sex and genital surgery must live in the self-identified gender for one year. After that they can apply to the National Board of Health and Welfare, and a certificate is required from the psychiatric gender team, supporting the application. Although the gender team tries to follow the ideal clinical program as shown in Figure 1–2, very often patients are referred back and forth between the specialists. Thus, a more realistic picture of the clinical work is shown in Figure 1–3.

The extended gender team at Karolinska University Hospital has regular meetings to discuss administrative issues such as waiting lists, new procedures, and, if needed, difficult cases. An advantage of a multidisciplinary team is that all professionals working with intervention, such as SLPs and surgeons, can be in close contact with the psychiatric team when needed. Many

patients are vulnerable because of affective and anxiety disorders. (Dhejne et al., 2016). Thus, SLPs meet and can have a relatively long contact with patients who may also be depressed or have anxiety disorders. It is a great advantage that the SLP, or a surgeon, can get support from a psychiatrist, psychologist, or other mental health professionals, if needed. Sometimes the psychiatric team needs to be informed, for example, by an SLP, that a patient is not emotionally stable during a period when the patient does not have regular contact with the psychiatric team.

Once a year, the extended gender team at Karolinska University Hospital organizes a day to educate the general public, patients, family members, trans organizations, and health care personnel about gender dysphoria, assessments, treatments, and recent research. Representatives from each professional area participate with short lectures, thus reflecting that the work with transgender patients within health care is multidisciplinary.

Voice Assessments, Gender-Affirming Voice and Communication Therapy, and Pitch-Raising Surgery

As seen in Figure 1–2, patients are referred for voice assessment when the psychiatric evaluation has led to a decision about a gender dysphoria diagnosis, such as Transsexualism (F64.0) or, since 2015, the diagnoses "Other Gender Identity Disorders" (F64.8) and "Gender Identity Disorders Not Otherwise Specified" (F64.9). That means that some patients are rather early in their transition process when they first meet the SLP. Some individuals may not yet present themselves in accordance to their self-identified gender role, or may not have thought about their voice much, whereas others have been living in the self-identified gender for a long time and may experience voice dysphoria. Our clinical experience is that it is of value, for both the patient and the SLP, to meet early in the process for information, a baseline voice recording, vocal hygiene instructions, and if needed, a plan for voice and communication therapy and/or follow-up. The clinical procedure and therapy programs at Karolinska University Hospital, as described by Södersten, Nygren, Hertegård, and Dhejne (2015), follow the chapter about Voice and Communication Therapy in SOC 7 (Coleman et al., 2012), as well as WPATH's Companion Document for Voice and Communication (Davies, Papp, & Antoni, 2015). When nonbinary individuals are referred because of voice dysphoria, they go through part of the voice assessments described below. Since no questionnaires or therapy programs are yet developed for this group, assessment and therapy are individually designed until research data are available.

Voice Assessment for Transgender Women

The voice assessment includes: (a) an interview to obtain demographic data; (b) patient self-evaluations using the Transsexual Voice Questionnaire, TVQ^{MtF} (Dacakis, Davies, Oates, Douglas, & Johnston, 2013), and the Voice Handicap Index (VHI) if the transgender woman shows signs of a voice disorder (Jacobson et al. 1997; Ohlsson & Dotevall, 2009); (c) audio recordings carried out according to a standard setting in a sound-treated booth, as well as (d) videolaryngostroboscopy, optimally carried out before the voice therapy starts. If the patient is concerned by a prominent thyroid cartilage, the shape of the larynx is video-recorded from the front and the side of the neck, during rest and swallowing.

Audio Recordings for Transgender Women

The speech material used for the audio recordings are: (a) reading of a standard text and narrating to a series of pictures in habitual voice, comprising a Speech Range Profile (SRP) visualized in Figure 1–4A and B; (b) sustained vowels; (c) reading of the standard text in a loud voice and heard over pink noise presented through headphones at a level of 70 dBA; (d) a Voice Range Profile (VRP), as seen in Figure 1–4C, performed to document the physiological voice range for frequency and sound pressure level (SPL) described by Ternström, Pabon, and Södersten (2016). We follow the guidelines by Hallin, Fröst, Holmberg, and Södersten (2012), which have also been used in other studies of transgender individuals (Holmberg, Oates, Dacakis, & Grant, 2010; Sanchez, Oates, Dacakis, & Holmberg, 2014).

For transgender women, the recordings are carried out before and after gender-affirming feminizing voice and communication therapy (see Figure 1–4), and after 6 months follow-up. A VRP is not recorded again after voice therapy, since it is not expected to change. If pitch-raising surgery is performed, recordings are done before and after surgery (see Figure 1–5), and at follow-up, optimally after 3, 6, and 12 months.

Voice Assessment for Transgender Men

As for transgender women, the assessment for transgender men includes an interview and self-evaluations of the voice related to gender identity, although no reliable or valid questionnaire yet exists. If the transgender man shows signs of a voice disorder, the VHI is used. Audio recordings are completed following the standard setting in a sound-treated booth. Transgender men are

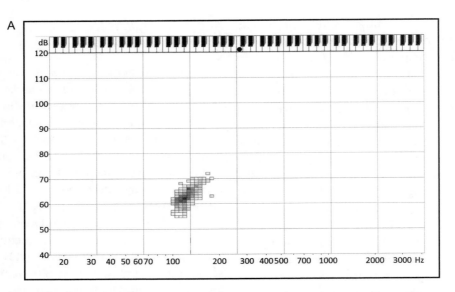

Figure 1–4. Speech Range Profiles from readings of a standard text and narration to pictures (**A**) before voice therapy and (**B**) after eight sessions of voice therapy for the same transgender woman. The x-axis shows fundamental frequency (in Hz) and the y-axis sound pressure level (in dB at 30 cm). The average f_0 increased from a male frequency of 120 Hz before therapy to a female frequency of 197 Hz after. The average sound pressure level, measured using L_{eq}, increased from 64 to 70 dB. Her Voice Range Profile is shown in (**C**) with min f_0 of 78 Hz indicated.

referred for videolaryngostroboscopy only if they have symptoms related to a voice disorder other than those related to the expected voice change during treatment with testosterone. Through the assessment, transgender men are screened for potential voice problems, so that voice therapy can be offered, if needed (Azul, Nygren, Södersten, & Neuschaefer-Rube, 2017; Nygren, Nordenskjöld, Arver, & Södersten, 2016).

Audio Recordings for Transgender Men

Audio recordings are done using the same speech material as for transgender women. The recordings of SRPs and VRPs are recommended to be carried out before hormone treatment once testosterone starts, after 3 or 6 months, and after 12 months (Figure 1–6) to follow the voice change during testosterone treatment (Deuster, Di Vincenzo, Szukaj, Am Zehnhoff-Dinnesen, & Dobel, 2016; Nygren et al., 2016).

Data Analyses of the Audio Recordings. The voice recordings for both transgender women and transgender men are analyzed audio-perceptually. The speech and voice range profiles are analyzed acoustically using fundamental frequency measures (average f_0, minimum f_0, and maximum f_0) and sound pressure level measures (L_{eq}, minimum and maximum SPL) following the recommendations by Hallin et al. (2012) and Ternström et al. (2016).

Gender-Affirming Voice and Communication Therapy for Transgender Women

Voice and communication therapy with the goal to feminize the voice to be congruent

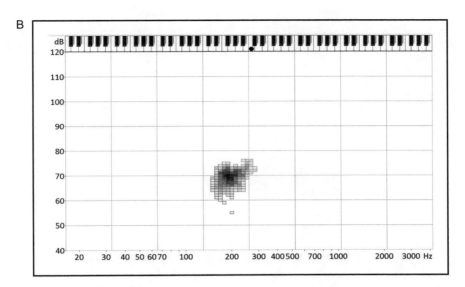

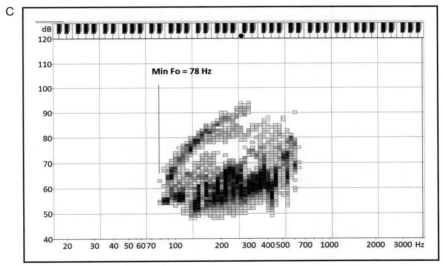

Figure 1–4. *(continued)*

with the person's self-identified gender is an important part of gender-affirming treatment. To be perceived as the self-identified gender has been acknowledged as a predictor for good outcomes and reduced gender dysphoria (Coleman et al., 2012; Smith, van Goozen, Kuiper, & Cohen-Kettenis, 2005; Van de Grift et al., 2016).

Voice therapy comprises breathing, relaxation, and vocal function exercises to in-crease vocal flexibility and prevent vocal fatigue (e.g., Angadi, Croake, & Stemple, 2017; Söderpalm, Larsson, & Almquist, 2004). To feminize the voice, it is necessary to adapt fundamental frequency, sound pressure level, voice quality, and articulation to reach a female-sounding voice. Specific chapters in this book (Chapters 7, 8, 10–13) give de-tailed information about voice and communication therapy. Although evidence for

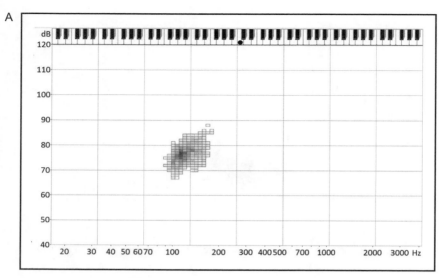

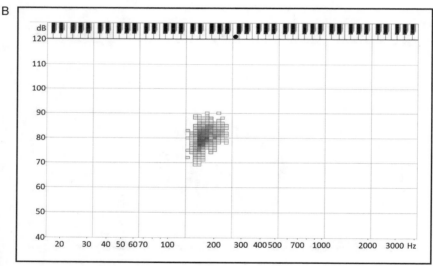

Figure 1–5. Speech Range Profiles (**A** and **B**) and Voice Range Profiles (**C** and **D**) before (**A** and **C**) and after (**B** and **D**) surgery with CTA for one transgender woman. The *x*-axis shows fundamental frequency (in Hz) and the *y*-axis sound pressure level (in dB at 15 cm). Average f_0 increased from a male frequency of 120 Hz (**A**) before surgery to 170 Hz after (**B**) and the sound level increased from 78 to 82 dB (15 cm). The desired increase in min f_0 from 78 Hz (**C**) to 131 Hz (**D**) is shown. Note also the decrease of max f_0 from 740 Hz to 440 Hz, which is not desired, as that reduces the frequency range.

feminizing voice and communication therapy is still scarce, there is an increasing number of publications supporting positive outcomes (for a review, see Oates, 2012; Oates & Dacakis, 2015; Chapter 6 in this book).

Pitch-Raising Surgery and Thyroid Chondroplasty

Surgery is an option after voice and communication therapy has been carried out.

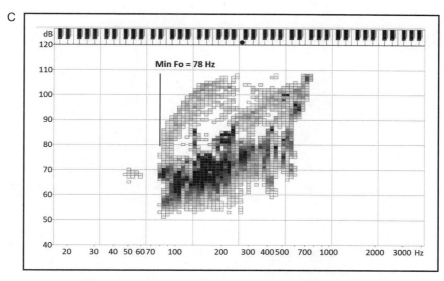

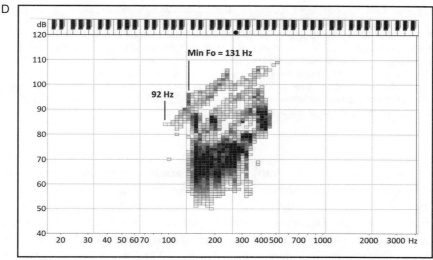

Figure 1–5. *(continued)*

The criteria for considering pitch-raising surgery are: (a) inability or great difficulties for the patient to modify pitch; (b) difficulties transferring a female pitch to everyday situations; (c) involuntary pitch drops when coughing and sneezing; and (d) severe vocal fatigue or strain when using a female voice. The decision is usually made during a joint meeting with the patient, the SLP, and the ENT-surgeon present. Audio recordings, data from acoustic analyses, patient's self-evaluations, and vocal fold status from videolaryngostroboscopy are available before and after voice and communication therapy, and form the basis for the discussion and decision.

Two surgical techniques have been used at Karolinska University Hospital over the years: cricothyroid approximation (CTA) and glottoplasty (GP), that is, an anterior web

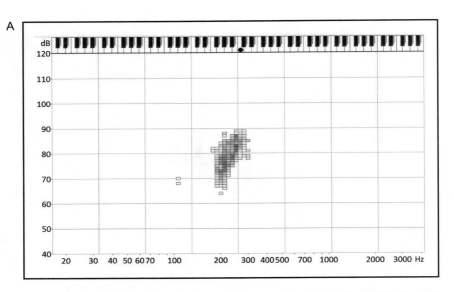

Figures 1–6. Speech Range Profiles (**A**, **B**, and **C**) and Voice Range Profiles (**D**, **E**, and **F**) for one transgender man before (**A** and **D**) testosterone treatment, after 3 months (**B** and **E**), and after 12 months (**C** and **F**). The x-axis shows fundamental frequency (in Hz), and the y-axis sound pressure level (in dB). The average f_0 decreased from a female pitch of 221 Hz (**A**) before treatment to 185 Hz (**B**) after 3 months, and to a male pitch of 103 Hz (**C**) after one year of testosterone treatment. In the Voice Range Profiles the min f_0 is indicated with a decrease from 175 Hz (**D**) before to 104 Hz (**E**) after three months, and to 73 Hz (**F**) after one year. Note that the L_{eq} data for figure (**C**) could be recalculated to 78 dB at 15 cm distance for comparison (+ 6 dB).

formation. Postoperative voice therapy is given at our hospital, since it is common that the voice becomes weaker and dysphonic and experiences a limited pitch range after surgery (e.g., Song & Jiang 2017). The postoperative voice therapy focuses mainly on vocal hygiene education and voice ergonomics, relaxed phonation, improving the voice quality if dysphonia occurs, and varying pitch to prevent a limited voice range.

In a systematic review by Van Damme, Cosyns, Deman, Van den Eede, and Van Borsel (2017), 20 studies were selected for analyses. CTA had been used in 8, anterior web formation in 6, and other techniques or combinations in 6. Among the results, a substantial rise in speaking f_0 after surgery was found for all techniques, and a majority of the patients were satisfied. An even more recent systematic review and meta-analysis

of 13 studies confirmed some of the findings by Van Damme et al. (2017), but also that the vocal fold shortening techniques appeared to result in a larger increase of speaking f_0 and less dysphonia (Song & Jiang, 2017). In a retrospective study, we recently analyzed data from 24 patients and compared long-term voice outcomes between CTA and GP, based on data from SRPs and VRPs and patients' subjective ratings (Kelly, Hertegård, Eriksson, Nygren, & Södersten, 2018). Both surgery techniques showed an increase of average f_0 after voice therapy and after surgery, and were stable after that, in agreement with results from other studies (Song & Jiang, 2017; Van Damme et al., 2017). There were statistically significant differences regarding VRP and self-rated data in favor of GP. Since a limited pitch range and hoarseness are common af-

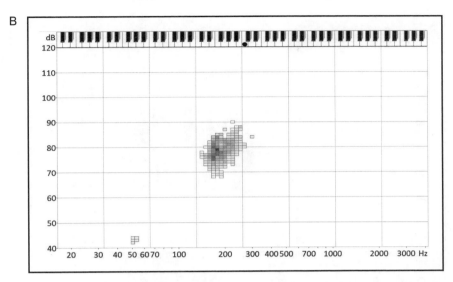

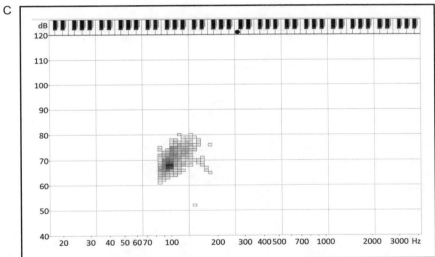

Figures 1–6. (continued)

ter pitch-raising surgery (Kelly et al., in press; Kim, 2017; Song & Jiang, 2017; Van Damme et al., 2017), postoperative voice therapy is strongly recommended.

Some transgender women need to reduce the prominent notch of their thyroid cartilage (Matai, Cheesman, & Clarke, 2003). The patients who ask for surgery are usually allowed it if the diagnosis of Gender Dysphoria has been given. Exclusion criteria are age <18 years (because the larynx may still grow), local infection, other local anatomical deviations, and special psychiatric conditions, such as dysmorphophobia.

Voice Therapy for Transgender Men

Performing voice recordings before the start of testosterone treatment and during treatment gives a great opportunity for the

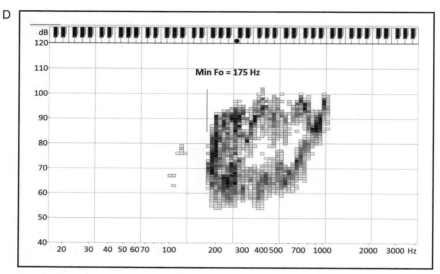

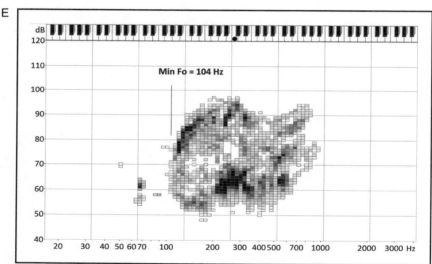

Figures 1–6. (*continued*)

patient and the SLP to follow the voice masculinization process. Testosterone treatment causes a masculinization of the voice, which is true for a majority of transgender men. Usually satisfaction with the voice gradually increases during the testosterone treatment (Deuster et al., 2016; Nygren et al., 2016). However, recent studies have shown that the number of individuals who experience vocal fatigue, vocal instability, difficulties projecting the voice or increased

loudness, and dissatisfaction with voice pitch or voice quality is not negligible (Azul, 2015; Azul et al., 2017). In one study, approximately 24% of transgender men engaged in a period of voice therapy according to results from a retrospective longitudinal study of 50 individuals (Nygren et al., 2016). This finding is in accordance with results from other studies that also emphasize that the need for voice therapy for transgender men should not be underesti-

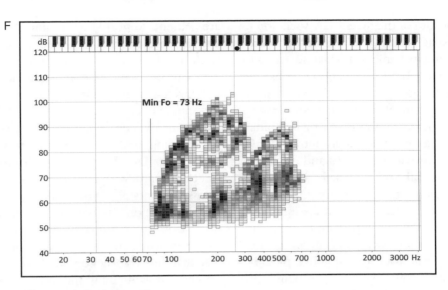

Figures 1–6. (continued)

mated (Cosyns et al., 2014; Nygren, 2014; Scheidt, Kob, Willmes, & Neuschaefer-Rube, 2004; Söderpalm et al., 2004; Van Borsel, De Cuypere, Rubens, & Destaerke, 2000).

Voice therapy for transgender men mainly includes exercises to reduce vocal fatigue and vocal instability, as well as exercises to lower the voice pitch, increase voice sound pressure level, project the voice, and improve voice quality (Nygren, 2014; Söderpalm et al., 2004). Patients' self-ratings of the voice, e.g., "satisfaction with the voice" related to their gender identity, are especially important when decisions about voice therapy are made, due to the heterogeneity of the transmasculine population (Azul, 2015; Papp, 2011). See Chapter 9 for further information about transmasculine clients' voices.

Educational Activities and Quality Enhancement of Care

To work with transgender individuals requires training to achieve the special competence needed, as stated in WPATH's SOC 7 (Coleman et al., 2012). The rapid development of the transgender field also requires *continuous* education and updates for colleagues within all professions who work with transgender women, transgender men, and non-binary individuals. Many initiatives for continuing education are taking place around the world, for example, papers written for ASHA's Special Interest Group in Higher Education (SIG 10).

The European Professional Association for Transgender Health (EPATH) was officially launched during the WPATH conference in Bangkok in February 2014. In March 2015, the first conference arranged by EPATH was held in Ghent in Belgium, and in April 2017 the second was arranged in Belgrade, Serbia. The goal of EPATH is to promote mental, physical, and social health and increase the quality of life among transgender people in Europe, and to ensure transgender people's rights for healthy development and well-being. The conferences arranged by EPATH and WPATH give very good updates on current research within the field of transgender health.

One aim of the Swedish Association for Transsexual Health (which is in the process of changing its name to Transgender Health) has been to develop a national consensus program for assessments and treatments for all disciplines involved in the medical care of patients who are transgender or non-binary. The association arranges an annual conference that provides updates and education, relevant for all, and especially for new colleagues entering the field. One part of the conference is that each profession meets and discusses issues important to its specific area. At another session, each professional group reports from its respective meetings to inform the other professions, which provides a multidisciplinary context. For example, the SLP group, with representatives from the six extended gender teams, has agreed on what should be included in voice assessment. Many countries today have similar regional or national organizations, including the United States, Australia, and Canada.

A National Quality Registry for Gender Dysphoria

When assessments and interventions within transgender health care are carried out in a systematic way, it is possible to build a bank of valuable data. Although the number of transgender individuals is increasing within health care in Sweden, and in other countries as well, they are still a small group compared with many other patient groups.

A system of national quality registries has been established in the last decade within the Swedish health and medical services. One national quality registry contains relevant data from specific patient groups such as waiting time for the first visit or to treatment, patient diagnosis, evaluation procedures, medical interventions, and outcomes after treatment. Especially important

are Patient Reported Outcome Measures and Patient Reported Experience Measures. Each registry is annually monitored so that data can be used for continuous learning, improvement, and research to create the best possible care. There are about 100 registries in Sweden today that receive central funding, and one is the new registry for Gender Dysphoria. A multidisciplinary steering board, with all specialists involved in assessments and gender-affirming medical interventions, as well as one representative from the national LGBT organization (the Swedish Federation for Lesbian, Gay, Bisexual and Transgender Rights) is in the process of launching the registry (Beckman & Sundin, 2017). The registry will be a unique source to ensure equal treatment throughout the country, and to provide data concerning patient satisfaction, life quality, and lifelong psychiatric and somatic health.

Concluding Remarks

The area of transgender and gender incongruence is changing remarkably fast in regard to political legislations, vocabulary and semantics, and societal opinions among the general public around the world. The number of individuals who seek medical help for gender dysphoria is growing rapidly in many countries, and the group is becoming increasingly more diverse. The view of gender as a binary classification is changing because gender identity has been shown to be much more multifaceted and complex. This creates special demands on the health care systems and specialists. Medical care needs to be adopted to meet each individual patient's special need for treatment. We find it necessary that specialists in the field collaborate in multidisciplinary teams to: (a) learn from each other; (b) help each other to follow and interpret the political, legislative, and cultural changes; (c) advocate for change; (d) conduct research; and (e) implement knowledge from new research into clinical practice.

References

American Psychiatric Association. (2013). *Diagnostic and Statistical Manual of Mental Disorders, Fifth Edition.* Arlington, VA: Author.

Angadi, V., Croake, D., & Stemple, J. (2017, Nov 3). Effects of vocal function exercises: A systematic review. *Journal of Voice.* p. ii: S0892-1997 (16)30446-5. doi:10.1016/j.jvoice.2017.08.031

Azul, D. (2015). Transmasculine people's vocal situations: A critical review of gender-related discourses and empirical data. *International Journal of Language and Communication Disorders, 50*(1), 31–47. doi:10.1111/1460-6984.12121

Azul, D., Nygren, U., Södersten, M., & Neuschaefer-Rube, C. (2017). Transmasculine people's voice function: A review of the currently available evidence. *Journal of Voice, 31*(2), 261.e9–261.e223. doi:10.1016/j.jvoice.2016.05.005

Beckman, U., & Sundin, M. (2017). *The national Swedish quality register for transgender health.* Oral presentation at the 2nd EPATH Conference, Belgrade, April 6–8, 2017.

Coleman, E., Bockting, W., Botzer, M., Cohen-Kettenis, P., DeCuypere, G., Feldman, J., . . . Zucker, K. (2012). Standards of care for the health of transsexual, transgender, and gender-nonconforming people, Version 7. *International Journal of Transgenderism, 13*(4), 165–232. doi:10.1080/15532739.2011.700873

Cosyns, M., Van Borsel, J., Wierckx, K., Dedecker, D., Van de Peer, F., Daelman, T., Laenen, S., & T'Sjoen, G. (2014). Voice in female-to-male transsexual persons after long-term androgen therapy. *Laryngoscope, 124*(6), 1409–1414. doi:10.1002/lary.24480

Dacakis, G., Davies, S., Oates, J., Douglas, J. M., & Johnston, J. R. (2013). Development and preliminary evaluation of the Transsexual Voice Questionnaire for male-to-female transsexuals. *Journal of Voice, 27*(3), 312–321. doi:10.1016/j.jvoice.2012.11.005

Davies, S., Papp, V. G., & Antoni, C. (2015). Voice and communication change for gender nonconforming individuals: Giving voice to the person inside. *International Journal of Transgenderism, (16)*3, 117–159. doi:10.1080/15532739.2015.1075931

Deuster, D., Di Vincenzo, K., Szukaj, M., Am Zehnhoff-Dinnesen, A., & Dobel, C. (2016). Change of speech fundamental frequency explains the satisfaction with voice in response to testosterone therapy in female-to-male gender dysphoric individuals. *European Archives of Oto-Rhino-Laryngology, 273*(8), 2127–2131. doi:10.1007/s00405-016-4043-0

de Vries, A. L., Noens, I. L., Cohen-Kettenis, P. T., van Berckelaer-Onnes, I. A., & Doreleijers, T. A. (2010). Autism spectrum disorders in gender dysphoric children and adolescents. *Journal of Autism and Developmental Disorders, 40*(8), 930–936. doi:10.1007/s10803-010-0935-9

Dhejne, C. (2017). *On gender dysphoria.* Doctoral dissertation. Published by Karolinska Institutet, Department of Department of Clinical Neuroscience. Stockholm, Sweden. Retrieved from https://openarchive.ki.se/xmlui/handle/10616/45580

Dhejne, C., Lichtenstein, P., Boman, M., Johansson, A. L., Långström, N., & Landén, M. (2011). Long-term follow-up of transsexual persons undergoing sex reassignment surgery: Cohort study in Sweden. *Plos One, 6*(2), e16885. doi:10.1371/journal.pone.0016885

Dhejne, C., Öberg, K., Arver, S., & Landen, M. (2014). An analysis of all applications for sex reassignment surgery in Sweden, 1960–2010: Prevalence, incidence, and regrets. *Archives of Sexual Behavior, 43*(8), 1535–1545. doi:10.1007/s10508-014-0300-8

Dhejne, C., Van Vlerken, R., Heylens, G., & Arcelus, J. (2016). Mental health and gender dysphoria: A review of the literature. *International Review of Psychiatry, 28*(1), 44–57. doi:10.3109/09540261.2015.1115753

Glidden, D., Bouman, W. P., Jones, B. A., & Arcelus, J. (2016). Gender dysphoria and autism spectrum disorder: A systematic review of the literature. *Sexual Medicine Reviews, 4*(1), 3–14. doi:10.1016/j.sxmr.2015.10.003

Hallin, A. E., Fröst, K., Holmberg, E. B., & Södersten, M. (2012). Voice and speech range profiles and Voice Handicap Index for males—methodological issues and data. *Logopedics Phoniatrics Vocology, 37*(2), 47–61. doi:10.3109/14015439.2011.607469

Holmberg, E. B., Oates, J., Dacakis, G., & Grant, C. (2010). Phonetograms, aerodynamic measurements, self-evaluations, and auditory perceptual ratings of male-to-female transsexual voice. *Journal of Voice, 24*(5), 511–522. doi:10.1016/j.jvoice.2009.02.002.

Jacobs, L. A., Rachlin, K., Erickson-Schroth, L., & Janssen, A. (2014). Gender dysphoria and co-occurring autism spectrum disorders: Review, case examples, and treatment considerations. *Lesbian, Gay, Bisexual and Transgender Health, 1*(4), 277–282. doi:10.1089/lgbt.2013.0045

Jacobson, B., Johnson, A., Grywalski, C., Silbergleit, A., Jacobson, G., Benninger, M. S, & Newman, C. W. (1997). The Voice Handicap Index (VHI): Development and validation. *American Journal of Speech-Language Pathology, 6*, 66–70.

Kelly, V., Hertegård, S., Erikkson, J., Nygren, U., & Södersten, M., (in press). Effects of gender-confirming pitch-raising surgery in transgender women. A long-term follow-up study of acoustic and patient-reported data. *Journal of Voice.*

Kim, H. T. (2017). A new conceptual approach for voice feminization: 12 years of experience. *Laryngoscope, 127*(5), 1102–1108. doi:10.1002/lary.26127.

Landén, M., Wålinder, J., & Lundström, B. (1996). Prevalence, incidence and sex ratio of transsexualism. *Acta Psychiatrica Scandinavica, 93*, 221–223. doi:10.1111/j.1600-0447.1998.tb09986.x

Matai, V., Cheesman, A., & Clarke, P. (2003). Cricothyroid approximation and thyroid chondroplasty: A patient survey. *Otolaryngology-Head and Neck Surgery, 128*(6), 841–847. doi:10.1016/S0194-59980300462-5

National Board of Health and Welfare. (2015). Good care of adults with gender dysphoria. National guidelines [Nationellt kunskapsstöd för vård och behandling av personer med könsdysfori]. Retrieved from http://www.socialstyrelsen.se/Lists/Artikelkatalog/Attachments/19798/2015-4-7.pdf

Nygren, U. (2014). *Effects of increased levels of androgens on voice and vocal folds in women with congenital adrenal hyperplasia and female-to-male transsexual persons.* Doctoral dissertation published by Karolinska Institutet. Department of Clinical Science, Intervention and Technology, Stockholm, Sweden. Retrieved from https://publications.ki.se/xmlui/bitstream/handle/10616/42326/Thesis_Ulrika_Nygren.pdf?sequence=3

Nygren, U., Nordenskjold, A., Arver, S., & Sodersten, M. (2016). Effects on voice fundamental frequency and satisfaction with voice in trans men during testosterone treatment—a longitudinal study. *Journal of Voice, 30*(6), 766.e723–766.e734. doi:10.1016/j.jvoice.2015.10.016

Oates, J. (2012). Evidence-based practice in voice therapy for transgender/transsexual clients. In R. Adler, S. Hirsch, & M. Mordaunt (Eds.), *Voice and communication therapy for the transgender/transsexual client: A comprehensive clinical guide* (pp. 45–68). San Diego, CA: Plural Publishing.

Oates, J., & Dacakis, G. (2015). Transgender voice and communication: Research evidence underpinning voice intervention for male-to-female transsexual women. *Perspectives on Voice and Voice Disorders. ASHA's Special Interest group (SIG 3), 25*(2), 48–58.

Ohlsson, A. C., & Dotevall, H. (2009). Voice Handicap Index in Swedish. *Logopedics Phoniatrics Vocology, 34*(2), 60–66. doi:10.1080/14015430902839185

Papp, V. (2011). The female-to-male transsexual voice: Physiology vs. performance in production. Doctoral dissertation, Rice University, Houston, Texas. Retrieved from https://scholarship.rice.edu/bitstream/handle/1911/70383/PappV.pdf?sequence=1

Pfäfflin, F. (2011). Remarks on the history of the terms identity and gender identity. *International Journal of Transgenderism, 13*(1), 13–25.

Reed, G. M., Drescher, J., Krueger, R. B., Atalla, E., Cochran, S. D., First, M. B., . . . Saxena, S. (2016). Disorders related to sexuality and gender identity in the ICD-11: Revising the ICD-10 classification based on current scientific evidence, best clinical practices, and human rights considerations. *World Psychiatry 15*(3), 205–211. doi:10.1002/wps.20354

Sanchez, K., Oates, J., Dacakis, G., & Holmberg, E. B. (2014). Speech and voice range profiles of adults with untrained normal voices: Methodological implications. *Logopedics Phoniatrics Vocology, 39*(2), 62–71. doi:10.3109/14015439.2013.777109

Scheidt, D., Kob, M., Willmes, K., & Neuschaefer-Rube, C. (2004). Do we need voice therapy for female-to-male transgenders? In B. Murdoch, J. Goozee, M. Whelan, & K. Docking (Eds), *Proceedings of the 26th International Association of Logopedics and Phoniatrics*, Brisbane, Australia.

Smith, Y. L., van Goozen, S. H., Kuiper, A. J., & Cohen-Kettenis, P.T. (2005).Transsexual subtypes: Clinical and theoretical significance. *Psychiatry Research, 137*(3), 151–160. doi:10.1016 /j.psychres.2005.01.00

Söderpalm, E., Larsson, A. K., & Almquist, S. (2004). Evaluation of a consecutive group of transsexual individuals referred for vocal intervention in the west of Sweden. *Logopedics Phoniatrics Vocology*, 29(1), 18–30.

Södersten, M., Nygren, U., Hertegård, S., & Dhejne, C. (2015). Interdisciplinary program in Sweden related to transgender voice. *Perspectives on Voice and Voice Disorders. ASHA's Special Interest group (SIG 3)*, 25(2), 87–97.

Song, T. E., & Jiang, N. (2017). Transgender phonosurgery: A systematic review and meta-analysis. *Otolaryngology–Head and Neck Surgery, 156*(5), 803–808. doi:10.1177/0194599817697050

Ternström, S., Pabon, P., & Södersten, M. (2016). The Voice Range Profile: Its function, applications, pitfalls and potential. *Acta Acustica united with Acustica, 102*(2), 268–283. doi:10.3813/AAA .918943

Van Borsel, J., De Cuypere, G., Rubens, R., & Destaerke, B. (2000). Voice problems in female-to-male transsexuals. *International Journal of Language and Communication Disorders, 35*(3), 427–442. doi:10.1080/136828200410672

Van Damme, S., Cosyns, M., Deman, S., Van den Eede, Z., & Van Borsel, J. (2017). The effectiveness of pitch-raising surgery in male-to-female transsexuals: A systematic review. *Journal of Voice, 31*(2), 244.e241–244.e245. doi:10.1016 /j.jvoice.2016.04.002

Van de Grift, T. C., Cohen-Kettenis, P.T., Elaut, E., De Cuypere, G., Richter-Appelt, H., Haraldsene, I. R., & Kreukels, B. P. C. (2016). A network analysis of body satisfaction of people with gender dysphoria. *Body Image, 17*(1), 184–190. doi:10 .1016/j.bodyim.2016.04.002

Winter, S., Diamond, M., Green, J., Karasic, D., Reed, T., Whittle, S., & Wylie, K. (2016). Transgender people: Health at the margins of society. *Lancet, 388*, 390–40 doi:10.1016/s0140-6736 (16)00683-8

Wålinder, J. (1971). Incidence, and sex ratio of transsexualism in Sweden. *British Journal of Psychiatry, 119*, 195–196.

World Health Organization. (2010). *International Statistical Classification of Diseases and Related Health Problems: ICD-10*. Geneva, Switzerland.

Zeluf, G., Dhejne, C., Orre, C., Nilunger Mannheimer, L., Deogan, C., Hoijer, J., & Ekeus Thorson, A. (2016). Health, disability and quality of life among trans people in Sweden—a Web-based survey. *BMC Public Health, 16*(1), 1–15. doi:10.1186/s12889-016-3560-5.

2

Psychotherapy and Support for Transgender Clients

Arlene Lev, Darren Cosgrove, and Timothy S. Crumley

Lucinda walked into the office looking crestfallen. Her hair, usually coiffed, was uncombed, and she was dressed in sweats and a T-shirt. Lucinda loved dressing up in beautiful fashionable clothing, and it had been a long time since she had been out in public looking so casual and disheveled. Actually, not since before her transition, when she was still living as a disgruntled man, who felt trapped in a life that was not her own, had she looked so miserable. This was the story she told: "I was out walking my dog. I walk my dog often in the early evening, sometimes a mile or so around the park. It has been many years since I've worried that someone would see me and think anything but that I was a well-dressed woman. I have been confident that I can pass easily. What happened is Oscar, my dog, got out of his collar. I have no idea how that happened. It never happened before. He started running, really fast, and we were very close to the street. So I yelled." She looked down. "I didn't think about it, I just yelled. My voice went into a deep masculine voice: 'OSCAR!' Everyone stopped and looked at me. The dog came running back, but everything else is a blur. A teenager started laughing. 'It's a man,' he said." Lucinda repeated it. "He called me an 'it.' He said I was a man. I'm not a man, but when I yelled for the dog, I sure sounded like one."

Introduction

There is a growing public awareness of the experiences of transgender people, in part due to the growing visibility of transgender celebrities and public debates surrounding bathroom access and military service. Accompanying this increasing social awareness is the common narrative that transgender people feel "trapped in the wrong body" and desire to live and express themselves as what many might consider the "opposite" sex; for Lucinda, this narrative accurately describes her life journey. Lucinda was assigned male at birth, and after years of struggling to understand a profound sense of gender dysphoria, she transitioned to living as a woman with the support of psychotherapy. For five years she has lived as a woman, utilizing female hormones which have helped her feminize her body. She prefers to live a "stealth" life, one where no one knows her history and where she can "pass" or blend easily into society. She thought she had accomplished her goal, until her dog slipped out of his collar.

For Lucinda, the traditional narrative of transition accurately fits her personal experience. However, other transgender people may not desire to pass, they may not experience themselves as "trapped in the wrong body," and many do not see their journey as moving from one side of a male/female binary to the "opposite" side. For such individuals, notions of a fixed essential, or binary gender fail to capture their lived experiences or sense of self as gender-fluid, non-binary, or otherwise outside a dichotomous conceptualization of gender as exclusively male or female. Transgender people are diverse in their gender identities and expressions, as well as their experiences and beliefs about being transgender. Therefore, any attempt to generalize transgender experiences, or the goals of those who come to therapy for "gender issues," is a fruitless effort at best, and problematically reductionistic at worst.

This chapter is offered as a summary, not of transgender experience, but rather of the diverse circumstances and needs that bring trans and gender nonconforming people to the offices of psychotherapists. Additionally, this chapter presents an invitation to the reader to consider the role that psychotherapy can play in collaborative care for trans people seeking voice modification. While each trans person's story is unique, and that unique experience presents a wide range of potential therapeutic needs and goals, these experiences are often unified by a common thread of needing to navigate a world of pervasive bias and oppression. As such, the need for access to health and human service professionals who understand and respect individuals' right to self-determination and gender diversity is of the utmost importance.

The authors of this chapter all work as psychotherapists and family therapists with transgender and gender diverse adults, adolescents, children, and their families. The lead writer is the Founder and Director of *Choices*

Counseling and Consulting in Albany, New York and is an educator and trainer on sexual orientation and gender issues through TIGRIS, the *Institute for Gender, Relationships, Identity, and Sexuality, Inc*. In addition to working as a psychotherapist, the second author has worked as a queer sexuality educator for 15 years and is currently a social work doctoral candidate engaging in participatory action research with non-binary young adults. The third author is also a psychotherapist and specializes in working with clients who identify as transgender and gender nonconforming. In addition, this author serves as the Clinical Director at an intensive residential, substance abuse rehabilitation facility in Albany, New York.

In an attempt to recognize their social positionality and the role that it plays in their relationship to the content presented in this chapter, all three authors wish to acknowledge their identities and experience as cisgender people and as white academics—noting that such experiences of privilege influence our perspectives.

Key Terminology

As an evolving construct and reflection of current cultural understanding, language is a changing, dynamic force. This is particularly true for terminology related to identity in general, and gender identity in particular. Given the process of understanding the self in relation to the world in which one exists, such language is often shifting, and is very much bound to cultural contexts. Nonetheless, the following terms are defined to reflect the authors' use of them in this chapter. We also include selected mental health terminology to assist in familiarizing the reader with our profession.

Transgender (or trans), as defined by Stryker (1994) is "an umbrella term that refers to all identities or practices that cross over, cut across, move between, or otherwise queer socially constructed sex/gender boundaries" (p. 251). In this chapter, we specifically use the term to refer to people who experience their gender as different from that which was assigned to them at birth. *Cisgender*, by contrast, refers to individuals whose gender identity and behavior "matches" their assigned sex at birth, and therefore refers to individuals who do not identify as transgender (Tate, Youssef, & Bettergarcia, 2014). *Cisgenderism* is the prejudice that privileges those individuals who identify with their assigned sex, while stigmatizing those who are transgender or gender nonconforming. Similarly, *cissexism* is the systemic discrimination that occurs against individuals who identify as transgender and which benefits individuals who identify as cisgender (McClearen, 2015).

When discussing the *gender binary*, the authors are referencing a socio-political system of gender that endorses only two possibilities—male *or* female—and sees these gender categories as discrete and mutually exclusive. Similarly, both transgender and cisgender people may hold binary gender identities (that is the exclusive identification as either a man or a woman) while not necessarily endorsing the idea that gender (as a system) *must* be exclusively binary. *Non-binary* gender identities are those held by individuals whose sense of their gender falls outside the strict, binary notions of gender being exclusively "male" or "female" (Richards et al., 2016). The term *gender nonconforming* may describe a person's gender identity, expression, and/or behavior when it differs from what is considered normative for their assigned biological sex within the context of their culture and historical period (Coleman et al., 2012).

A *health care provider* is a broad umbrella term for any professional in the health care industry, including physicians and behavioral health specialists. Professionals who provide psychological services or behaviorally focused therapeutic services are generally referred to as *mental health professionals*, and they can have diverse training and educational backgrounds. Behavioral health care is managed differently from country to country, university degrees are conferred utilizing varying academic standards, and national and statewide credentialing processes are also widely divergent; therefore, the nomenclature described below references providers in the United States, where people do not have universal access to health insurance.

Social workers are the largest group of professionals currently providing services in the helping professions; social workers generally hold master's-level degrees. *Psychologists* generally hold PhDs and have received advanced training in behavioral psychology, the study of the brain, and diagnostic testing. Both social workers and psychologists study human development and psychopathology; commonly social workers are most focused on adverse environmental conditions and how they impact individuals and communities, whereas psychologists specialize in human behavior, cognition, and the internal functioning of the mind. *Psychiatrists* are medical practitioners with advanced training in psychology, psychopathology, and human physiology, and are able to prescribe medication. Additionally, within the allied helping professions are many *mental health counselors, marriage and family therapists,* and *psychiatric nurse practitioners*, all who bring specialized perspectives as mental health professionals.

Social workers, psychologists, and many other mental health specialists can be licensed and capable of receiving insurance reimbursements in the United States. Other terms commonly used are *behavioral specialists, counselors,* and *psychotherapists,* which are general terms (versus titles or degrees) for those who work as mental health professionals. A mental health professional (as well as a health care provider in general) may be referred to as a *gender specialist* if that provider has significant experience working with transgender clients and gender identity–related issues and topics (Lev, 2009). Mental health providers not only offer therapy and advocacy to support transgender clients, they are also the primary referral source for physicians providing medical and surgical treatments.

The term *gatekeeper* refers to a power dynamic that is inherent in the therapist and client relationship, specifically when mental health professionals have the ability to block transgender clients from receiving medical care (Lev, 2009). When a client is seeking medical treatment or surgeries related to gender dysphoria, physicians, surgeons, and/or insurance companies often require an assessment performed by a mental health professional. Mental health providers are therefore situated "between" the physician and those requesting medical or surgical treatments and may therefore be seen as an arbitrary barrier in accessing medical care, hence the term "gatekeeper."

Lastly, *transgender-affirming (or trans-affirming) practices* refer to non-pathologizing clinical approaches that embrace diverse gender-related identities, expressions, and experiences as normative and healthy expressions of self. Additionally, trans-affirming practices acknowledge the power and layers of privilege inherent in the therapeutic working relationship between a client seeking services and a provider who can effectively support or reject a client's needs and identity.

Seeking Therapy

Of the nearly 6,500 transgender people who participated in a national survey, 75%

reported having sought psychotherapy for issues specifically related to their gender identity (Grant et al., 2011). Psychotherapy with transgender clients and the individual needs, goals, and desires that they bring to the therapeutic relationship are as diverse as trans people themselves. They may seek out therapy for the same reason cisgender people do: relationship struggles, depression, addiction, coping with a chronic illness, and so forth. However, trans people also seek out therapeutic assistance for specific issues related to gender. We identify four reasons transgender people seek out psychotherapeutic services: gender dysphoria, assessment and referral, coping with oppressive social systems, and transition-related struggles with family acceptance. Each of these concerns will be outlined below.

Gender Dysphoria

Many transgender clients seek out therapy because they are experiencing *gender dysphoria*, a term that describes the psychological discomfort some individuals experience between their assigned birth sex (often referred to as biological or natal sex) and their gender identity. The term was first coined by Fisk (1974), describing people who experience incongruence with their anatomical body coupled with dissonance regarding the gendered social expectations associated with their sexed body. Gender dysphoria can range from mild to severe, and can cause socio-emotional problems, mental health symptoms, and severe family and occupational challenges. Gender dysphoria can be treated medically with cross-sex hormone therapy and various surgical procedures that can provide lasting relief. Gender dysphoria can also be ameliorated through various socially adaptive measures, involving clothing choices, mannerisms, and pronoun and name changes that can establish a cross-gender, and legal, identity (Coleman et al., 2012; Lev, 2016).

The person seeking therapy for gender dysphoria may have felt dysphoric for years, the dysphoria may have increased over time, or they may have only begun to experience this (sometimes not until adulthood). People experiencing gender dysphoria are often also experiencing other psychosocial challenges—they may be depressed or anxious; sometimes they are abusing alcohol or other substances to cope with their dysphoria. For such individuals there can be feelings of hopelessness about their future, and they can have trouble imagining living a life where they have more comfort in their gender expression (Lev, 2013).

The term "gender dysphoria" is the same nomenclature used diagnostically in the *Diagnostic and Statistical Manual of Mental Disorders, Fifth Edition* (DSM-5) (American Psychiatric Association, 2013). When discussing diagnosis, Gender Dysphoria will be capitalized; otherwise it is used in a more general sense to describe human discomfort caused by gender dissonance and or anatomical discordance.

Assessment and Referral

Helping individuals to determine the best way to address the concerns that bring them to therapy, or the goals that they wish to accomplish, can involve a comprehensive assessment completed by a psychotherapist knowledgeable about gender diversity. Although physicians can provide their own assessments for medical or surgical care, few have either the time or the training, and therefore request referrals from gender specialists (Coleman et al., 2012). In fact, many people seek out a therapist solely because they need the requisite paperwork as part of their referral for gender affirming medical and surgical treatments.

Although some transgender individuals without dysphoria may seek transition related care, such services are often sought by those experiencing some degree of discomfort with their body, or how others perceive their body and gender in social situations. Medical transition allows for the opportunity to feel more comfortable in one's body and can improve one's quality of life and mental health (de Vries, McGuire, Steensma, Wagenaar, Doreleijers, & Cohen-Kettenis, 2014; Keo-Meier et al., 2015; Newfield et al., 2006). Masculinizing or feminizing one's body may aid in the ability to move through the world not only with a greater internal sense of gender congruence, but also in such a way that enhances the ability to be seen as one's experienced gender (Coleman et al., 2012). Such changes can significantly lessen the experience of gender dysphoria. Further, given the pervasive nature of transphobia and the alarming rates of social and health disparities—including violence, harassment, and job discrimination (James et al., 2016; Nuttbrock et al., 2012)—access to such care is often a matter of both physical safety and social functioning.

While access to gender-affirming medical care can vary in different geographical areas (urban versus rural settings), and from one state to the next, individuals seeking hormones and surgeries are often required to meet with a mental health provider for evaluation and/or referral to care. An increasing number of medical providers are offering services utilizing an *informed medical consent model*. This allows physicians to initiate hormonal treatment without a referral from a mental health provider based on their own assessment of the client's ability to understand the effects of hormonal therapy. Many doctors do not feel they have the time or skills to provide a thorough mental health exam; therefore, surgical treatments almost always require a psychological evaluation by a mental health provider.

Furthermore, many insurance companies often will not pay for services without comprehensive mental health exams preceding care. The assessment is commonly sent in the form of a letter referring the client from the mental health practitioner to the medical provider.

The requirement for assessment and referrals is a subject of professional and community debate. Requiring psychological assessment presumes medical gatekeeping and challenges the concept of trans-affirming care. Therefore, it is common for clients seeking such services to find themselves in the offices of a psychotherapist despite the fact that many may not be seeking (or needing) psychological support. While some are open to the counseling process, others experience frustration with the nature of gatekeeping that can present barriers to medically necessary care. On the other hand, some people who seek out a therapist only to receive a medical referral may have a positive experience in therapy and choose to remain after they have received their letters of referral. This next stage of counseling may offer the opportunity to engage in an ongoing psychotherapeutic process. For those who choose to not continue in psychotherapy, it is hoped that the positive experience they have will enable them to seek out therapy at another point in their lives, should they ever need it.

Coping with Oppressive Social Systems

Collazo, Austin, and Craig (2013) explain that "pervasive discrimination and victimization are among the most salient issues impacting the lives of transgender individuals and should be explored thoroughly and sensitively" (p. 231). As such, therapists are encouraged to consider their transgender and gender nonconforming clients from a holistic perspective. To be specific, none of our clients' identities or experiences exist independently of the influence of the sociocultural and political environment in which they live. And so, while many of the clients who come to psychotherapy may not be struggling with their gender identity or dysphoria at all, they may be negotiating oppressive systems that are taking a toll on their mental health (Nuttbrock et al., 2010). This can include pervasive cissexism, hostile work environments, or the threat of violence on the streets. It may surprise such clients to find that the therapeutic process can be helpful in providing them with support, as well as potential advocacy.

Transition-Related Struggles and Family Acceptance

Another reason for seeking therapeutic services is for support coping with family acceptance and rejection. Transition can present challenges for family members who may struggle with a spouse, partner, parent, or child who is transitioning. The focus of trans-affirming therapy with individuals in transition is often on issues of coming out to family or assisting them in coping with their family's reactions (Giammattei, 2015; Malpas, 2015).

The spouses of transgender people may seek therapeutic services (individual or group counseling) to cope with transition-related changes in their lives. Couples counseling can provide support to partners who are navigating issues related to transition and relationship identity. Similar services may also be beneficial for transgender people seeking assistance with coming out to their children (regardless of their age) and negotiating family roles and interpersonal and relational dynamics. Although not all gender specialists provide family counseling, it is our philosophy that family systems therapy can help address the changes that may occur in family dynamics (Lev, 2004).

As noted, trans clients seek therapy for all the reasons that other people do: anxiety, insomnia, learning disabilities, loneliness, cancer, jealousy, grief, infertility, trauma, and so forth. Sometimes these issues are bound up with gender dysphoria, or their trans identity, and sometimes they are not particularly relevant, except in a holistic way, in that we all must bring all parts of ourselves to the therapeutic encounter for it to be successful.

Diagnosis, Standards of Care, and the Politics of Access

The specific mechanics of accessing gender-affirming medical care can vary depending upon state policies, insurance guidelines, and one's ability to pay for care; it is important to note that there is not always a trans-affirmative provider accessible to all clients needing care. In recent years, clinical and medical guidelines have been refined to address many of these complex issues (Coleman et al., 2012). The following offers an overview of these topics.

The Politics of Care

Diagnostic systems, by their nature, label trans people as being disordered or diseased. In doing so, they pathologize the individual, overlooking the larger social problems caused by a rigid and exclusively binary understanding of gender (Burdge, 2007; Markman, 2011; Spade, 2003). In utilizing diagnostic approaches, it is the trans individual, not society at large, that is problematized (Lev, 2013). With these concerns in mind, the role that diagnosis plays in the procurement of medical and surgical services for transgen-

der people has been an issue of intense conflict and engaged discourse among and between trans people and care providers for the past 15 years (De Cuypere et al., 2010; Ehrbar, 2010; Lev, 2004, 2013). The very acts of assessment and diagnosis can put mental health providers in the role of gatekeepers, determining what transition-related doors will open or close for clients, and access is often governed not only by state and insurance guidelines, but also by providers' own biases or assumptions regarding gender (Whitehead et al., 2012).

As discussed previously, some trans clients may seek medical transition as a means to best express their gender identity, even if they do not report significant distress regarding specific physical characteristics. Spade (2003) discusses the ways in which many providers expect specific distressed narratives as evidence of the necessity for transition-related care: what Prosser (1998) referred to as a *transsexual narrative*. Furthermore, Spade critiques the tendency for these expectations to be rooted in binary assumptions around gender, in such a way that trans clients are expected to not only be deeply troubled by their bodies but also endorse a strong desire to identify as the "opposite" sex. Lev (2004) said these narratives are "not inaccurate," they are just not "inclusive" (p. 215). Spade (2003) reflects upon the pressure trans people face to present false narratives of struggle and easily digestible articulations of their genders, in order to gain access to the care they need and desire.

While problems with diagnoses abound, a diagnosis is often required within our current medical system in order for trans people to access services. With an increasing number of insurance companies paying for transition-related care, it is possible that without a diagnosis many trans people would not be able to safely or affordably access the care they need (Lev, 2013). In this vein, mental health providers and voice therapists alike should be knowledgeable of the service barriers often faced by their clients. Such barriers may often be related to economic disparity and injustice, and trans people, especially trans people of color, experience disproportionately high rates of unemployment and poverty (James et al., 2016). Combined, these factors suggest not only that therapists can be seen as gatekeepers but that accessing such providers' services, in and of themselves, can be a financial impossibility.

Diagnosis

The purpose of diagnosis is to recognize and organize human pain and suffering in an effort to best treat it within the framework of current psychological knowledge. However, when navigating diagnostic labeling, it is necessary to also recognize the societal and political forces impacting sexual and gender minorities and the creation of consistently high levels of chronic stress, on both macro and micro levels. Members of stigmatized minority groups experience high levels of prejudice and discrimination and consequently are at increased risk for negative outcomes and maladaptive behaviors. This is referred to as minority stress (Institute of Medicine, 2011; Meyer, 1995).

The DSM-5 diagnosis for Gender Dysphoria describes the psychological pain experienced by those who are transgender and have anatomical dissonance; however, how much of what is described as the effects of minority stress and what is solely related to gender dysphoria remains an area of continuing debate. Most agree that the current DSM-5 is an improvement over the previous diagnostic manuals (Lev, 2013). The term Gender Dysphoria (which replaced Gender

Identity Disorder) more accurately describes the emotional pain and suffering *some* transgender people experience, and removes the label of the word "disorder" as applied to any expression of gender identity. However, there are people who are transgender who do not experience dysphoria; indeed, their desire for transition can be better described as euphoric. The language of the DSM-5 is significantly less sexist and has shifted the focus away from binary gender categories; the DSM-5 describes transitioning to an "other gender (or some alternative gender different from one's assigned gender)," allowing for multiple expressions of gender outside of male/female categories. Changes in the DSM often influence the larger established organizations like the World Health Organization and the International Classification of Diseases to reform diagnostic manuals, processes that are under way as of this writing. Nonetheless, Whitehead et al. (2012) make an important point that the ideologies that guide clinicians do not simply flow from diagnostic criteria, but rather "are authored in practice" (p. 398). Therapists can pathologize clients without a diagnosis and can also minimize the stigma of diagnosis while utilizing them to pave the way for treatment. Generally speaking, the DSM-5 diagnosis for Gender Dysphoria is noted as part of a medical referral for treatment.

Standards of Care

The World Professional Association of Transgender Health (WPATH) is the only international, interdisciplinary, non-profit, professional organization devoted to promoting evidence-based trans-affirmative clinical care and research, education and training, and advocacy, especially within public policy, in support of transgender health. In 2012, WPATH revised the Standards of Care (SOC), which are clinical and medical guidelines developed for professionals who provide transgender care. The Standards of Care 7th edition is identified as flexible clinical guidelines which distinguish between gender nonconforming behavior and gender dysphoria, and clearly state the need to de-pathologize transgender identities (Coleman et al., 2012). These guidelines lessen the role of gatekeeping by removing any requirement for psychotherapy and outlining a clear assessment and referral processes for people seeking care.

Although the new diagnostic criteria in the DSM recognizes that not all trans people experience gender-related distress, the diagnostic category of Gender Dysphoria presents a challenge to people wishing to engage in some degree of medical transitioning but not having a history of significant conflict with their present body. The SOC 7 addresses these concerns by providing a provision for an informed consent model, and an increasing number of medical providers are offering services in this way. Although seen as a political victory in increasing access to care and avoiding utilization of unnecessary services, such a practice is far from universal. It also assumes that clients starting medical treatments have had sufficient psychoeducation to understand the changes that will ensue.

Best Practices in Psychotherapy

Despite the problems related to diagnosis, pathologizing, and gatekeeping, good psychotherapy has been found to be both a useful and an affirming tool for many seeking trans-affirming medical care, especially when the clients themselves seek out therapy (Singh & dickey, 2017). Such work can help address the psychological and emotional needs that are directly or secondarily related to one's gender experience. Work with a psychotherapist can be beneficial as one navigates coming out at work and school and to family and loved ones. Psychotherapists can provide access to psychoeducation, family and group couple counseling, and case management when necessary. They can assist in medical and legal referrals, as well as advocate for their clients and the transgender community at large.

As a result of the gatekeeping role therapists have been placed in (and that some practitioners actively engage in), it is safe for providers to assume that clients will come to therapy with certain assumptions and concerns about gatekeeping and psychotherapy. Trans-affirming providers should address these expectations with clients early in their work together, including an explicit discussion of the stigma experienced in the health care systems, to acknowledge that client assumptions are often well founded, while working to build a therapeutically effective and affirming relationship.

Affirmative Therapy

Best practices with transgender and gender nonconforming people include utilizing affirmative therapy techniques (APA, 2015; Carroll, Gilroy, & Ryan, 2002; Lev, 2004; Singh & dickey, 2017). Austin and Craig (2015) describe trans-affirming practice as "a non-pathologizing approach to clinical practice that accepts and validates all experiences of gender" (p. 21). This approach requires acknowledgment of the role power and privilege play in any therapeutic relationship. Carroll, Gilroy, and Ryan (2002) encourage those working with trans clients to consider that "counselors, supervisors, and researchers should recognize that they may not only have a role in alleviating the emotional distress of clients who challenge the binary gender system but may also be responsible for contributing to or exacerbating it" (p. 133).

When a client who identifies as transgender is meeting with a provider for the first time, the clinician should discuss the client's right to autonomy, explaining that the client is the only one who is truly positioned to determine their gender. The clinician can also explain that there are questions that must be asked to gain a better sense of the client and their internal experience; however, the provider also makes it clear that these questions are not meant to challenge the client's identity. Client-centered techniques, including unconditional positive regard, active listening, and demonstration of empathy, are key components of affirmative therapy and best practices with transgender and gender nonconforming clients (Riley, Wong, & Sitharthan, 2011).

Additionally, Austin and Craig (2015) describe the following opening statement as being trans-affirming, and one that may help build trust with the client early in therapy:

> *Welcome, I'd like to take a moment to share my approach to practice with you. In keeping with clinical practice that is affirming and inclusive, I embrace a trans-affirmative approach in which all experiences of gender are acknowledged and validated. I aim to create a space for clients to safely explore, understand, and inhabit their unique experiences of gender. (p. 22)*

Such statements, in conjunction with consistent use of clients' self-identified pronouns and name, lay the groundwork for the creation of a safe space where clients can explore and share their internal experiences and gender identity.

While thoughtful, intentional, and reflective initial statements and conversations are meant to empower the client in the therapeutic process (and break down gatekeep-

ing in the working relationship), it is important to remember that clients may continue to hold assumptions about the nature of psychotherapy, given the general bias and cisgenderism they experience in the world. The American Psychological Association (APA, 2015) encourages providers to "recognize how stigma, prejudice, discrimination, and violence affect the health and well-being of transgender and gender nonconforming people" (p. 838). In doing so, providers will build rapport and trust by examining the relational process of ongoing therapeutic work between client, therapist, and society at large.

Working with the Spectrum of Gender

By centering the experience of clients as the basis and starting point for therapy, providers must trust in an individuals' understanding of their own gender. While clinicians may invite clients to examine their inner landscape and sense of self, such inquiries are not rooted in the motivation to challenge or dismissively question a client's gender. Instead, such work should invite the opportunity for the healthy, curious, and affirming process of holistic self-inquiry. For such exploration to occur, clinicians must recognize their own gender-related biases and assumptions and work toward the development of personal paradigms that honor and respect all genders—including those that fall within and those that challenge the binary. In practice, this includes recognizing that some trans clients comfortably identify as male or female, while others may "experience extreme intrapsychic pressure to pick either a 'male' or 'female' body or gender identity" (Burdge, 2007, p. 247).

Providers should be prepared to provide psychoeducation regarding gender identity as a continuum existing within social and political frameworks and support the notion that gender identity can take various forms, or, indeed, no form at all (Burdge, 2007 citing Swann & Herbert, 1999; Coleman et al., 2011). Affirmative models require less direction from the therapist and more of a supportive presence through the use of verbal and non-verbal cues (as mentioned earlier), open-ended questions, as well as language from the therapist that does not assume a client's experience, identity, or self-description (such as pronouns). In short, the therapist applies similar, client-centered approaches to all clients regardless of gender identification.

Feminist Approaches to Psychotherapy

Feminist therapy offers a critical lens through which the practitioner and client can collectively examine the social and environmental factors that are linked to oppression, particularly that which is related to gender (Coady & Lehmann, 2007). Practice rooted in feminist theory is often action oriented. It is not sufficient to work toward individual change. Rather, as a socialist-collectivist theory (Payne, 2015), the focus of change is structural and systems based. Ultimately, while feminist social work is interested in improving the individual circumstances of clients, there is a broader interest in changing the environmental conditions that produce gendered oppression (as well as classism, homophobia, racism, etc.).

As an empowerment-based approach, feminist theory has been applied to psychotherapy in an effort to break down hierarchical roles between therapist and client, and to support women in examining stereotypical and limiting societal beliefs. Over time, it has matured into a broad-based

systemic theory that examines the limitations imposed on all marginalized people, and the constrictions of gender roles within a cross-cultural context. It can be a powerful lens through which to work with transgender and gender nonconforming people as they explore gender-based expectations and intersectionality in transition.

With an emphasis on transformative work, therapists taking a feminist approach are as concerned with process as they are with outcomes, and thus there is an emphasis on consciousness raising among individuals and groups, as well as a development of egalitarian relationships between client and therapist (Corey, 2012). Within this therapeutic context, clients are seen as the experts and take the lead in interpreting, assessing, and ultimately solving their own presenting problem (Coady & Lehmann, 2007; Corey, 2012). Feminist-based therapy is seen as an appropriate practice approach for addressing a wide range of issues that stem from oppression. Nonetheless, some clients engage in mental health services unwillingly (such as those who may be court mandated) or with pressing and immediate needs that may not permit the time or interest it takes to effect broad social restructuring (Coady & Lehmann, 2007; Payne, 2015). In cases such as these, the therapist should be mindful that although the client's problems may originate from social inequality and oppression, the therapist should prioritize the focus of work on the client's most pressing goals and needs (Coady & Lehmann, 2007).

Transgender-Affirmative Cognitive Behavioral Therapy

While client-centered techniques are crucial, Austin and Craig (2015) describe a more direct, Cognitive-Behavioral approach that focuses on issues impacting transgender clients specifically. These interventions can be used to assist trans clients in identifying, challenging, and ultimately replacing negative self-beliefs and underlying schemas. The key here is to identify and focus on thoughts and beliefs that center around external messages, and those that allow for a negative self-concept. As negative self-perceptions are challenged, more realistic and affirming perceptions are suggested and entertained by the client, where the client ultimately develops a more positive view of gender identity and the self as a whole (Austin & Craig, 2015). As a result, this approach may be more directive and structured in nature compared with approaches that may be more client centered by default.

Group Therapy

In addition to and in conjunction with individual therapy, group therapy is often a key component for a transgender and gender nonconforming person in therapy. According to Carlozzi (2017):

> Social support is very important for reducing the sense of isolation that many transgender persons experience. Many report that they first sought information and support for themselves on the internet, describing how comforting it was to find out there were other people like them. (p. 46)

Research has found that connectedness with others/contact with those who have similar experiences is important to both trans youth and adults (Riley, Sitharthan, & Clemson, 2013; Singh, 2013; Singh, Hays, & Watson, 2011). As described by Heck, Croot, and Robohm (2013), group therapy focused on issues pertaining to transgender clients can allow for peer-to-peer advice and feedback.

Group-based work allows transgender individuals who may otherwise feel isolated to connect with those who have similar experiences, as well as those who may have more knowledge in addition to these experiences. An example highlighted in the literature is the topic of transitioning, where clients are able to provide each other with advice and support on the "how," "when," and "to what extent" regarding coming out to friends, family, and co-workers, along with other aspects of transitioning (Heck, Croot, & Robohm, 2013). Although transgender groups can be peer led, therapeutic group discussions are overseen by a mental health professional who acts as a facilitator and who may "step in" as needed to promote a positive therapeutic environment. Group therapy may also focus on and address discrimination experienced by transgender clients, as well as discussions around how such experiences can be (and have been) navigated. Moreover, group therapy allows clients to build a face-to-face support network they may otherwise miss out on.

Family Systems Therapy

In addition to individual and group counseling, family therapy is another key component of best practices when working with transgender and gender nonconforming clients. Family Systems Therapy, a specific therapeutic modality, is recommended, as this perspective explores, identifies, and challenges internal processes, communication patterns, and dynamics between and within family members (Giammattei, 2015; Lev, 2004; Malpas, 2015). Lev (2004) points out that, just as transgender clients navigate their own developmental stages and coming-out process, so do their families. As a result, family systems therapy can further support transgender clients by supporting their families in various ways.

Specifically, clients may use therapy as a space to come out to family members (Lev, 2004). They may bring family members into therapy to have the discussion in a space that feels neutral and safe, with the mental health provider present as a supportive third party. Following the meeting, clients and their family members may process their reactions, experiences, and expectations with the therapist. Family members, along with the client, may share fears, concerns, and expectations for a transition process. Such exchanges may provide clients with some relief from having to play the "educator" role.

Other focuses of family therapy may include the impact that parents coming out and their transition will have on their children, as well as planning for such disclosure. It also fits when a child reports experiences related to gender dysphoria and families seek counseling to determine how they can best (and safely) support their child (Lev, 2004).

Narrative Therapy

Narrative therapy, developed by Michael White and David Epston, focuses on the stories people internalize and tell about their lives within the context of societal discourses. White and Epston (1990) say that "in striving to make sense of life, persons face the task of arranging their experiences of events in sequences across time in such a way as to arrive at a coherent account of themselves and the world around them" (p. 10). Transgender people, and others who are outside of the socially approved gender binary, have often spent lifetimes trying to understand their own life stories amid the pathologizing accounts available as part of the public discourse and the emerging

stories shared within the transgender community. Additionally, they must negotiate the gatekeeping within the mental health community to actualize their identity. They may have been told that therapists want to hear a particular narrative, and indeed this remains true in far too many clinical contexts. Discovering, identifying, and naming themselves is a psychological process—a process because too often the stories they have about themselves, the ones they have told themselves about who they are, were actually written by others. In the language of narrative therapy, through listening, the goal is to help clients *re-author* their lives. "The process of constructing a life narrative is never a solitary experience; narratives and life stories take place within communities of shared experiences, as part of the social discourse" (Lev, 2004, p. 221), which includes the therapeutic dialogue.

Narrative therapy is non-pathologizing, client centered, and collaborative, and assists people in separating the problems they are experiencing from who they are—what is referred to as *externalizing* the problem. It is an excellent form of therapy to use with clients who are coming out and struggling to understand who they are. Providers can reduce the effects of minority stress when they take a client-centered approach encouraging clients to share their life stories. When such sharing occurs, providers can tune in to client experiences by suspending their preconceived assumptions and preventing personally preferred outcomes from getting in the way of meeting clients where they are (Carroll, Gilroy, & Ryan, 2002; Freedman & Combs, 1996; Meyer, 1995).

Self-Reflection and Education

Another element of best practices involves recognizing and addressing therapists' biases.

Providers are encouraged to seek out the most up-to-date information and research on working with transgender and gender nonconforming people and their families, as well as strive to work in ways that are gender affirmative (APA, 2015; Coleman et al., 2012; Harper et al., 2013). WPATH offers a set of expectations and SOCs when working with transgender and gender nonconforming people (Coleman et al. 2012). Additionally, the APA (2015) offers guidelines for best practices in therapy that state that psychoeducation is key for providers in preventing biased and negative outcomes, specifically where the client's goals are not the primary focus. Specifically, guideline 4 of the Guidelines for Psychological Practice with Transgender and Gender Nonconforming People states, "Psychologists are aware of how their attitudes about and knowledge of gender identity and gender expression may affect the quality of care they provide to transgender and gender nonconforming people and their families" (APA, 2015).

Regardless of training and amount of experience, providers are not immune to their own internal biases and societal forces that impact our clients' lives. Examples of bias that can impact the therapeutic relationship, and even serve to harm the client, include but certainly are not limited to, the following. First, providers may believe gender is dichotomous, and thus believe transgender and gender nonconforming clients seek to become the "opposite" gender. Such beliefs may, and will, have a negative impact on clients who identify as a gender other than male or female, identify with multiple genders, or identify with no gender at all. Additionally, the belief that transgender clients strive to engage in certain (specific) treatments, and in a certain order (e.g., taking hormones before desiring surgery), allows for dangerous, unsafe working relationships and environments for clients. Providers who attempt to impose medical treatments or even suggest that there are "correct steps" in seeking such services are making assumptions about client needs that may not be true.

To understand our clients, we must first begin to understand the societal, historical, and cultural contexts in which they live, external factors that we as providers often contribute to without full awareness. Providers across the medical spectrum benefit their clients when they seek out information and knowledge regarding the "political, historical, and psychological contexts in which transgendered clients live" (Carroll, Gilroy, & Ryan, 2002, p. 133). The Standards of Care (Coleman et al. 2012) and American Psychological Association (2015) echo this responsibility of therapists working with transgender and gender nonconforming people. Providers are strongly advised to develop an understanding of the barriers and societal events, in addition to daily obstacles that transgender and gender nonconforming clients face, as this will allow the provider to better empathize with the client, engage in the client's worldview, and challenge one's own views and perceptions.

Advocacy

As noted in the previous paragraph, trans-affirming providers must understand how to be supportive of clients, as well as understand that many of the stressors impacting this population are external. As noted by Carroll, Gilroy, and Ryan (2002, p. 133), "In this paradigm shift, the focus is not on transforming transgendered clients but rather transforming the cultural context in which they live." Trans-affirming providers should support their clients in navigating societal dynamics and external stressors, as well as advocating for their clients when possible and appropriate. Consistent and thorough advocacy is key when it comes to best practices with transgender and gender nonconforming clients (Riley, Wong, & Sitharthan, 2011).

Such advocacy will take various forms. Providers may be called upon to be advocates in schools and work environments, or other institutions where cisgenderism permeates. This can take the form of training and workshops at job sites, developing trans-affirming policies within schools, or writing letters in support of a client's claim for Social Security Disability when needed. Clinically based advocacy may include, but certainly is not limited to, writing referral letters for mental health and medical treatments and including the client's family in therapy to address family-related dynamics and stressors if these interventions are desired by the client. Therapists can also play an active role in advocating for transgender rights and access to health care on a more general, institutional level (such as writing letters to Congress). Providers can exercise their power in advocating, communicating, and coordinating additional services for their clients, including making referrals for voice and communication training.

The Integration of Mental Health Counseling and Voice and Communication Training

It has been rare that voice training was a part of integrated systems of care. In the past, voice and communication modification was viewed as an adjunctive treatment for transgender care, although it is now included in the SOC version 7 and is being integrated into holistic treatment. Historically mental health services were also viewed as adjunctive. In the Standards of Care v6, treatment was referred to as "triadic," referring to hormones, surgery, and what was then referred to as the "real-life experience,"

the expectation that transgender people should live in their affirmed identity for a year before any medical treatments would be provided (Lev, 2009). Assumptively, the therapist, acting as a gatekeeper to medical providers, would be the overseer of the real-life test. Although the current SOC has abandoned the language of triadic care, most people, including both providers and clients, still see medical treatments as the primary focus of treatment (Lev, 2004). However, for many clients, especially trans women, both psychotherapy and voice training can be an essential component of their overall transition plan.

It is our belief that trans people are often best served by integrated systems of care within a framework of collaborative services (Feldman & Goldberg, 2006; Lev & Wolf-Gould, in press; Schechter, 2009). The value of collaborative care in the medical field has been researched, with evidence showing success (Woltmann, 2012). By definition, collaborative care is an integrated care system—including providers from two or more parallel health systems—that requires an ecological and systems perspective (Seaburn et al., 1996). Gagne (2005) emphasized that collaborative care is not a fixed, static approach, but an adaptable viewpoint that strengthens accessibility and delivery of services. This is our vision for psychotherapy and voice training—collaborative and integrated partnerships in treating trans clients.

For collaboration to be effective, there must be a "framework of common objectives" (von Trotsenburg, 2014), and the highest level of care is generally thought to be possible only in integrated models housed within the same physical location (Feierabend & Bartee, 2004). This is most easily attained through multidisciplinary clinics that offer medical and mental health services under one roof. In addition, some institutions are able to provide educational, advocacy, and legal services. Models for integrated care are currently being developed in the United States working with gender nonconforming and transgender youth (Hsieh & Leininger, 2014; Sherer, Rosenthal, Ehrensaft, & Baum, 2012; Tishelman et al., 2015). As noted in Chapter 1, it is possible to work with collaborative systems *across institutions, clinical discipline, and specialty*, developing true interdisciplinary treatment teams (Ducheny, Hendricks & Keo-Meier, 2017; Lev & Wolf-Gould, in press).

Moreover, working within a collaborative system is crucial with trans clients. For instance, should it become obvious that a client is distressed about their voice, then a referral to a voice specialist may be indicated. This should be a routine referral for all gender specialists, and they should have access to voice therapy referrals (including online resources in areas where local voice specialists may not be available). Conversely, many trans people who eschew therapeutic services might be receiving treatment from voice specialists and it may become obvious that they are experiencing anxiety or depression as they negotiate their transition. Voice therapists can be very helpful in paving the way to help trans clients who are frightened or resistant to therapy access appropriate trans-affirmative clinicians.

An example of case management via a multidisciplinary approach (where a psychotherapist assists a client in obtaining voice therapy) could involve the following.

Jos who identifies as non-binary, is seeing a psychotherapist in private practice. They are exploring Jos's internal experiences around gender. During this process Jos has established that they are not comfortable with their current voice. They identify that they would likely experience more comfort, relief, and confidence if their voice were of a self-defined form. The psychotherapist, in addition to processing the client's current experiences and expectations for what an ideal voice would sound and be like, explores options for a voice therapy referral and advocates on behalf of Jos. With Jos's consent, the therapist sends out a referral letter and begins correspondence with a local voice specialist, discussing how Jos will benefit from voice therapy, specifically as they practice and experience a voice that is more in-line with their identity and self-expression.

Overall, the importance of a multidisciplinary approach is supported within clinical practice guidelines from several major professional organizations, including WPATH (Coleman et al., 2012), the American Academy of Child and Adolescent Psychiatry (Adelson et al., 2012), the AAFP (2015), the American Academy of Family Physicians jointly with the American Academy of Physician Assistants (AAPA, 2011), and the Endocrine Society (Hembree et al., 2017). Interdisciplinary collaboration, however, is rarely a part of formal education, regardless of one's profession. A guideline for how multidisciplinary teams can provide optimal treatment has been highlighted by the "six C's": *care, compassion, competence, communication, courage,* and *commitment* (Ndoro, 2014). *Communication* can be especially challenging in the busy-ness of the medical and therapeutic community. The practice of collaborative care requires attention to relationship issues between providers, extra time to make contact, and discipline to maintain coordination with fragmented and stressful organizations.

Closing Thoughts

Historically, medical and psychological treatments for transgender and gender nonconforming people have been based on the framework of treating transgender people within a pathologizing medical model. The emphasis on diagnoses—and a dichotomous view of gender through which many providers have come to understand trans people—has reinforced the adherence to masculine and feminine stereotypes in order to be deemed eligible for transition-related care. As practitioners, policy makers, service consumers, and advocates push for increasingly affirming care, we must critically examine whether or not our work reifies oppressive gender paradigms or deconstructs them. We must ask ourselves if our efforts maintain systems of cissexism through the encouragement of adaptation to one's environment—or do we work with those we serve to create different, more affirming environments?

As providers, we must recognize that although the aforementioned gender-confirming medical services and voice therapy may be important parts of many transgender people's expression of self and their ability to "pass," transition-related goals vary widely. Many people share the desires and goals that Lucinda presented at the start of this chapter. Her experiences, and those of clients like her, must be held with the utmost respect. For other clients, passing may be perceived as a form of assimilation into cisgender norms (Hines, 2006). They may enter our offices seeking therapy and perhaps desiring transition-related health care, yet they may present narratives that reject binary or essentialist notions of gender. Their gender and gender-related goals, like Lucinda's, should be affirmed and respected. Maintaining an awareness of the range of trans experiences and abandoning the notion of a single "normative" transition trajectory are essential in all phases of the therapeutic relationship and affirming care for trans clients. We must be ready to support clients as they navigate the often tumultuous waters of service access.

We must also remain cognizant of the fact that trans health care does not exist in a bubble. Our services are interwoven with complex multidisciplinary fields. Furthermore, our clients navigate these systems and their relationships with us, through the lens of many intersecting identities and experiences. Our trans clients are not *just trans*. Our clients, like all people, carry gendered experiences as well as racial and ethnic identities and religious and cultural experiences and may move through the world with both seen and unseen disabilities. Providers must recognize that our clients do not come to us with singular or silo'ed experiences but are living within an intricate web of both privileged and subjugated identities. We must tune in to the experiences of sexism, homophobia, racism, classism, and other forms of dominance that both we and our clients bring to our work together. Our clients' identities and experiences, like our own, are rich, complex and intersectional. We cannot expect our work to be any less.

References

Adelson, S. L., Walter, H. J., Bukstein, O. G., Bellonci, C., Benson, R. S., Chrisman, A., . . . Medicus, J. (2012). Practice parameter on gay, lesbian or bisexual sexual orientation, gender-nonconformity, and gender discordance in children and adolescents. *Journal of American Academy of Child and Adolescent Psychiatry, 51,* 957–974.

AAFP (American Academy of Family Physicians). (2011, February). Family physicians and physician assistants: Team-based family medicine—a joint policy statement of the American Academy of Family Physicians and the American Academy of Physician Assistants (AAPA). Retrieved January 24, 2018, from http://www.aafp.org/dam /AAFP/documents/practice_management/admin _staffing/AAFP–AAPAJtPaper.pdf

American Psychiatric Association. (2013). Diagnostic and statistical manual of mental disorders (DSM-5). American Psychiatric Pub.

APA (American Psychological Association). (2015). Guidelines for psychological practice with transgender and gender nonconforming people. *American Psychologist, 70(9),* 832–864, doi: 10.1037/a0039906.

Austin, A., & Craig, S. L. (2015). Transgender affirmative cognitive behavioral therapy: Clinical considerations and applications. *Professional Psychology, Research and Practice, 46*(1), 21–29.

Burdge, B. J. (2007). Bending gender, ending gender: Theoretical foundations for social work practice with the transgender community. *Social Work, 52*(3), 243–250.

Carroll, L., Gilroy, P. J., & Ryan, J. (2002). Counseling transgendered, transsexual, and gender-variant clients. *Journal of Counseling and Development, 80,* 131–139.

Carlozzi, A. (2017). Counseling transgender persons and their families. *Counseling Today, 60*(2), 44.

Coady & Lehmann (Eds.). (2007). Theoretical perspectives for direct social work practice: A generalist-eclectic approach (2nd ed.). New York, NY: Springer.

Coleman, E., Bockting, W., Botzer, M., Cohen-Kettenis, P., DeCuypere, G., Feldman, J., . . . Zucker, K. (2012). Standards of care for the health of transsexual, transgender, and gender nonconforming people, 7th Version. *International Journal of Transgenderism, 13,* 165–232.

Collazo, A., Austin, A., & Craig, S. L (2013). Facilitating transition among transgender clients: Components of effective clinical practice. *Clinical Social Work Journal, 41,* 228–237.

Corey, G. (2012). *Theory and practice of counseling and psychotherapy*. Boston, MA: Cengage Learning.

De Cuypere, G., Knudson, G., & Bockting, W. (2010). Response of the World Professional Association for Transgender Health to the proposed DSM 5 criteria for gender incongruence. *International Journal of Transgenderism, 12*(2), 119–123.

de Vries A. L., McGuire J. K., Steensma T. D., Wagenaar E. C., Doreleijers T. A., & Cohen-Kettenis P. T. (2014). Young adult psychological outcome after puberty suppression and gender reassignment. *Pediatrics, 134*(4), 696–704.

Ducheny, K., Hendricks, M. L., & Keo-Meier, C. L. (2017). TGNC-affirmative interdisciplinary collaborative care. In A. A. Singh & l. m. dickey (Eds.), *Affirmative counseling and psychological practice with transgender and gender nonconforming clients* (pp. 69–94). Washington DC: American Psychological Association.

Ehrbar, R. D. (2010). Consensus from differences: Lack of professional consensus on the retention of the gender identity disorder diagnosis. *International Journal of Transgenderism, 12*(2), 60–74.

Feierabend R. H., & Bartee, Z. L. (2004). A collaborative relationship between a community mental health center and family practice residency program. *Families, Systems, and Health, 22,* 231–237.

Feldman, J. L., & Goldberg, J. M. (2006). Transgender primary medical care. *International Journal of Transgenderism, 9,* 3–34.

Fisk, N. M. (1974). Editorial: Gender dysphoria syndrome—the conceptualization that liberalizes indications for total gender reorientation and implies a broadly based multi-dimensional rehabilitative regimen. *Western Journal of Medicine, 120*(5), 386–391.

Freedman, J., & Coombs, G. (1996). *Narrative therapy: The social construction of preferred realities*. New York, NY: W. W. Norton and Co.

Gagne, M. (2005). What is collaborative mental health care? An introduction to the collaborative mental health care framework. *Canadian Collaborative Mental Health Initiative*. Retrieved November 9, 2017, from http://www.shared-care.ca/files/02-Framework-EN.pdf.

Giammattei, S. V. (2015). Beyond the binary: Trans-negotiations in couple and gamily therapy. *Family Process, 54*(3), 418–434.

Grant, J. M., Mottet, L., Tanis, J., Harrison, J., & Herman, J. L. (2011). *Injustice at every turn: A report of the National Transgender Discrimination Survey*. National Center for Transgender Equality and National Gay and Lesbian Task Force. Retrieved from http://www.thetaskforce.org/static_html/downloads/reports/reports/ntds_full.pdf

Harper, A., Finnerty, P., Martinez, M., Brace, A., Crethar, H. C., Loos, B., . . . Hammer, T. R. (2013) for the ALGBTIC LGBQQIA Competencies Taskforce. Association for Lesbian, Gay, Bisexual, and Transgender Issues in Counseling competencies for counseling with Lesbian, Gay, Bisexual, Queer, Questioning, Intersex, and Ally individuals. *Journal of LGBT Issues in Counseling, 7*(1), 2–43.

Heck, N. C., Croot, L. C., & Robohm, J. S. (2013). Piloting a psychotherapy group for transgender clients: Description and clinical considerations for practitioners. *Professional Psychology: Research and Practice,* pp. 1–7. doi: 10.1037/a0033134.

Hembree, W., Cohen-Kettenis. P. T., Gooren, L. J., Hannema, S. E., Meyer, W. J. 3rd., Murad, M. H., . . . T'Sjoen, G. G. (2017). Endocrine treatment of gender-dysphoric/gender-incongruent persons: An Endocrine Society clinical practice guideline. *Journal of Clin Endocrinology and Metabolism, 102*(11), 1–35.

Hines, S. (2006). What's the difference? Bringing particularity to queer studies of transgender. *Journal of Gender Studies, 15*(1), 49–66.

Hsieh, S., & Leininger, J. (2014). Resource list: Clinical care programs for gender-nonconforming children and adolescents. *Pediatric Annals, 43,* 238–244.

Institute of Medicine. (2011). *The health of lesbian, gay, bisexual, and transgender people: Building a foundation for better understanding*. Washington, DC: The National Academies Press.

James, S. E., Herman, J. L., Rankin, S., Keisling, M., Mottet, L., & Anafi, M. (2016). *The Report of the 2015 U.S. Transgender Survey*. Washington, DC: National Center for Transgender Equality.

Keo-Meier, C. L., Herman, L. I., Reisner, S. L., Pardo, S. T., Sharp, C., & Babcock, J. C. (2015). Testosterone treatment and MMPI-2 improvement in transgender men: A prospective controlled study. *Journal of Consulting and Clinical Psychology, 83*(1), 143–156.

Lev, A. I. (2004). *Transgender Emergence: Counseling gender-variant people and their families*. New York, NY: Taylor and Francis.

Lev, A. I. (2009). The ten tasks of the mental health provider: Recommendations for revision of the World Professional Association for Transgender Health, Standards of Care. *International Journal of Transgenderism, 11*(2), 74–99.

Lev, A. I. (2013). Gender dysphoria: Two steps forward, one step back. *Clinical Social Work Journal, 41*(2), 288–296

Lev, A. I. (2016). Gender dysphoria. In N. A. Naples (Ed-in-Chief), *Wiley-Blackwell encyclopedia of gender and sexuality studies* (pp. 987–990). Oxford, UK: Wiley-Blackwell.

Lev, A. I., & Wolf-Gould, C. (in press). Collaborative treatment across disciplines: Physician and mental health counselor coordinating competent care. *Gender Affirmative Model: An interdisciplinary approach to supporting transgender and gender expansive Children*. Washington, DC: American Psychological Association.

Malpas, J. (2015). Can couples change gender? Couple therapy with transgender people and their partners. In J. J. Bigner & J. L. Wetchler (Eds.), *Handbook of LGBT-affirmative couple and family therapy* (pp. 69–85). New York, NY: Routledge.

Markman, E. (2011). Gender identity disorder, the gender binary, and transgender oppression: Implications for ethical social work. *Smith College Studies in Social Work, 81*(4), 314–327.

McClearen, J. (2015). The paradox of Fallon's fight: Interlocking discourses of sexism and cissexism in mixed martial arts fighting. *New Formations: A Journal of Culture/Theory/Politics, 86*, 74–88.

Meyer, I. H. (1995). Minority stress and mental health in gay men. *Journal of Health and Social Behavior, 36*, 38–56.

Ndoro, S. (2014). Effective multidisciplinary working: The key to high-quality care. *British Journal of Nursing, 23*(13), 724–727.

Newfield E., Hart, S., Dibble, S., & Kohler, L. (2006). Female-to-male transgender quality of life. *Quality of Life Research, 15*(9), 1447–1457.

Nuttbrock, L., Hwahng, S., Bockting. W., Rosenblum, A., Mason, M., Macri, M., & Becker J. (2010). Psychiatric impact of gender-related abuse across the life course of male-to-female transgender persons. *Journal of Sex Research, 47*(1), 12–23.

Payne, M. (2015). *Modern social work theory* (3rd ed.). Chicago, IL: Lyceum Books.

Prosser, J. (1998). *Second skins: The body narratives of transsexuality*. New York, NY: Columbia University Press.

Richards, C., Bouman, W. P., Seal L., Barker M. J., Nieder, T. O., & T'Sjoen, G. (2016). Non-binary or genderqueer genders. *International Review of Psychiatry, 28*(1), 95–102.

Riley, E., Sitharthan, G., Clemson, L., & Diamond, M. (2013). Recognising the needs of gender-variant children and their parents. *Sex Education, 13*(6), 644–659.

Riley, W. K., Wong, T., & Sitharthan, G. (2011). Counseling support for the forgotten transgender community. *Journal of Gay and Lesbian Social Services, 23*(3), 395–410.

Schechter, L. S. (2009). The surgeon's relationship with the physician prescribing hormones and the mental health professional: Review for Version 7 of the World Professional Association for Transgender Health's *Standards of Care, International Journal of Transgenderism, 11*, 222–225.

Seaburn, D. B., Lorenz, A. D., Gunn, W. B., Gawinski, B. A., & Mauksch, L. B. (1996). *Models of collaboration: A guide for mental health professionals working with health care practitioners*. New York, NY: Basic Books.

Sherer, I., Rosenthal, S. M., Ehrensaft, D., & Baum, J. (2012). Child and adolescent gender center: A multidisciplinary collaboration to improve the lives of gender nonconforming children and teens. *Pediatrics in Review 33*, 273–276.

Singh, A. A, (2013). Transgender youth of color and resilience: Negotiating oppression and finding support. *Sex Roles, 68*(11/12), 690–702. https://doi.org/10.1007/s11199-012-0149-z

Singh, A. A., & dickey, l. m. (2017). *Affirmative counseling and psychological practice with transgender and gender nonconforming clients*. Washington, DC: American Psychological Association.

Singh, A. A., Hays, D. G., & Watson, L. S. (2011). Strength in the face of adversity: Resilience strategies of transgender individuals. *Journal of Counseling and Development, 89*(1), 20–27. https://doi.org/10.1002/j.1556-6678.2011.tb00057.

Spade, D. (2003). Resisting medicine, re/modeling gender. *Berkeley Women's Law Journal, 18*, 15.

Stryker, S. (1994). My words to Victor Frankenstein above the village of Chamounix: Performing transgender rage. *GLQ: A Journal of Lesbian and Gay Studies, 1*(3), 237–254.

Tate, C. C., Youssef, C. P., & Bettergarcia, J. N. (2014). Integrating the study of transgender spectrum and cisgender experiences of self-categorization from a personality perspective. *Review of General Psychology 18*(4): 302–312.

Tishelman, A. C., Kaufman, R., Edwards-Leeper, L., Mandel, F. H., Shumer, D. E., & Spack, N. P. (2015). Serving transgender youth: Challenges, dilemmas, and clinical examples. *Professional Psychology: Research and Practice, 46*(1), 37–45.

von Trotsenburg, M. (2014). Building a center for gender dysphoria research and transgender health care: The road from wishful thinking to reality. In B. Kreukels, T. Steensma, & A. de Vries (Eds.), *Gender dysphoria and disorders of sex development: Progress in care and knowledge* (pp. xvii–xix). New York, NY: Springer.

White, M., & Epston, D. (1990). *Narrative means to therapeutic ends*. New York, NY: W. W. Norton.

Whitehead, J. C., Thomas, J., Forkner, B., & LaMonica, D. (2012). Reluctant gatekeepers: "Transpositive" practitioners and the social construction of sex and gender. *Journal of Gender Studies, 21*(4), 387–400.

Woltmann, E., Grogan-Kaylor, A., Perron, B., Georges, H., Kilbourne, A. M., & Bauer, M. S. (2012). Comparative effectiveness of collaborative chronic care models for mental health conditions across primary, specialty, and behavioral health care settings: Systematic review and meta-analysis. *American Journal of Psychiatry, 169*(8), 790–804.

3

The Role of the SLP in Counseling

Richard K. Adler and Jack Pickering

Introduction

Counseling involves the establishment of an effective interpersonal relationship within which people are empowered to change and grow, becoming more autonomous, self-directing, and responsible. Counselors in collaboration with their clients and significant others help change feelings, attitudes, and thoughts that may prevent or restrict positive, personal growth (Corey, 2009; Ivey, Ivey, & Zalaquett, 2010). In transgender health, the mental health counselor plays a primary role in supporting people who are exploring gender identity, including those going through gender transition (WPATH, 2011). This important role is described in the previous chapter.

Counseling is also a role played by many helping professionals and can even be extended to families, friends, and supportive partners in the community. Speech-language pathologists (SLPs) are among the helping professionals who apply counseling skills to support people, specifically those with communication disorders and differences (Flasher & Fogle, 2012; Holland & Nelson, 2014; Luterman, 2008). Flasher and Fogle (2012) mention that there is a social science literature that describes counseling theories and skills that SLPs can utilize in order to support the people with whom they work. The literature is quite robust. This chapter will highlight some of the evidence and suggest how it can be applied to people who are transgender seeking voice and communication modification.

The notion that SLPs should counsel is not new. Charles Van Riper, as stated in Riley (2002), once said, "It is not enough to know the kind of disorder a person has, one must know the kind of person who has the disorder" (p. 1). He went on to say that one way of looking at speech and voice output is the identification and exhibition of the 'self.' Berry and Eisenson (1956) stated that "speech may be considered defective if the speaker is excessively self-conscious or apprehensive about objectively small deviations . . . in his manner of speaking" (p. 1). More recently, texts in voice disorders have described the role of counseling in voice therapy (Andrews, 2006; Aronson & Bless, 2009, Boone, MacFarlane, & Von Berg, 2005), and a recent taxonomy for voice therapy includes counseling as a specific, indirect intervention approach for people experiencing voice disorders (Van Stan, Roy,

Awan, Stemple, & Hillman, 2015). These observations provide a strong rationale for the application of counseling skills by speech-language pathologists.

It is important to note that counseling in speech-language pathology is not an optional approach or set of strategies that may or may not be used in certain circumstances. Rather, it is an essential component of clinical service delivery. The Scope of Practice of the American Speech-Language-Hearing Association (ASHA, 2016b) describes the SLP's counseling role, which includes empowering individuals and families affected by developmental and acquired communication disorders as well as speech, language, and voice differences. When counseling, SLPs engage clients in collaborative interactions related to their speech, language, communication, and swallowing disorders, and these interactions promote understanding and acceptance. Therefore, counseling skills can be applied with gender diverse people to help them adapt to, cope with, and modify feelings, attitudes, and thoughts that create barriers to change, that is, progress in voice and communication training. As SLPs, we strive for positive development, maturity, improving function, and improving skills.

Luterman (2008) describes two broad types of counseling performed by speech-language pathologists and audiologists: (a) informational counseling and (b) personal-adjustment counseling. Informational counseling includes the education and resources provided to clients and families that help to empower them and provide a rationale for assessment and therapy, including voice and communication training. Informational counseling can also include referral information for support groups and other resources. Personal-adjustment counseling includes the application of counseling theories and approaches to help clients change their feelings and thinking, particularly when

the feelings and thoughts create a barrier to progress.

Luterman (2008) makes it clear that personal-adjustment counseling is challenging for SLPs and audiologists but needs to be incorporated into the fabric of assessment and intervention. We are not psychotherapists and need to understand our counseling role and the boundaries that exist that may require referral to a mental health professional. Nonetheless, we are fully capable of applying the evidence in counseling to support clients who seek our services (Flasher & Fogle, 2012). By doing so, SLPs more effectively treat the whole person and address the impact of a disorder or difference by: (a) developing goals and capitalizing on strengths; (b) increasing autonomy, self-direction, and responsibility; and (c) modifying contextual factors to reduce barriers and enhance facilitators (World Health Organization, 2013).

The SLP plays a vital role in helping clients who identify as gender diverse produce a safe, healthy voice that is congruent with their gender identity. This requires both informational and personal-adjustment counseling provided by the SLP. The array of counseling approaches to meet these requirements provides clinicians with strategies and tools to support people who are transgender.

Attributes of and Foundational Skills for the SLP-Counselor

Survey research indicates that people in the transgender community often do not feel comfortable interacting with unfamiliar health care professionals (Kelly & Robinson, 2011), limiting access and restricting opportunities for positive change. As a result, SLPs need to exhibit the attributes of an effective helping professional and practice effective listening skills in order to foster trust and encourage client motivation to engage in voice and communication training (Hancock & Haskins, 2015).

Corey (2009) describes a wide range of counseling approaches available to mental health counselors, some of which are described in the prior chapter, and the importance of integrating these approaches to be an effective counselor. Prior to describing the theories, though, he states the importance of the counselor himself or herself as the most important "tool" in fostering change. In other words, the person counseling is as important as the approach used to counsel. With this thought in mind, there are three qualities or attributes of an effective counselor (Flasher & Fogle, 2012; Ivey, Ivey, & Zalaquett, 2010; Rogers, 1957) initially described by Carl Rogers:

- Congruence—engaging in interactions in a genuine way; communicating that we, as counselors, are in touch with our own feelings and thoughts.
- Unconditional positive regard—listening to the client without judgment regardless of the client's actions or behaviors; attending to the positive components of a client's story.
- Empathy—attempting to understand the client from his or her experience and point of view. It is important to note that clinicians must be careful in their application of empathy because a listener-helper cannot really understand another's experience; however, clinicians can still try to walk with clients as they engage in their journey.

These qualities are central to person-centered counseling, the first of five counseling approaches to be discussed later in this chapter. These qualities are clearly relationship-oriented and can be enhanced when the clinician is collaborative, caring,

and confident. Of course, collaboration in this context does not mean making decisions for clients, but rather empowering them to set and achieve their own goals. Clinicians in this case provide an opportunity for client empowerment and problem solving by using active listening skills, that is, skills associated with effective interviewing. While interviewing and counseling are different, the application of interviewing skills can support the SLP's counseling role by enhancing client-clinician rapport, developing trust, and providing an opportunity for the client to tell his/her story. Ivey, Ivey, and Zalaquett (2010) describe the following active listening skills:

- Attending behavior—the reinforcing ways we interact with clients using our facial expression, body language, words, and tone of voice. It is important that we communicate acceptance and openness during our clinical interactions and follow the client's lead during our clinical conversations.
- Asking open and closed questions—Our questions help us begin an interaction and maintain an effective flow during the conversation. Questions communicate to the client our desire to interact and understand.
- Observation skills—We need to tune in to our client's communication, both verbal and non-verbal. What we see and hear will shape our feedback, particularly if we sense conflict or stress in the client's interaction. Our observational skills allow us to be with our client in the moment.
- Encouraging, paraphrasing, summarizing—Here, we make statements that lead our clients to trust that we are truly listening and interested in what they say. These statements prompt the client, facilitate continued interaction, clarify understanding, and organize our thinking. We are not parroting back exactly what clients say,

but using these strategies to aid in understanding and let clients know we are with them.

■ Reflecting and validating feelings—It is important for SLP-counselors to acknowledge and address our client's feelings, both spoken and unspoken. We can reflect the client's "feeling" words and make statements that help us know where the client is from an emotional perspective.

As an SLP, we know that the client/clinician relationship is vital to progress and reaching goals set forth within an empathic environment (Rogers, 1951, 1961). This speaks directly to transgender clients who seek out accepting and empathetic professionals to help in their transition plan. Riley (2002) described "an approach to counseling that focuses on the client-clinician relationship" (p. 6). She states that according to Carl Rogers, "the basic assumption presented is that clients have the ability to find their own solutions in an accepting, empathic environment" (p. 6).

The attributes of congruence, unconditional positive regard, and empathy support relationship building and, as noted earlier, are underlying principles of Rogers' person-centered counseling. The application of these skills can help the client "know" that the clinician is interested, supportive, and sensitive to his or her needs. In the context of voice disorders, Behrman (2006) described Motivational Interviewing (MI) as an approach used to enhance an individual's adherence to change. MI is described as person centered, suggesting that the client is an expert in respect to his or her experience, needs, feelings, and thinking. The client's expertise and ultimately desire and responsibility to change are fostered by the clinician's interaction. Attributed to the work of Miller and Rollnick (2002), MI follows four guiding principles:

■ Expressing empathy
■ Developing discrepancy
■ Rolling with resistance
■ Supporting self-efficacy

In order to address these guidelines, MI encourages clinicians to apply the following strategies during clinical interactions (Behrman, 2006):

■ Asking open-ended questions
■ Affirming listening reflectively
■ Summarizing
■ Eliciting change talk

While the first four guidelines are consistent with active listening, "eliciting change talk" refers to a clinician's active process of reflecting and summarizing what the client has said in past sessions that reflects movement toward behavior change. This later step in MI uses clients' own words and actions to help them transition from resistance, a lack of adherence to intervention, to a plan of action that will lead to compliance and positive change. As we attempt to foster clients' responsibility to change their voice and communication, MI may be helpful for those people who seem resistant to the work required to change their voice and communication. It is a sensitive, non-threatening way that we can listen and facilitate client motivation.

Approaches to Counseling for the SLP

Holland and Nelson (2014, p. 13) list the intent of counseling with communication disorders as a series of goals for our clients, goals that apply to the voice and communication differences explored with transgender clients. While influenced in large part by Positive Psychology (Seligman, 2002), a number of other counseling approaches are reflected in these goal statements. Below, each goal is listed and followed by a description of how it fits within the context of transgender voice and communication.

- *To grieve what has been lost.* Gender diverse clients may express the loss of their gender assigned at birth, in favor of the gender they feel more appropriately encompasses who they truly are; therefore, they are eager to use the voice that is congruent with their new gender identity.
- *To understand what has happened as fully as possible.* Transgender clients want to understand their new role in life and in society as they get to know themselves in their preferred gender; the newly learned voice and communication skills help the transgender client achieve this.
- *To develop coping strategies and to increase resilience.* Many gender diverse people struggle with voice training in order to align the newly learned voice parameters with their new gender identify. One of our roles as an SLP is to use counseling techniques to help the transgender client achieve an authentic voice and communication pattern.
- *To make peace with the disorder.* Once they understand that their issue is a voice difference and not a disorder, clients who are transgender often have said they feel at peace with their new identity. A previous transfeminine client had told one of the authors that "having a voice difference and not a disorder makes me feel better; I don't need a disorder to deal with while I transition. I hear enough of that from my psychotherapist."
- *To make sensible adaptations to the disorder.* Transgender clients do not necessarily make adaptations but rather they have expressed their "new way of speaking and presenting themselves to the world."

Transgender clients are eager to use their new voice and communication skills in real-life situations and are relieved that they will not be misgendered (sometimes referred to as "read") as much in the future.

- *To capitalize on strengths in order to minimize weaknesses.* Transgender clients have explained that after voice training, they feel a sense of strength in who they are to all who meet them. "The new voice and communication parameters make me feel stronger as a woman."
- *To live as fully as possible despite impairment.* Although we do not purport the idea that voice and communication training for the transmasculine or transfeminine client is related to an impairment, transgender clients often feel despair, but not usually for their new voice or gender identity, but rather for not being able to have done this earlier in their lives or not having family supporting them.

These goals provide useful guidelines for clinicians supporting people whose feelings and thinking create a barrier to change, and a variety of counseling approaches can be applied to meet the goals. Corey (2009) encourages counselors to integrate approaches to maximize their counseling role, keeping in mind the effectiveness of any approach relies on the development of a strong interpersonal relationship, as described earlier and in the previous chapter on psychotherapy. SLPs can assist transgender and gender nonconforming clients through the integrated application of counseling approaches, each of which helps foster change. Among the approaches described by Holland, Corey, and others, five approaches will be described below:

- Person-centered counseling
- Existential counseling

☐ Cognitive-behavioral therapy
☐ Narrative Therapy
☐ Positive Psychology

Person-centered counseling. The key features of person-centered counseling have already been introduced in this chapter (see the section "Attributes of and Foundational Skills for the SLP-counselor"). Furthermore, Quinn (2012) proposes a "person centered" approach to the treatment of multicultural clients following the principles of Carl Rogers. Riley (2002) states that it is important to recognize the "clinician as counselor, connecting with the client, guiding the client to feel independent and self-confident as the basis for dealing with clients with communication disorders," (p. 7). Her principles are based on Rogers' writings that state that "the self-actualizing individual is open to and aware of experiences, is free of defense responses, lives in harmony with others, can perceive experiences realistically, has self-esteem, and can adapt to new situations" (p. 7). She further states that a state of congruence develops between the client's perception and the reality of the situation. This is the beginning of the client/clinician relationship that has to be developed first for counseling to be effective.

Existential counseling. According to Mulhauser (2016), "clients who view their problems as challenges of living rather than symptoms of psychopathology, and clients who are genuinely attracted to increasing self-awareness . . . will be well-served by existential counseling," (from http://www.counselingresource.com). Exploring the client's reality, known as phenomenology, is the cornerstone of this type of counseling. SLPs do not have to learn how to psychoanalyze or adopt this specific philosophical method but might embrace this as a way of exploring challenges and barriers to the client, including grieving and loss, mentioned

by Holland and Nelson (2014) in the beginning of this section.

Transgender voice and communication training fits into this scheme perfectly. After all, leading a more meaningful life is truly embracing the existential way of understanding ourselves. Many of our transgender clients have mentioned that they feel guilty and experience a sense of loss during transition. Some share religious reasons for this and some report that they were plagued by family discord. According to Spillers (2007), although people generally accept no responsibility for causing their communication disorder, some clients feel a sense of guilt, and in the case of transgender clients, this guilt may be very deeply rooted. But looking at transgender voice and communication as a difference, instead of a disorder, empowers clients to accept the new way of using voice and enables them to continue transition without guilt. The SLP can guide the client through this. We are leading the client through voice and communication training, which requires the SLP to be fully invested in training, including counseling, and to listen with empathy and without judgment as clients go through their transition. This is the SLP embracing the existential approach to counseling. For some of the people we work with, it will be helpful to encourage them to discuss these existential feelings with their mental health counselor. In addition, support groups are a frequent component of existential counseling and can be very important to the transmasculine or transfeminine client.

A basic premise of existential counseling is looking at reality, the relationship of reality and the individual's awareness of reality. To understand the existential style of counseling, one must ask 'what is therapeutic interaction?' Kierkegaard, an existential philosopher, looked at the clinician as a person with values and expectations. It is very important to look at the clinician's ability to communicate these characteristics to the client and family, if they are involved. After all, what is therapy? It is an interactive process with the outcome of producing positive change. Counseling can be looked at in the same way. As stated earlier, positive, helping relationships are the essence of counseling. As SLPs, we are involved in facilitating trusting interpersonal relationships; our intent is to promote growth in another person.

Cognitive-behavioral therapy. There are a number of cognitive-behavioral therapies that share a similar thread: unhelpful (sometimes referred to as distorted or faulty) thinking leads to emotional and behavioral problems (Bloom, 2010; Corey, 2009; Flasher & Fogle, 2012; Luterman, 2008). In other words, the way we think about an event or life circumstance can affect the way we feel and behave. Often, ways of thinking are based on long-held beliefs that are learned over time. The goal of cognitive-behavioral therapy is to identify unhelpful thinking and replace it with more effective, flexible thinking. This often requires the clinician to confront the client when thinking is not rational. Careful attention to the client's language can often uncover distorted thinking, and changes in language (what the client says) can often support behavior change.

Flasher and Fogle (2012) summarize four cognitive distortions that impact the way we think about things and events and that affect a client's motivation to change:

- Catastrophizing—the belief that, no matter what, the worst thing will happen in a given event of circumstance. Clients who are transgender may believe that they will be misgendered and ridiculed if they try to use their voice to order coffee or ask for help while shopping.

- "I should" statements—a tendency toward perfection or an inability to accept flaws. A client who is transgender may believe that he or she cannot speak in public until the voice is "just right."
- Dichotomous thinking—viewing a circumstance as either one thing or another, without seeing a middle ground or continuum. A client who is transgender may believe that a listener's reaction to his or her voice will be either good or bad, with no potential for a neutral, non-judgmental reaction.
- Overgeneralization—the belief that if something is true in one situation it will be true in similar circumstances. A client who is transgender may not shop for a dress in one store because of a negative experience in another.

Ylvisaker and Feeney (2005), working with people after traumatic brain injury, described the implementation of advanced organizers and scripts like Goal-Plan-Do-Review and hard/easy to help modify an individual's language and, ultimately, thinking about challenging everyday situations. Positive self-talk ("I can do this!") prior to an interaction or situation can also be used to support success. For a person who is transgender, an advanced organizer in the shape of a flow chart can be constructed that provides the client with an opportunity to list strategies to use (a) prior to a conversation, (b) while engaging in the conversation, and (c) after the conversation is completed. Positive language can be incorporated into the organizer. Examples might include:

- Before I speak, I will take two or three relaxing breaths and use positive self-talk.
- When I talk, I will use good eye contact and speak with more forward resonance (see Chapter 11).
- After I am done talking, I will review the interaction, listing three things that went well.

A newer cognitive-behavioral approach that has been described in the literature on stuttering (Beilby, Byrnes, & Yaruss, 2012) is called Acceptance and Commitment Therapy (ACT). Attributed to Hayes, Strosahl, and Wilson (1999), ACT is described as the management of experiential avoidance and emotional instability. ACT attempts to decrease frustration through acceptance and a focus on valued living. Beilby, Byrnes, and Yaruss (2012, p. 290) describe six core processes of this approach:

- Self-concept: the process of developing flexibility in how one views himself or herself. The way we view ourselves is a thought that triggers an emotional response, such as avoidance. ACT introduces alternative responses like willingness and acceptance.
- Defusion: the process of promoting behavioral flexibility, recognizing that thoughts are thoughts, not facts.
- Acceptance: the process of embracing emotional and cognitive events without attempting to change them.
- Mindfulness: the process of developing a perspective on the present and extending this perspective into everyday life rather than dwelling on thoughts and experiences in the past.
- Values: the process of clarifying aspects of life that are most meaningful to the client and considering resources that are available to the person that can be directed toward achieving personal goals and away from behaviors like avoidance.
- Committed action: the process of following through with goals and future quality-of-life priorities.

The above processes may be useful for people who are transgender and gender diverse if they are avoiding communication opportunities or frustrated by their voice and communication skills at a given time in therapy. These processes would also be helpful if clients are placing too much value on producing a "perfect voice" or thinking that there is only one way to accomplish their goals. Mindfulness provides an opportunity for clients to experience the moment without judgment, whether that moment includes breathing, exploring self-confidence, or mentally visiting a safe, comfortable space. Distracting or negative thoughts are acknowledged but allowed to move on while attention is refocused on the present moment (Boyle, 2011; Davis & Hayes, 2012; Shapiro & Carlson, 2009).

Narrative therapy. Associated with White and Epston (1990), narrative therapy allows clients to explore their story, externalizing problems and creating a more positive sense of self. The primary benefit of narrative therapy is to separate the problem from the person, which generates hope and decreases blame. Bloom (2010) describes some of the techniques that are used in narrative therapy:

- Externalization and deconstruction—Identity maps are used to: (a) map the influence of a problem on the person's life, and (b) map the influence of the person's life on a problem. These activities, which can focus on clients' personal attributes, goals, and strengths, show clients that they are much more than the problem or the challenge that they face.
- Searching for unique outcomes—In this approach, the client and clinician discuss times when the problem was successfully confronted or when the client was resourceful in responding to a challenge. The client can use these unique outcomes to develop a solution story, an alternative re-story.
- Alternative stories and re-authoring—The clinician listens for instances in clients' communication when they were

successful, resourceful, and ready to change. These reflect a move away from the original problem-oriented narrative. Sharing these instances with clients supports their alternative, re-story. Client competencies and positive actions are documented for the individual's new story.

■ Documenting the evidence—In this technique, the clinician writes letters to the client about changes that have been made from session to session. Letters can: (a) reconnect the client to the positive aspects of a session, (b) summarize the changing influence a problem or challenge has had on the client, and (c) document unique outcomes and exceptions to the problematic story that emerged from the session. These letters reinforce the client's choice to change on an ongoing basis.

Positive Psychology. Martin Seligman, in his book *Authentic Happiness* (2002), describes Positive Psychology as an approach to clinical intervention that focuses on strengths and assumes that people want to live lives with meaning and purpose. He and his colleagues created this theory as a response to other, more typical, theories that focus on the negative challenges that accompany disorder. Instead, Positive Psychology focuses on the benefits of personal attributes like optimism, resilience, wisdom, and creativity. As an approach to counseling, Positive Psychology is highly collaborative and designed to create a positive and organized sense of self and an optimistic vision of the future for our clients, even in light of significant change.

Using Positive Psychology, clients can achieve wellness and a more optimistic perspective through a number of activities, including: (a) making a gratitude visit, (b) listing three good things in life, and (c) describing yourself at your best. The following gratitude activities have been applied in a group context at the end of transgender voice and communication sessions:

■ Completing a thank you note that expresses gratitude toward an important person

■ Discussing something that a client is grateful for from the session

■ Writing down and describing an accomplishment, a hobby, or a strength

■ Making a plan to list three positive things that happen over the next week

In his book *Flourish*, Seligman (2011) presents a Theory of Well-Being using the acronym PERMA. Holland and Nelson (2014) apply PERMA to counseling in communication disorders, and it has merit in addressing the communication differences that are the focus of transgender voice training. The acronym is briefly described below.

P: Positive Affect—The good feelings attached to past experience and positive expectations for the future contribute to well-being.
E: Engagement—The ability to become fully involved in those things that are happening "in the moment" is important for an individual's well-being.
R: Relationships—Involvement with others and experiencing a sense of belonging are ways of enhancing well-being.
M: Meaning—The ability to serve beyond oneself and to advocate for others contributes to an individual's well-being.
A: Accomplishment—The opportunity to succeed and to feel good about meeting one's goals enhances well-being.

In transgender voice and communication, the PERMA model has been applied in a number of ways:

■ The gratitude activities mentioned above influence positive feelings.

- A client did a hair and makeup "class" that provided a context for practicing communication while engaging in an activity that was meaningful.
- Group therapy encourages shared, peer feedback and encourages relationship building. Recently, members of a transgender voice and communication group started going out for coffee after each group session.
- A transgender woman in a voice and communication program lobbied for changes in a county-level anti-discrimination statement to include gender identity and gender expression. Interactions related to her advocacy work were practiced in therapy.
- Clients in a transgender program went into a college class and taught students about the transgender experience, enhancing the students' cultural competence and providing a strong sense of accomplishment for the clients.

The application of the PERMA model provides a way of including meaningful, functional activities for clients who are transgender. Client-centered conversation, rather than de-contextualized therapy activities, can be a chance to both practice voice and communication skills and discuss aspects of the clients' lives that are meaningful and rewarding and provide hope for the future. The use of videos to encourage self-advocacy, engagement in group therapy, and creative project-based activities that extend beyond a single session all have potential to help clients who are transgender experience enhanced well-being, optimism, and self-confidence.

Becoming a Micro-counselor

No matter which approach an SLP uses, Ivey, Ivey, and Zalaquett (2009) and Ivey and Moreland (1997) suggested the concept of

micro-counseling when a teachable moment occurs even in the course of a therapy session. We suggest that the SLP become a "micro-counselor." This is achieved through effective interviewing and effective interpersonal communication skills developed by the SLP over time. Micro-skills counseling may be achieved by the following:

- Video-taping sessions to analyze client/patient and your own behaviors.
- Identifying helping skills you use and the clients' need to express themselves.
- Becoming aware of your client's attending skills such as active listening as well as your own eye contact, body language, and so forth.
- Summarizing for the client what was learned or what will be learned at the next session or sets of sessions.
- Analyzing your own vocal tone and rate and volume of your speech.
- Becoming aware of Proxemics (the way you position yourself and the client/patient in the room).
- Paraphrasing without adding your own prejudices; listening without judgment.
- Using verbal encouragement.
- Reflective listening: non-verbal behaviors are a major part of communication; there might be mixed messages from the client's verbal versus non-verbal behaviors such as conflicts, contradictions, and incongruities; encourage paraphrasing or summarizing.
- Using positive language during interactions.

Realizing that SLPs are trying to demystify counseling for the transgender client, and for themselves, your counseling may take five minutes during one session or it can take an entire session. Throughout training, you want to make sure your verbal and non-verbal signals are in sync so as not to confuse, frighten, or anger the client. It is time to get over the complexity of a counseling moment by practicing; that makes you a better counselor when it is needed. With that said, clinicians should be mindful to be very disciplined about their counseling role because sessions can "run away" if not monitored. Clients may need boundaries and reminders that voice is the primary area of focus for the session (personal communication Hirsch, September 28, 2017). Furthermore, some topics may be better explored with the individual's mental health counselor, as described in the previous chapter.

Voice "Windows": A New SLP Approach to Counseling

Borrowing from personal computer vocabulary, Adler (2017) purports a theory of "Windows of the Voice." This paradigm outlines the stages transgender clients progress through as they learn their new voice and communication skills as well as understand their empowering role in the entire journey. Adler teaches the "Windows of Your Voice" to all of his transgender clients to prepare them for their empowerment and self-advocacy and to prepare them for counseling that will be part of each session. However, this framework will change over time, addressing the person's feelings, attitudes, and thinking along the way. Table 3–1 lists the eight windows that a client will experience when participating in voice and communication training.

Understanding the variety of windows of the client's voice will help the SLP be a more effective therapist as well as counselor for the transgender client. Counseling plays a significant role in guiding the client through these stages to be most successful. Window 1: *Brain Voice vs. Inner Voice*: The SLP will hear the client say, "I hate the way my voice sounds" and that is the "brain voice" telling him/her from past ex-

Table 3–1. Windows of the Voice

Windows	Meaning
Window 1	Brain Voice vs. Inner Voice
Window 2	Mindful of Risks
Window 3	Modeling
Window 4	Developing the Real You
Window 5	Believability
Window 6	Ancillary Voice Usage
Window 7	Embracement
Window 8	Confidence/Poise

periences versus "My voice sounds feminine sometimes, but I want my voice to match just me as a woman." That is the inner voice ("inside our head voice") telling us that the client can change with help (from the SLP). We are striving for a change in feelings and thinking about voice and communication and paying greater attention to the productive inner voice. After all, isn't this the heart and soul of the counseling that we do with our transgender clients?

Window 2 works on the client to be *mindful of risks*. The client has to be brave enough to try the new voice techniques and the actual new "inner" voice that is now "out" by trying it in a variety of places. In other words, they need to take the risk of knowing they might be "read" but continue to plough through to eventually feel comfortable with the voice that all others hear. This helps build a client's self-esteem and worth. One of Adler's clients, who will be called Kate, transitioned into a beautiful, confident woman. She could have been a twin of the country singer Shania Twain. However, she felt her voice sounded like a man's despite a pitch range of 160 to 210 Hz that is clearly in the female range. She took a risk by agreeing to go with me to a restaurant, department store, and a movie box office to use her new voice and communication skills. She was never mistaken for a male; this shows that voice is perceptual and that skills can be effectively taught. Kate took a risk and developed confidence that her new voice was acceptable to others identifying her as a woman.

Window 3, or *Modeling*, allows the client to continue to take risks, learn to model the therapist, and learn techniques that will help create the new "inner voice"; being aware of why it sounds good and why modeling is important; and being aware that there are reasons for why it comes out 'wrong,' and feeling open to discussing it with the SLP and those in her circle of family and friends/allies. Many clients feel awkward trying, for instance, Resonant Voice Therapy or Vocal Function Exercises that are very effective with transgender clients. But after a short time, they realize how they help them achieve a voice and communication pattern that matches their gender identity. Practice then becomes easier and less frightening. And successful practicing comes from the client modeling the clinician as new techniques are presented. The SLP helps guide the client past the awkwardness of these exercises.

Developing the Real You is what Window 4 encourages. The SLP will help the client empower him/herself to own the new voice; learn what makes the client's voice unique to us and to others; and use the new voice even if it feels awkward in various situations, knowing that the voice is now the "real you."

The SLP can offer the transgender client a new word or Window 5: *Believability*. Through counseling and encouragement, the SLP will help the client believe in his/her new voice and believe it is the "real you" that is speaking. Overall, it is a process of empowering the client to be confident and assured that others "believe" your voice as well; it is helpful in achieving authenticity.

Helping clients change feelings and think about their transition and their voice and communication skills is a positive outcome of counseling.

The new voice that is developing in the transgender client also carries over into ancillary voice usage. Window 6, or *Ancillary Voice Usage*, teaches the client how to cough, clear the throat, and change the secondary aspects of voice to match the communication intent for a variety of emotions. Knowing this will empower the client to know and accept that there will be some moments that are "read" by others and yourself because the voice did not come out as the client intended. Cisgender individuals have days when they sound more masculine or more feminine in everyday situations. Discussing this with a client is very helpful.

The SLP can offer the transgender client another new term for Window 7: *Embracement*. This is an empowering word for the new voice user. It tells the client to embrace who you are now; the woman/man/gender nonconforming individual. A range of progress and failure come to people in all aspects of their lives, not just voice. The client, knowing that he/she can change the voice in some ways, is based on the situation in which the client finds him/herself. Embracement is the final stage to complete the empowerment journey. And changing the voice will ultimately bring a state of congruence to the new, authentic self.

Finally, Window 8: *Confidence/Poise*, helps the client move on with life feeling confident every day that the voice is the "real you." The SLP guides the client to "spread the word" to others, being confident that if you "fall back," that doesn't mean the end-all; the client will bounce back and once again embrace the newly established voice and communication skills. Developing these skills will help the SLP guide the client through all eight window stages.

Conclusion

As noted in this chapter, speech-language pathologists have an array of counseling skills and approaches that can be used to support people who are transgender. Person-centered counseling, existentialism, cognitive-behavioral therapy, narrative therapy, and Positive Psychology each have principles and ideas that we can utilize to develop effective relationships, empower the people with whom we work, and support change in thinking and feeling. The new "Windows" approach serves as a framework for achieving these important outcomes.

Existentialism and the "Windows" approach teaches us that we have the freedom to make life as we would like to have it and we are responsible for establishing our own reality and fulfilling our own destiny (Spillers, 2007; Yalom, 1980). To a transgender person, this means fulfilling the desire to express gender identity and develop a voice and communication system that is consistent with that presentation.

The integrated application of these counseling approaches and the use of strategies mentioned earlier can support positive change in our clients' feelings, attitudes, and thinking, particularly in relation to voice and communication. As SLPs, we need to have the confidence to use counseling tools, recognizing that referral to and collaboration with a mental health counselor may be necessary to fully engage in our SLP-counselor role. Given the psychosocial issues that face many clients who are transgender, taking on the role of counselor provides a context to develop client trust and responsibility. Through the application of counseling approaches, we may also help foster increased client self-confidence and a greater willingness to take risks as communicators. Miars (2002) describes existential authenticity as a "cornerstone to a positive view of life." He further states that "authenticity recognizes the individual's ultimate freedom and responsibility to choose how to live in the world" (p. 3).

References

Adler, R. (2017). The SLP as counselor for the transgender client. *SIG 10: Perspectives in Higher Education*, Vol. 2. Rockville, MD: ASHA.

Adler, R., Hirsch, S. & Mordaunt, M. (2012). *Voice and communication therapy for the transgender/transsexual client: A comprehensive clinical guide* (2nd ed.). San Diego, CA: Plural Publishing.

American Speech-Language-Hearing Association. (2010). *Preferred practice patterns for the profession of speech-language pathology*. Available from http://www.asha.org/policy.

American Speech-Language-Hearing Association. (2016a). *Code of ethics* [Ethics]. Available from http://www.asha.org/policy.

American Speech-Language-Hearing Association. (2016b). *Scope of practice in speech-language pathology* [Scope of practice]. Available from http://www.asha.org/policy/.

Andrews, M. L. (2006). *Manual of voice treatment* (3rd ed.). Clifton Park, NY: Thompson Delmar Learning.

Aronson, A. E., & Bless, D. M. (2009). *Clinical voice disorders* (4th ed.). New York, NY: Thieme Medical Publishers, Inc.

Behrman, A. (2006). Facilitating behavioral change in voice therapy: The relevance of Motivational Interviewing. *American Journal of Speech-Language Pathology, 15*(2), 215–225.

Beilby, J. M., Byrnes, M. L. & Yaruss, J. S. (2012). Acceptance and Commitment Therapy for adults who stutter: Psychosocial adjustment and speech fluency. *Journal of Fluency Disorders, 37*(4), 289–299.

Berry, M., & Eisenson, J. (1956) *Speech disorders: Principles and practices of therapy* (2nd Edition). New York, NY: Appleton-Century-Crofts.

Bloom, C. (2010). Finding the psychotherapeutic harmonies embedded within Mark Ylvisaker's holistic approach to executive function rehabilitation. *Journal of Behavioral and Neuroscience Research, 8*(1), 60–69.

Boone, D. R., McFarlane, S. C., & Von Berg, S. L. (2005). *The voice and voice therapy* (7th ed.). Boston, MA: Pearson, Allyn and Bacon.

Boyle, M. (2011). Mindfulness training in stuttering therapy: A tutorial for speech-language pathologists. *Journal of Fluency Disorders, 36,* 122–129.

Corey, G. (2009). *Theory and practice of counseling and psychotherapy* (8th Edition). Belmont, CA: Brooks/Cole Cengage Learning.

Davies, S., Papp, V. G., & Antoni, C. (2015). Voice and communication change for gender nonconforming individuals: Giving voice to the person inside. *International Journal of Transgenderism, 16*(3), 117–159.

Davis, D., & Hayes, J. (2012). What are the benefits of mindfulness? *American Psychological Association, 43*(7), 64.

DiLollo, A., & Neimeyer, R. A. (2014). *Counseling in speech-language pathology and audiology: Reconstructing personal narratives.* San Diego, CA: Plural Publishing.

Flasher, L. V. & Fogle, P. T. (2012). *Counseling skills for speech-language pathologists and audiologists* (2nd ed.). Clifton Park, NY: Delmar-Cengage Learning.

Hancock, A., & Haskin, G. (2015). Speech-language pathologists' knowledge and attitudes regarding lesbian, gay, bisexual, transgender, and queer (LGBTQ) populations. *American Journal of Speech-Language Pathology, 24*(2), 206–221.

Hayes, S. C., Strosahl, K. D., & Wilson, K. G. (1999). *Acceptance and Commitment Therapy: An experiential approach to behavior change.* New York, NY: Guilford Press.

Holland, A. L., & Nelson, R. L. (2014). *Counseling in communication disorders: A wellness perspective* (2nd ed.). San Diego, CA: Plural Publishing.

Ivey, A. E., Ivey, M. B., & Zalaquett, C. P. (2010). *Intentional interviewing and counseling: Facilitating client development in a multicultural society* (7th ed.). Belmont, CA: Brooks/Cole Cengage Learning.

Ivey, A. E., & Moreland, J. R. (1997). *Microcounseling: Innovation in interview training* (3rd ed.). Alexandria, VA: Microtraining Associates.

Kelly, R., & Robinson G. (2011). Disclosure of membership in the lesbian, gay, bisexual, and transgender community by individuals with communication impairments: A preliminary Web-based survey. *American Journal of Speech-Language Pathology, 20*(2), 86–94.

Kierkegaard, S. (1985). *Fear and trembling* (A. Hannay, translator). New York, NY: Penguin.

Kierkegaard, S., Hong, H. V., & Hong, E. H. (2000). *The essential Kierkegaard.* Princeton, NJ: Princeton University Press.

Luterman, D. (1984). *Counseling the communicatively disordered and their families.* Boston, MA: Little, Brown.

Luterman, D. (2008). *Counseling persons with communication disorders and their families* (5th ed.). Austin, TX: Pro-Ed.

May, R. (1953). *Man's search for himself.* New York, NY: W. W. Norton & Co.

McLeod, S. (2014). *Carl Rogers.* Retrieved December 3, 2016, from http://www.simplypsychology .org/carl-rogers.html

Miars, R. D. (2002). Existential authenticity: A foundational value for counseling. *Counseling and Values, 46,* 3.

Miller, W. R., & Rollnick, S. (2002). *Motivational interviewing: Preparing people for change* (2nd ed.). New York, NY: Guilford Press.

Mulhauser, G. *An introduction to Existential Counselling.* Retrieved December 5, 2016, from http: counselingresource.com

Muller, J. (1995). *Kierkegaard's philosophy: Self-deception and cowardice in the present age.* Lanham, MD: University Press of America.

Pierce, L. M. (2016). Overwhelmed with the burden of being myself: A phenomenological exploration of the existential experience of counselors-in-training. *Journal of Humanistic Counseling, 55*(2), 136–150.

Quinn, A. (2012). A person-centered approach to multicultural counseling competence. *Journal of Humanistic Psychology, 53*(2), 202–251.

Raskin, N. J., Rogers, C. R., & Witty, M. C. (2008). Client-centered therapy. In R. Corsina & D. Wedding (Eds.). *Current psychotherapies.* Belmont, CA: Thomson Higher Education.

Riley, J. (2002). Counseling: An approach for speech-language pathologists. *Contemporary Issues in Communication Science and Disorders, 29,* 6–16.

Rogers, C. (1951). *Client-centered therapy: Its current practice, implications, and theory.* London, UK: Constable.

Rogers, C. R. (1957). The necessary and sufficient conditions of therapeutic personality change. *Journal of Consulting Psychology, 21.* Retrieved February 14, 2017, from http://www.shoreline .edu/dchris/psych236/Documents/Rogers.pdf

Rogers, C. R. (1961). *On becoming a person: A psychotherapist's view of psychotherapy.* New York, NY: Houghton Mifflin.

Rogers, C. R. (1980). *Way of being.* Boston, MA: Houghton Mifflin.

Rogers, C. (1995). *Client-centered therapy: Its current practice, implications and theory.* Philadelphia, PA: Trans-Atlantic.

Seligman, M. (2002). *Authentic happiness: Using the new positive psychology to realize your potential for lasting fulfillment.* New York, NY: Free Press.

Seligman, M. (2011). *Flourish.* New York, NY: Free Press.

Shapiro, S., & Carlson, L. (2009). *The art and science of mindfulness integrating mindfulness into psychology and the helping professions.* Washington, DC: American Psychological Association.

Shipley, K. G. (1997). *Interviewing and counseling in communicative disorders: Principles and procedures* (2nd ed.). Boston, MA: Allyn & Bacon.

Spillers, C. S. (2007). An existential framework for understanding the counseling needs of clients. *American Journal of Speech-Language Pathology, 16*(3), 191–197.

Van Riper, C. (1963). *Speech correction: Principles and methods* (4th ed.). Englewood Cliffs, NJ: Prentice-Hall, Inc.

Van Riper, C. (2017). *Counseling.* Retrieved September, 30, 2017 from https://quizlet.com/174202035/counseling-flash-cards/

Van Stan, J. H., Roy, N., Awan, S., Stemple, J., & Hillman, R. E. (2015). A taxonomy of voice therapy. *American Journal of Speech-Language Pathology, 24*(2), 101–125.

White, M., & Epston, D. (1990). *Narrative means to therapeutic ends.* New York, NY: W. W. Norton and Company.

World Health Organization. (2013). How to use the ICF: A practical manual for using the International Classification of Functioning, Disability and Health (ICF). Exposure draft for comment. Retrieved August 2, 2017, from http://www.who.int/classifications/drafticfpracticalmanual2.pdf?ua=1.

WPATH. (2011). Standards of Care Version 7. Retrieved December 28, 2016, from http://www.wpath.org/site_page.cfm?pk_association_webpage_menu=1351&pk_association_webpage=3926

Yalom, I. D. (1980). *Existential psychology.* New York, NY: Basic Books.

Ylvisaker, M., & Feeney, T. (2005). School success after brain injury: Behavioral, social, and academic issues. In *The child with cerebral palsy, acquired brain injury and developmental delay: A family-based approach to neurodevelopment.* New York, NY: Taylor and Francis Publishers.

4

Medical Considerations

Linda Gromko and Kevin Hatfield

A word from the chapter authors: As we launched into this project, it became apparent that the topic of Medical Considerations was far too broad for a single chapter. With forty years of combined experience in providing direct medical care to transgender individuals (young children to elders), we appreciate that therapies, terminology, and attitudes change over time. We recognize that this information will be elementary for many readers, but advanced for others. We respectfully ask that you take what is useful for you and your patients, and utilize the resources cited to guide you further.

—L. Gromko, MD and K. Hatfield, MD

Introduction

Over recent years, transgender and gender non-conforming individuals have sought health care in record numbers, and yet the 2011 National Transgender Discrimination Survey of 6,000 transgender individuals found 30% delayed seeking care due to prior disrespect and 50% had to teach their providers about their own health care (Grant et al., 2010). Certainly, the increased visibility of transgender people in the mainstream media has contributed to an increased awareness of the presence and needs of this population. In turn, the Internet has helped transgender people learn about the idealized trans health care that is available in institutions such as the University of California San Francisco, Fenway Medical Center in Boston, and Vancouver Coastal Health in British Columbia, among others.

Information from the World Professional Association for Transgender Health (WPATH) is available online (WPATH.org). Specific WPATH Standards of Care are available to patients and health care providers. As of this writing, the current published Standards of Care is SOC-7. The newest SOC-8 guidelines are now being drafted for late 2018 publication. A unique United States Professional Association for Transgender Health (USPATH) has been convened to reflect the growing body of knowledge, expertise and leadership that care providers in the United States bring to the international organization. WPATH holds international conferences biannually; regional conferences are held in the United States, as USPATH. While WPATH provides more formally vetted guidelines for worldwide health care professionals, individuals have often found published academic university affiliated guidelines, lay literature, online support networks, and YouTube videos to be sources of useful assistance as well.

Traditionally, health care providers have not received formal training in transgender medicine. Several medical schools have begun to offer transgender medical content. The University of Washington, for example, offers an annual quarter-long elective on the medical and surgical aspects of transgender health. Additionally, the University of Washington offers an LGBT pathway for medical students, permitting interested students to select clerkship rotations in LGBT-focused clinical settings. New York University and the University of California San Francisco are among other medical schools that have developed transgender medicine coursework. Academically sponsored fellowships in transgender surgery are now being offered for the first time in New York City and Philadelphia.

While medical education remains at an early stage of development nationwide—and many professional schools have yet to offer any training at all, transgender patients expect their health care providers to be informed about their specific medical issues, as well as be becoming culturally competent when working with Transgender/Gender Diverse patients (Grant et al., 2010).

We hope that this chapter will help clinicians and trainers understand some of the salient and overriding medical needs of the transgender and gender non-conforming population.

What Is Gender and What Is Gender Identity?

Most simply, gender reflects whether a person was born a boy or a girl. Today, this is often described as "Assigned Male at Birth" (AMAB) or "Assigned Female at Birth" (AFAB). We often hear the terms "natal male" or "natal female." The terms "genetic male" and "genetic female" imply that we are indeed aware of the karyotyping or chromosomal makeup of an individual (it is very pertinent to remark that the transgender community's endorsement of terms changes over time. Appropriate terminology today may be obsolete or even offensive tomorrow). See Table 4–1 for definitions of the basic terminology.

Gender *identity* refers to how people see *themselves*. For example, a "cis-gender male" is born male and identifies himself as

Table 4–1. Definitions for Basic Terms

Basic Definitions to Help Health Care Providers Working with Transgender/Gender-Variant Populations	
Term	**Definition**
Gender	Biological definition and refers to whether a person was born male or female or intersex (beyond the scope of this chapter). Gender is based on anatomy and/or genetic makeup.
Gender identity	How a person defines themselves, i.e., male or female, somewhere in between or "without" gender. The term "gender incongruence" is used to describe the circumstance where gender and gender identify are divergent.
Gender expression	Refers to an individual's choice of clothing, style of grooming, behavior, and tenor of social interactions that convey masculinity, femininity, both, or neither.
Sexual orientation	Refers to who a person is attracted to—and is independent of gender, gender identity, and gender expression.

male. The cis-gender male experiences gender congruence or synchrony. A *transgender* male, however, was assigned female at birth and identifies or *affirms* their gender as male, in what is experienced as gender incongruity.

An increasing number of people do not align with the "gender binary" at all (Ehrensaft, 2011). These people may define themselves as "gender non-binary"—identifying as neither male *nor* female. They may define themselves as "gender fluid." Some people identify as agender—not identifying with *any* specific gender. You may also hear the terms "male of center" or "female of center"; where a person lies on the gender continuum is defined by that individual *only*.

Gender identity is highly personal—defined only by the person involved. Needless to say, such definitions are critically important to individuals. Health care professionals are encouraged to make every effort to use the definitions accepted by a specific client—and to use the pronouns that a person finds acceptable. As an example, many gender non-binary people may use the pronouns "they" or "them." Simply asking, "What would you like to be called," or "What pronouns do you use" can convey enormous respect to our patients.

What Is Sexual Orientation?

Sexual orientation refers to who we are *attracted* to in a sexual manner. Like gender orientation, sexual orientation may be seen as a continuum with people being attracted to people of their own gender (be that their birth gender or their identified gender), the opposite gender, both, or neither. Sexual orientation is considered to be a separate concept from gender orientation. Some say that "gender is who you *are*, sexual orientation is who you *love* (Erikson-Schroth,

2014). Most importantly, gender identity, gender expression, and sexual orientation are defined *only* by a specific person—for themselves.

What Is Gender Dysphoria?

Gender dysphoria is commonly defined as an overarching understanding of oneself as being *other* than the birth gender—*and feeling distress related to that*. Gender dysphoria may be ameliorated by a variety of modalities: hormone therapy, voice training, surgical interventions to masculinize or feminize, psychotherapy, family therapy, and so forth.

The recognition and treatment of anxiety and depression is of particular importance, as nearly half of all transgender individuals report having attempted suicide at some time in their lives (Mizock & Hopwood, 2016). Supportive modalities include the prescription of appropriate antidepressants and/or anxiolytics, cognitive behavioral therapy, support groups, and crisis intervention (Trans Lifeline services, for example, may be accessed by telephone or text).

While gender dysphoria can be enormously discomfiting, it is important to remember that not all transgender individuals report gender dysphoria. Gender dysphoria can be minimized by the approaches listed above—all intended to help individuals find greater gender congruence for themselves. Again, it is the client/patient who defines which therapies and interventions are appropriate individually for them.

When Does Biological Gender Differentiation Begin?

Early in pregnancy, all fetuses look essentially the same. Then, at about 10 weeks into a pregnancy, male fetuses begin to make the hormone testosterone—programmed by the DNA in their chromosomes (XY). Female fetuses (XX) do not. As a result of testosterone, a male fetus develops a penis and scrotum, whereas a female fetus develops a clitoris and external labia—all from structures that began as being virtually identical. The gonads, that is, testicles for males and ovaries for females, develop within the abdominal cavity, with testes descending into the scrotal sac during the mother's pregnancy. Understanding that males and females develop from homologous embryologic structures, that is, the same raw materials, is helpful to clinicians and patients wanting to better understand the techniques of gender-affirming surgeries (Mizock & Hopwood, 2016).

At puberty, all individuals begin to elaborate dominant sex hormones: testosterone from the male testes, or estrogen and progesterone from the female ovaries. This is preceded by adrenarche: the secretion of DHEA and androgenic steroids by the zona reticularis of the adrenal glands common to both genders. Adrenarche is heralded by body odor and axillary hair growth. While not yet puberty, adrenarche signals that puberty will occur over the next one to two years.

In treating gender dysphoria in older adolescents and adults, we essentially shift the dominant sex hormone in an individual's hormonal milieu by prescribing "cross sex hormones" (or simply stated, "cross hormones"). By administering exogenous estrogen and testosterone suppressors to a natal male, the circulating testosterone is greatly reduced. By administering exogenous testosterone to a natal female, the circulating estradiol (estrogen) is reduced. During the administration of cross hormones, the body's natal hypothalamic-pituitary axis is temporarily modified. Natal gonads respond by secreting less testosterone in a

natal male, or less estrogen in the natal female. Do note that while the hypothalamic-pituitary axis is modified *temporarily* during hormone administration, the effects of cross hormone administration (e.g., development of facial hair, lowering of the voice with testosterone, breast development with estrogen) are likely to be permanent.

When Do Individuals Become Aware of Gender Dysphoria?

It is widely recognized that many children are aware of gender dysphoria between the ages of 3 and 5. Others become acutely aware of dysphoria—even to a point of panic and suicidality—as puberty approaches. With the onset of periods for natal girls or the deepening of the voice for natal boys, puberty is the time when transgender children seem to realize that they are *not* going to grow up in their affirmed gender—at least not without significant medical and/or surgical interventions. It is during this time when unsupported youth experience high levels of anxiety, isolation, academic struggles, and even suicidal ideation (Reisner et al., 2015).

In older youth, we hear accounts of "things not feeling right" until a young person learns about the entity of being gender variant. For some of these youth, knowing that there is a "name" for their feelings provides comfort, along with a path toward gender synchrony.

Many individuals may report an awareness of gender dysphoria but are not aware of available treatment. Others are fully aware that treatment—medical, surgical, and so forth—is available, but they cannot pursue these options due to a variety of economic, family, or career-related factors. We have seen people seek treatment after the death of parents or a spouse, for example. And we have seen people whose gender dysphoria was so profound that they came to realize that they simply could not go on living without making the transition to their affirmed gender.

What Medical Treatment Is Available for Gender Dysphoria?

For young children, treatment for gender dysphoria generally consists of supporting family and community affirmation of a child's social transition (no hormone therapy is needed because pre-pubescent children are very much alike, having yet to elaborate dominant sex hormones). Affirming a social transition may include supporting a child's adaptation of a gender-congruent appearance in clothing and hair and using appropriate names and pronouns. It may include advocacy in a child's school to ensure that a child is supported in "presenting" with appropriate gender expression and called by the correct names at school. A recent University of Washington study, published in the journal *Pediatrics*, demonstrated that such children develop healthfully in a variety of parameters when parental support is abundant (Olson, Durwood, DeMeules, & McLaughlin, 2016).

For early adolescents, hormonal manipulation is available in the form of puberty blockers (histrelin subdermal implants or depo-leuprolide injections). Puberty blockers *temporarily* interrupt the hypothalamic-pituitary axis, signaling the pituitary gland to block secretion of FSH (follicle stimulating hormone) and LH (luteinizing hormone)—both of which ordinarily stimulate the testicles or ovaries to secrete their respective hormones (testosterone or estrogen/progesterone).

The use of puberty blockers in transgender adolescents by the Dutch was first published in 2006. In the United Stated, histrelin and depo-leuprolide have been utilized for many years in the treatment of precocious puberty, that is, when puberty begins at *very early* ages in children. This information is reassuring to clinicians and parents, in that long-term safety of puberty blockers has been established (Hembree et al., 2017).

In transgender children, puberty blockers are typically used at Tanner Stage 2. There are five Tanner Stages. Stage 1 is pre-pubertal. Tanner Stage 2 is recognized by the development of the natal testicle to a length of at least one inch, or the development of a breast "bud" under the areola of a natal female's breast. The later Tanner Stages, that is, through Tanner Stage 5, correspond with further adolescence progressing into adulthood.

Puberty blockers (histrelin or depo-leuprolide) put the puberty process on "pause," allowing a gender dysphoric child to "buy some time" by preventing the inevitable secondary sex changes of puberty. Young adolescents of both genders continue to grow in height. But the natal male child will not experience the deepening of voice, facial hair growth, or maturation of the genitals. Similarly, the natal female will not begin periods or experience further breast or genital development while being treated with a puberty blocker.

It is important to know that puberty blockers can be stopped at any time. When a blocker implant is removed or blocker injections are halted, puberty continues on as it was genetically programmed to do. Thus, puberty blockers provide children and families considerable flexibility. A blocker does nothing irreversible; it simply allows time for children and families to move toward further gender treatment if and when it is appropriate. But started early in the sub-group of gender dysphoric children who are "insistent, consistent, and persistent" (Meier & Harris, n.d.) the blocker/cross hormone regimen eliminates development of secondary sex characteristics that are so distressing to this group—and so difficult and costly to remedy in later life (de Vries, Steensma, Doreleijers, & Cohen-Kettenis, 2011; Delemarre-van de Waal, & Cohen-Kettenis, 2006; Hembree et al., 2017).

What Are the Effects Produced by Cross Hormones and How Are They Administered?

For natal females wishing to transition male (or moving toward the male spectrum), testosterone may be used in the form of custom-compounded creams, gels, transdermal patches, or most commonly, injections. Transition is rapid, often heralded by a drop in vocal pitch within the first few months and continuing for at least 12 months (Nygren et al., 2016). This effect can be slowed when patients (especially adolescents) need or desire slower escalation of the testosterone dose. Individuals who sing often request slower dose escalation in an attempt to preserve greater vocal range. This method, along with careful and sustained practice, has shown to be beneficial (Adler, Constansis, & Van Borsel, 2012; Constansis, 2008). Body hair becomes more coarse and plentiful, and scalp hair may recede in a typically male pattern. Patients are informed that balding may occur on testosterone. Facial hair growth varies greatly, as does the loss of scalp hair. Skeletal muscles bulk if a patient participates in strength training activities. Sexual appetite and the desire for food increase. The clitoris enlarges, and vaginal tissues become drier. Monthly menstrual cycling typically stops within three to six

months depending on the dose of testosterone. Clinicians are careful to remind their trans male patients that safe sex includes contraception for those having sexual contact with people who produce sperm. Despite menstrual cessation, unexpected pregnancies have been reported.

Natal males transitioning female (or toward the female spectrum) often begin their treatment with a testosterone suppressant to decrease the levels of testosterone in the bloodstream, and thereby decrease testosterone effects such as body hair growth and erectile function. (Note: testosterone blockers are different than the puberty blockers discussed earlier). The blood pressure medication spironolactone and sometimes finasteride are commonly used in the United States, although cyproterone acetate is used elsewhere in the world—all available in tablet form.

Estradiol (estrogen) is available as patches, oral tablets dissolved sublingually, and injections. The loss of morning or "random" erections is an early change. Breast bud development and nipple sensitivity occur within a month or two, with maximum breast development generally expected within three years. Body hair becomes sparser and skin becomes softer. Estradiol generally has no effect on facial hair; nor does it usually restore prior loss of scalp hair.

Unlike their trans male counterparts, trans females do not experience a change in vocal range (Edgerton, 1974). A persistently male voice becomes a source of particular distress, especially when clients are misgendered or "sir'd" (mistaken for male) on the phone. As described throughout this book, regular practice of "speaking female" and ongoing professional vocal training are the non-invasive approaches which can produce impressive natural results. Although it requires a great deal of effort, and range of time, it is far less expensive than vocal surgery. Surgical treatments for vocal feminization are aimed at shortening and/or thinning the functioning vocal cords—for example, by laser technology. Such surgeries are invasive, expensive, and rarely covered by insurance. Additionally, these procedures carry risks of temporary and/or permanent hoarseness, and in some cases require a patient to avoid speaking for six weeks or more after surgery (Anderson, 2014; Casado et al., 2015; Gross, 1999; Remacle et al., 2011). Chapter 5 provides additional information about voice feminization surgery.

Individuals transitioning toward their affirmed gender tend to experience a sense of calm. Some providers attribute this to the fact that patients are acting on their gender goals, but certainly there are hormone receptors in the brain that may be directly responsible. Steroid rage is rarely observed in trans males maintaining physiologic levels of testosterone. An increase in mood range, the tendency to cry more easily, or even a degree of mood lability are not uncommon to see in trans females on physiologic doses of estradiol. Trans women may welcome these changes as confirmation that the hormone treatments are having the desired effect.

Monitoring blood levels of estradiol and testosterone is easily performed, though clinicians are urged to monitor in a consistent manner. It is recognized that a drug reaches a pharmacologic "steady state" in the body after five half-lives worth of medications have been administered. With injections, we obtain nadir or trough levels right before the sixth injection; random levels provide less meaningful information. (Note that injected hormones may be given weekly, monthly, or at 10-day intervals.) Blood levels in patients using oral medications, creams/gels, or patches may be taken after a patient has achieved a steady state in roughly two to four weeks.

Do Hormone Treatments Have Dangers?

All medications carry both risks and benefits. Individuals seeking to masculinize (trans males) may experience the following testosterone related risks:

- Increased weight
- Increased risk of sleep apnea
- Worsening of cholesterol values (elevated total and LDL cholesterol, lower HDL)
- Elevated red blood cell count with risk of "sludging" of cells, i.e., as in polycythemia

Individuals taking estradiol may experience:

- Increased risk of deep vein thromboses (clots) in the lower extremities or pelvis
- Increased risk of pulmonary emboli if a clot travels to the pulmonary circulation. Note that blood clot risks are higher in smokers, in individuals who are mistakenly taking ethinyl estradiol [oral contraceptive form] instead of estradiol [bio-identical], and in patients with thrombophilias (a hereditary or acquired tendency to form blood clots). While the actual risks of developing a pulmonary embolism are small, pulmonary emboli can be lethal.
- Increased risk of gall bladder disease
- For patients taking spironolactone as a testosterone suppressant, reversible kidney failure can occur in patients taking certain blood pressure medications (ACE inhibitors or ARBs) in addition to spironolactone. Individuals with marginal kidney function should be monitored carefully and are generally cautioned not to use spironolactone.

What Surgical Treatment Is Available for People Experiencing Gender Dysphoria?

While the majority of transgender individuals actually do not have gender-affirming surgery, options are becoming more elegant—and functional. For example, in years past, sexual responsiveness was sacrificed in vaginoplasty (creating a vagina). Newer techniques provide for excellent appearance, vaginal depth that allows for penetration if desired, and full orgasmic function.

Surgical Treatments for Trans Women

- Facial Feminization Surgery (FFS) incorporates a variety of procedures that may minimize jaw and brow prominences, reposition the frontal hairline, reshape the nose, and/or reduce the size of the thyroid cartilage. The latter shaves the Adam's apple only and is not intended to alter the vocal cord structures. That said, experts report cases where permanent vocal changes have occurred in some patients.
- Voice surgery (described elsewhere in this book) involves shortening the vocal cords to produce a higher vocal frequency.
- Breast augmentation surgery enhances the breast development produced by hormone administration.
- Orchiectomy removes the testicles only, reducing the need for testosterone blockers, but not impacting the appearance of the external genitalia (except for creating the appearance of an empty scrotal sac).
- Vaginoplasty is a complex, though commonly performed, surgery during which the testicles are removed, the glans penis is dissected and restructured to fashion a clitoris, the urethra is shortened and relocated below the neoclitoris, and the vagina is constructed from inverted penile tissue and sometimes grafted scrotal tissue. Where inadequate tissue exists, tissue grafts from the hip area may also be utilized. Post-operative vaginal dilation, done in a conscientious manner by the patient, is critical to prevent the neovagina from closing.

Surgical Treatments for Trans Men

- Chest reconstruction ("top surgery") removes female breasts, with an outcome suggesting a "cut" or muscular pectoralis appearance. (Most trans males who have top surgery will have used chest binders earlier in transition. A binder might be described as a sleeveless Spandex T-shirt, fitting so snugly that patients may complain of breathing restriction that limits their athletic activity.)
- Metoidioplasty utilizes the basic concept that a clitoris exposed to testosterone will enlarge and appear as a phallus. Severing the supporting ligaments of the clitoris allows the phallus to protrude. Combined with urethral extension, a trans man is able to urinate standing up—through the phallus. A metoidioplasty may be followed by scrotoplasty with testicular prostheses.
- When penetrative intercourse is desired, a more extensive, multi-surgery phalloplasty builds a longer phallus using tissue derived from the radial forearm, the anterior thigh, or the latissimus dorsi area of the patient's back. In phalloplasty, the patient's ovaries, uterus, and fallopian tubes are removed; the perineal opening is usually closed in a procedure called vaginectomy. Another procedure for creating a phallus is that of the pedicle flap; a "handle" of tissue is

created from the soft tissue of the lower abdomen, released and repositioned in the correct location.

In both metoidioplasty and phalloplasty, orgasmic function is maintained by the preservation of clitoral tissue. In phalloplasty, for example, the clitoris may be positioned inside the base of the neophallus, or just below it. Erections in phalloplasty are made possible by the inclusion of a semi-rigid, malleable rod within the phallus, or the use of implantable devices such as those used in natal males with erectile dysfunction (Gromko, 2015).

What Do Our Transgender Patients Need from Us as Clinicians?

Clearly, gender transitions can be complicated—particularly when all aspects, that is, psychotherapy, medical and surgical treatments, and vocal training are considered. Yet, when asked what they would have done differently, most of our patients reply, "I would have done it earlier." Because most of us did not receive formal training in transgender health, we may find our clients to be our best teachers (James et al., 2016). At the bare minimum, we can reciprocate by providing personal respect: careful listening, conscious use of appropriate names and pronouns, and the integrity to admit our own lack of formal training with the added commitment to find the necessary information our patients require.

References

Adler, R. K., Constansis, A. N., & Van Borsel, J. (2012). Female-to-male transgender/transsexual considerations. In R. K. Adler, S. Hirsch, & M. Mordaunt (Eds.), *Voice and communication therapy for the transgender/transsexual client: A comprehensive clinical guide* (pp. 153–186). San Diego, CA: Plural.

Adler, R. K., Hirsch, S., & Mordaunt, M. (2012). *Voice and communication therapy for the transgender/transsexual client: A comprehensive clinical guide* (2nd ed.). San Diego, CA: Plural Publishing.

Anderson, J. A. (2014). Pitch elevation in trangendered patients: Anterior glottic web formation assisted by temporary injection augmentation. *Journal of Voice, 28*(6), 816–821.

Casado, J. C., O'Connor, C., Angulo, M. S., & Adrián, J. A. (2015). Wendler glottoplasty and voice-therapy in male-to-female transsexuals: Results in pre and post-surgery assessment. *Acta Otorrinolaringologica Espanola, 67*(2), 83–92.

Constansis, A. N. (2008). The changing female-to-male (FTM) voice. *Radical Musicology, 3*, 1–18.

de Vries, A. L., Steensma, T. D., Doreleijers, T. A., & Cohen-Kettenis, P. T. (2011). Puberty suppression in adolescents with gender identity disorder: A prospective follow-up study. *Journal of Sexual Medicine. 8*(8), 2276–2283.

Delemarre-van de Waal, H. A., & Cohen-Kettenis, P. T. (2006). Clinical management of gender identity disorder in adolescents: A protocol on psychological and paediatric endocrinology aspects. *European Journal of Endocrinology, 155*(suppl 1), S131–S137.

Edgerton, M. T. (1974). The surgical treatment of male transsexuals. *Clinics in Plastic Surgery, 1*(2), 285–323.

Ehrensaft, D. (2011). *Gender born, gender made: Raising healthy gender-nonconforming children.* New York, NY: The Experiment.

Erikson-Schroth, L. (2014). *Trans bodies, trans selves: A resource for the transgender community.* New York, NY: Oxford University Press.

Grant, J. M., Mottet, L. A., Tanis, J., Harrison, J., Herman, J., & Keisling, M. (2010). *Injustice at every turn: A report of the National Transgender Discrimination Survey* [Internet]. National Center for Transgender Equality and National Gay and Lesbian Task Force.

Gromko, L. (2015) *Where's my book: A guide for transgender and gender non-conforming youth, their parents, and everyone else.* Seattle WA: Author.

Gross, M. (1999). Pitch-raising surgery in male-to-female transsexuals. *Journal of Voice, 13*(2), 246–250.

Hembree, W. C., Cohen-Kettenis, P. T., Gooren, L., Hannema, S. E., Meyer, W. J., Murad, M. H, . . . Sjoen, G. G. T. (2017). Endocrine treatment of gender-dysphoric/gender-incongruent persons: An Endocrine Society clinical practice guideline. *Journal of Clinical Endocrinology Metabolism*, *102*(11), 3869–3903.

James, S. E., Herman, J. L., Rankin, S., Keisling, M., Mottet, L., & Anafi, M. (2016). *The Report of the 2015 U.S. Transgender Survey*. Washington, DC: National Center for Transgender Equality.

Meier, C., & Harris, J. (n.d.). American Psychological Association fact sheet: Gender diversity and transgender identity in children. Retrieved February 21, 2018, from http://www.apadivisions.org/division-44/resources/advocacy/transgender-children.pdf

Mizock, L., & Hopwood, R. (2016). Conflation and interdependence in the intersection of gender and sexuality among transgender individuals. *Psychology of Sexual Orientation and Gender Diversity, 3*(1), 93–103.

Morley, J. E. (2016). Overview of the endocrine system. *Merck Manual, Professional Version.* Retrieved February 17, 2018, from http://www.merckmanuals.com/professional/endocrine-and-metabolic-disorders/principles-of-endocrinology/overview-of-the-endocrine-system

Nygren, U., Nordenskjold, A., Arver, S., & Sodersten, M. (2016). Effects on voice fundamental frequency and satisfaction with voice in trans men during testosterone treatment. *Journal of Voice, 30*(6): 766.e23–766.e34.

Olson, K. R., Durwood, L., DeMeules, M., & McLaughlin, K. (2016). Mental health of transgender children who are supported in their identities. *Pediatrics, 137*(3) e20153223; doi: 10.1542/peds.2015-3223.

Reisner, S. L., Vetters, R., Leclerc, M., Zaslow, M. A., Wolfrum, S., Shumer, D., & Mimiaga, M. J. (2015). Mental health of transgender youth in care at an adolescent urban community health center: A matched retrospective cohort study. *Journal of Adolesc Health*, 56(3), 274–279.

Remacle, M., Matar, N., Morsomme, D., Veduyckt, I., & Lawson, G. (2011). Glottoplasty for male-to-female transsexualism: Voice results. *Journal of Voice, 25*(1), 120–123.

5

Voice and Communication Modification: Historical Perspective

Jack Pickering and McKenzee Greene

Introduction

It has been a little more than 40 years since the first report of voice and communication modification for a person who is transgender. In that initial paper, Kalra (1977) presented a case study at the American Speech-Language-Hearing Association (ASHA) convention in Chicago that described voice modification for a trans woman. A year later, Bralley and his colleagues published an article in the *Journal of Communication Disorders* on the impact of voice modification on a trans woman (Bralley, Bull, Gore, & Edgerton, 1978). These case studies have been followed by a growing body of literature describing clinical service delivery in transgender voice and communication modification, as well as increasing research evidence to support intervention for people who are transgender, particularly trans women. While the next chapter provides a detailed description and careful analysis of the research evidence in transgender voice and communication training, what follows is a historical perspective, from Kalra's ground-breaking study to the present.

This historical perspective will be broken up into two time periods: (a) before 2006, the year that this book was first published and (b) after 2006. This division reflects the relatively slow, steady growth in the professional literature prior to 2006, contrasted by a more rapid and significant increase in research and service delivery since that time. It is worth noting that the recent growth in voice and communication services over the past decade coincides with a rapidly changing social, political, and cultural landscape for people who are transgender and gender nonconforming, as well as an evolving understanding and re-conceptualization of gender. Both of these developments have and will continue to impact the nature and extent of practice for speech-language pathologists (SLPs) working with people who are gender diverse, which will in turn influence the direction of clinical research in voice and communication training.

As part of the following historical perspective, this chapter will include a review of the literature on client self-reported voice and communication satisfaction, including the development of and research on the Transsexual Voice Questionnaire (TVQ^{MtF}; Dacakis et al., 2013). There will also be a brief description of the current evidence for surgical procedures to modify the vocal anatomy and therefore the voice of people who are transgender. The chapter will conclude with a summary of voice and communication services at the present time, services that are evolving and expanding with the significant changes being realized in transgender health and gender studies. From a practical, clinical standpoint, this means that caseloads will include a broader range of gender diverse clients, including adolescents who are increasingly requesting voice and communication training (see Chapter 17).

Historical Perspective: Before 2006

The Early Research

After Kalra (1977) and Bralley et al. (1978), a small number of case reports and small-N studies were found in the professional literature prior to 2006. The research focused primarily on vocal characteristics and resonance, the two areas of clinical practice that continue to be emphasized with trans women. Early treatment studies with trans women indicated that intervention can facilitate the safe increase in average speaking fundamental frequency (f_0) to levels that are consistent with cisgender women (Dacakis, 2000; Mount & Salmon, 1988; Söderpalm, Larsson, & Almquist, 2004). Dacakis (2000) found a positive correlation between the number of sessions and the greater increase of f_0, suggesting that more treatment sessions provided a greater likelihood of maintaining a higher f_0.

Early research on voice and communication modification also found that increases in speaking fundamental frequency alone were not necessarily enough to positively impact listener perception of gender for trans women, including changes in inflection. Specifically, more upward inflection and less level inflection patterns supported the perception of a female speaker (Gelfer & Schofield, 2000; Wolfe, Ratusnik, Smith, & Northrop, 1990). The influence of resonance was also considered in the early research (Gelfer & Mikos, 2005; Gelfer & Schofield, 2000; Mount & Salmon, 1988), with evidence indicating that increasing resonance (formant) frequencies, especially F2, may positively impact the perception of gender in trans women. The relative contributions of fundamental frequency and resonance frequencies were also considered in these early studies, something of considerable interest to researchers and clinicians at the present time.

Van Borsel, De Cuypere, and Van den Berghe (2001) investigated the interaction between physical appearance and vocal perception of trans women. Results indicated that physical appearance, including nonverbal communication, appeared to be a more positive indicator for being perceived as feminine, while voice alone seemed to be less significant to this perception. Interestingly, a similar study with trans men suggested that there was no significant interaction between voice and appearance, so gender perception based on these two factors was influenced differently for people transitioning from female to male (Van Borsel, de Pot, & De Cuypere, 2009). Collectively, the early research in transgender voice and communication suggested that intervention for trans women supported gender transition but that raising pitch alone was not enough.

As more research emerged on the effectiveness of voice and communication modification, the role of client voice and communication satisfaction was also being investigated. Byrne, Dacakis, and Douglas (2003) investigated a group of 21 trans women's communication satisfaction, including pragmatic language abilities. Results of this study indicated that communication satisfaction was positively related to satisfaction with voice, length of time in the gender reassignment program, perceived communication ability, and pitch. Furthermore, the transgender participants' self-perceptions were significantly more negative than the self-perceptions of the study's 21 cisgender women who served as control participants. These findings indicated that self-perceived pragmatic language and satisfaction with voice may provide clinicians with pertinent information about the overall communication satisfaction of their clients. Since the publication of this study, research on client self-reported voice and communication satisfaction has increased substantially and will be included later in the chapter.

There was one pre-2006 study that investigated voice change in trans men (Van Borsel, De Cuypere, Rubens, & Destaerke, 2000). Initially, 16 trans men were surveyed about their perception of voice change after hormone therapy. While most of the participants were satisfied with their voice change, some expressed unexpected results in regard to the timing and extent of the change (e.g., difficulty singing, being perceived as a female speaker at times). In the same research study, Van Borsel et al. (2000) completed a longitudinal analysis of voice change in two trans men during and after hormone therapy, which resulted in a reduction in f_0 to gender-neutral levels, reduced fundamental frequency range, and no change in perturbation. Based on this investigation, Van Borsel et al. (2000) indicated that some trans men may experience voice problems during and after hormone

treatment, so SLPs may have a role in voice assessment, education, and therapy for some trans men. For a thorough review of the literature on trans male speakers and a description of voice and communication modification, see Chapter 9.

Describing Transgender Voice and Communication Modification

As the early research emerged, so too did published descriptions of voice and communication services for trans women. Oates and Dacakis (1983) wrote the first description, which was based primarily on studies of gender differences in communication and on the limited research on transgender voice and communication available at that time. Oates and Dacakis (1983) recommended that voice modification should include changes in fundamental frequency, with attention given to prosody, intensity, voice quality, resonance, articulatory precision, vocabulary, and conversational style and content. Vocal health and nonverbal communication were also mentioned as factors to consider when working with the transgender population. Two laryngeal surgeries were also discussed for modifying fundamental frequency, procedures that were experimental at the time.

Fourteen years after their article outlining considerations for voice modification, Oates and Dacakis (1997) wrote a thorough review of the research in transgender voice and communication using literature describing: (a) differences between men's and women's voices; (b) perceptual characteristics of voice that affect gender identification; (c) vocal characteristics associated with transgender voice; (d) stereotypes regarding men's and women's voices; and (e) laryngeal surgery to modify fundamental frequency (and thus the pitch) of trans women. In their extensive reference list, only five research studies were found that addressed treatment efficacy for transgender individuals. Despite Oates and Dacakis' caution that research on treatment effectiveness was very limited, recommendations that emerged from the literature review continue to be implemented in voice and communication programs around the world.

Oates and Dacakis (1997) suggested that voice services for trans women should address: (a) increasing fundamental frequency to at least 155 Hz (a gender-neutral frequency); (b) increasing resonance (formant) frequencies; (c) decreasing intensity; (d) increasing a breathy voice quality; and (e) modifying intonation patterns (more shifts in intonation, fewer level intonation patterns, and less extensive downward intonation patterns). Articulation of speech sounds, rate, vocabulary, and communication style and content were also noted as aspects of communication that could be targeted in treatment, based on the available research on gender-based communication differences and stereotypes.

In addition to the characteristics of voice and communication that should be targeted in therapy, Oates and Dacakis (1997) suggested important steps in intervention, including careful assessment of communication throughout the treatment process, collaboration with the client to establish goals, and attention to the production of voice and language in the client's real world. They also suggested giving attention to non-verbal vocalizations, like coughing and laughing, as important aspects of voice training. This systematic, multidimensional approach to voice and communication modification for trans women continues to be implemented in their clinical program at LaTrobe University in Melbourne, Australia (Dacakis, 2008; Oates & Dacakis, 2017), and

research from the program has had a significant impact on service delivery in transgender voice and communication.

After the publication of Oates and Dacakis (1997), two additional articles were published that described voice and communication modification (Freidenberg, 2002; Gelfer, 1999). Gelfer (1999) outlined a hierarchical approach to voice services that began with establishing a target pitch, effective use of inflection, and production of a vocal quality that is "light and clear" (p. 203). Biofeedback, using a Visi-Pitch or other tools, was suggested in order to habituate the target pitch. In addition to vocal characteristics, Gelfer emphasized the production of resonance, with the ultimate goal of a natural, female voice. In later stages of the program, language and non-verbal communication were included. Treatment ended when the clinician and client agreed that an acceptable female voice had been achieved.

Freidenberg (2002) also described voice and communication modification for trans women, summarizing Gelfer's (1999) hierarchy and providing additional information on aspects of intervention, like life experience, the transition process, standards of care, and influential professionals (like mental health counselors) who provide care for clients in the transgender community. Freidenberg urged clinicians to prepare carefully for work with transgender clients, as their voice and communication intervention is being done in the context of a broader transition process. Attention to cultural and gender differences and stereotypes was included. Freidenberg ended with an observation that client satisfaction sometimes appears at odds with improvements in acoustic-perceptual features of voice. This apparent mismatch has become a theme of recent research on transgender voice and communication.

As these specific descriptions of voice and communication modification were being published, SLPs and students studying communication disorders started seeing references to transgender voice and communication in general textbooks on voice disorders and voice therapy (see Aronson, 1990; Challoner, 1986; additional sources include Andrews, 1999; Boone, McFarlane, & Van Berg, 2005; Stemple, Glaze, & Gerdeman, 1995). It was not until 2006 that Adler, Hirsch, and Mordaunt published the first comprehensive text on the assessment and intervention of transgender speakers, the first edition of this book. The book continues to serve as an important guide for SLPs interested in working with individuals in the transgender community. The publication by Adler, Hirsch, and Mordaunt (2006) coincided with the beginning of a substantial increase in research, resources, and service provision for transgender speakers that continues to this day.

Historical Perspective: After 2006

A Brief Review of the Evidence

Since the first edition of Adler, Hirsch, and Mordaunt (2006), there has been a significant increase in the professional literature in transgender voice and communication, including evidence to support some aspects of training for trans women. Research since 2006 has focused on the aspects of voice and resonance mentioned previously (e.g., Gelfer & Tice, 2013; Gelfer & Van Dong, 2013; Gorham-Rowan & Morris, 2006; Hancock, Colton, & Douglas, 2014; McNeill, Wilson, Clark, & Deakin, 2008; Van Borsel, Janssens, & De Bodt, 2009), including the

relative contribution of voice and speech characteristics to changes in gender perception for trans women (e.g., Gallena, Stickels, & Stickels, 2017; Gelfer & Bennett, 2013; Hancock & Garabedian, 2013; Hardy et al., 2016; King, Brown, & McCrea, 2012; Leung, Oates, & Chan, 2018; Skuk & Schweinberger, 2014). The most recent of these studies is a systematic review and meta-analysis. Based on a data set of 38 articles, Leung, Oates, and Chan (2018) determined that pitch, resonance, loudness, articulation, and intonation contributed to listener perception of gender, providing evidence that supports the targets frequently described for transfeminine voice and communication training.

In addition to this research, aerodynamic and physiological studies of voice have emerged (e.g., Holmberg, Oates, Dacakis, & Grant, 2010; Palmer, Dietsch, & Searl, 2012), and aspects of articulation and language have been described (e.g., Hancock, Stutts, & Bass, 2015; Schwartz & LaSalle 2008; Van Borsel & De Maesschalck, 2008). Finally, Hancock and Helenius (2012) published a case study about voice and communication modification with an adolescent client. These examples do not represent an exhaustive list of studies, but reflect the growing research on transgender voice and communication modification since 2006. Other important topics have been described in the literature, such as trans male speakers (Azul, 2015, 2016; Azul, Arnold, & Neuschaefer-Rube, 2018; Azul, Nygren, & Sodersten, 2017; Block, 2017; Davies, Papp, & Antoni, 2015; Irwig, Childs, & Hancock, 2017; Nygren et al., 2016), which will be explored in detail in Chapter 9. Research on client self-reported voice and communication satisfaction has increased substantially and will be included later in the chapter, as will vocal fold and laryngeal surgeries.

The existing evidence supporting voice and communication modification for trans women was recently discussed by Oates and Dacakis (2015) and is described in more detail in the next chapter. To summarize briefly, Oates and Dacakis (2015) indicated that there is strong evidence to support raising fundamental frequency to approximately 180 Hz and increasing resonance (formant) frequencies to the levels of cisgender females. Other evidence, less convincing according to the literature, indicates that trans women benefited from therapy that:

■ increased variability in fundamental frequency,
■ increased the speaker's high and low fundamental frequency,
■ reduced intonation patterns that are level or falling,
■ decreased vocal intensity and effort, and
■ incorporated a breathy voice quality.

In their article, Oates and Dacakis (2015) acknowledged the still limited but growing evidence base in transgender voice and communication modification. They also recognize that the traditional binary construct of gender is changing, which means that some transgender speakers may be interested in goals that focus on vocal flexibility (for example), not a specific increase or decrease in one or more vocal characteristics. In addition to the growing literature in transgender voice and communication described by Oates and Dacakis (2015), there is an expanding set of resources for clinicians serving people in the transgender community (for example, see "Providing Transgender Voice Services" on the ASHA website: http://www.asha.org/Practice/multicultural/Providing-Transgender-Transsexual-Voice-Services/). One important source of support for practicing clinicians and clients is the World Professional Association for Transgender Health (WPATH).

World Professional Association for Transgender Health

WPATH (http://www.wpath.org) is a multidisciplinary, international organization that promotes evidence-based care, education, research, advocacy, public policy, and respect in transgender health. Incorporated in 1979 as the Harry Benjamin International Gender Dysphoria Association (HBIGDA), the organization changed its name to the World Professional Association for Transgender Health in 2007. WPATH sponsors a biennial symposium and publishes the *International Journal of Transgenderism*, both important vehicles for understanding and disseminating information on transgender health. The last two symposia, in Bangkok and Amsterdam, included specific educational strands in voice and communication.

WPATH is made up of professionals from a wide variety of disciplines, including medicine, psychology, law, social work, counseling, psychotherapy, family studies, sociology, anthropology, sexology, and speech and voice therapy. WPATH provides opportunities for professionals from various specialties, including speech-language pathology, to communicate across disciplines in the context of research on gender identity and the treatment of gender dysphoria (Adler, 2015). WPATH has a Board of Directors and is made up of 19 committees, including the Standing Committee on Voice and Communication (WPATH, 2017).

HBIGDA and later WPATH started publishing Standards of Care (SOC) in 1979. While speech-language pathologists, speech-language therapists, and speech-voice clinicians (among the international titles) have been working for decades on voice and communication with people who are transgender, WPATH finally included voice and communication intervention in the Standards of Care version 7 in 2011 (Coleman et al., 2012; WPATH, 2017). Consideration for including a speech-language pathologist on the standards writing committee began after the Oslo Symposium in 2009, and Richard Adler joined the writing committee shortly thereafter. It was at this time that WPATH added Speech and Voice (eventually changed to Voice and Communication) to the list of treatments that would be included in the new Standards of Care (Adler, 2015).

Generally speaking, Version 7 of the SOC includes language that is more flexible than in the past, allowing for more individualization of services. Attempts were also made to move away from a strict medical, disease-oriented model of transgenderism (Gender Identity Disorder vs. Gender Dysphoria). As in past versions, the mental health counselor maintains a strong presence in facilitating health care services, like hormone therapy, surgery, and so forth. However, Version 7 makes it clear that the person who is transgender has the primary responsibility for their care (not a physician or counselor) in the context of an interdisciplinary team. While SLPs regularly work within interdisciplinary teams, many professionals in a transgender team are less familiar with practicing clinicians and may be more difficult to access in our present health care system (Adler, 2015; Coleman et al., 2012; WPATH, 2017).

In regard to voice and communication, the newest version of the Standards of Care suggests a holistic program of voice and communication modification, developed collaboratively between client and clinician. Individual and group treatment can be considered, and services need to extend

beyond the modification of pitch. Clinicians should have a firm understanding and experience in voice therapy because of the nature of the intervention. The SOC include a statement about voice feminization surgeries for people who are transgender, including important cautions for individuals trying to modify their voice via surgery (Coleman et al., 2012; WPATH, 2017).

According to the standards, SLPs working with people who are transgender should focus on a variety of communication areas, depending on the client's needs. These areas include:

- Vocal Health
- Voice: Pitch, Intonation, and Volume
- Resonance
- Articulation
- Language: Pragmatics, Syntax, Semantics
- Non-verbal communication
- Real-Life Experiences/Authenticity/Safety

About the time that Version 7 of the SOC was being developed, WPATH created the Standing Committee on Voice and Communication. Past and present members of the committee represent countries from around the world, including Australia, New Zealand, Canada, Sweden, the United Kingdom, and the United States. One of the first tasks of the committee was to generate goals and objectives (Adler, 2015), which are found at http://www.wpath.org/site_page.cfm?pk_association_webpage_menu=1347&pk_association_webpage=3908 (retrieved September 9, 2017). The goals are as follows:

- **GOAL 1:** To create an international network of professionals with expertise in the voice and communication issues experienced by gender variant children, adolescents, and adults.

- **GOAL 2:** Develop and promote the Standards of Care.
- **GOAL 3:** Develop and promote voice and communication services.
- **GOAL 4:** Reduce discrimination against gender variant people on the basis of their voice and communication characteristics.

It is worth noting that the next version of the SOC, Version 8, is being considered and the writing committee has been developed. Like Version 7, the newest iteration of the Standards will include voice and communication.

WPATH's Companion Document and Other Recent Developments

In addition to the aforementioned goals and objectives, the Standing Committee on Voice and Communication wrote a companion document that further delineates the roles and responsibilities of SLPs working with speakers who are transgender and gender non-binary (Davies, Papp, & Antoni, 2015). The document is published in *The International Journal of Transgenderism* and is included on the organization's website (http://www.wpath.org) alongside the Standards and other resources for practicing clinicians. In the companion document, Davies, Papp, and Antoni (2015) describe: (a) the scope and limitations of voice and communication intervention; (b) evidence-based practice; (c) the implications of an evolving gender spectrum; (d) speech and voice assessment; (e) components of a program for voice feminization; (f) issues of access to service; (g) voice feminization surgery; and (h) voice masculinization.

Among the treatment-related strategies described in the document, vocal warm-up and stretching are encouraged and motor learning principles are noted. The applica-

tion of evidence-based practice approaches for voice therapy are also considered, including Vocal Function Exercises (VFE; Stemple, Glaze, & Klaben, 2010), Resonant Voice Therapy (RVT; Verdolini-Marston, Burke, Lessac, Glaze, & Caldwell, 1995), and semi-occluded vocal tract techniques (SOVT; Kapsner-Smith, Hunter, Kikham, Cox, & Titze, 2015). Language, including pragmatics, and non-verbal communication are noted in the document as potential areas for intervention, but need to be considered relative to social and behavioral contexts. Therefore, the emphasis on language and non-verbal communication is likely to vary depending on client need, and may not be necessary within a client's plan (Davies, Papp, & Antoni, 2015).

In addition to the companion document (Davies, Papp, & Antoni, 2015), there have been other activities that specifically address the committee's goals, including the publication of eight articles on transgender voice and communication modification in the ASHA Special Interest Group's (SIG) *Perspectives in Voice and Voice Disorders* in March and July 2015. These papers addressed a variety of topics, including the research evidence supporting treatment (Oates & Dacakis, 2015), challenges in service delivery (Antoni, 2015; Azul, 2015), cultural competence (Hancock, 2015), interdisciplinary intervention (Sodersten, Nygren, Hertegard, & Dhejne, 2015), and WPATH as a resource (Adler, 2015; Davies, 2015; Pickering, 2015). There has also been the inclusion of papers on voice and communication at regional WPATH-associated conferences, like the Australia and New Zealand Professional Association for Transgender Health (ANZPATH), European Professional Association for Transgender Health (EPATH), Canadian Professional Association for Transgender Health (CPATH), and United States Professional Association for Transgender Health (USPATH).

In the United States, ASHA's Special Interest Group 3, Voice and Voice Disorders, sponsored an invited presentation on transgender voice and communication modification at the 2015 convention in Denver (Adler & Pickering, 2015). While presentations on transgender voice and communication have been included at ASHA conventions since Kalra's 1977 case study, a brief search for transgender-related talks at recent ASHA conventions indicated a steady increase from 7 presentations in 2014, to 9 in 2015, and 15 in 2016. Among the 31 presentations, treatment outcomes, primarily in case studies, and service delivery models were reflected most frequently. Professional development activities in the United States, described by Hirsch, Helou, and Block, and in the United Kingdom by Antoni, were part of a presentation at the 2016 WPATH Biennial Symposium in Amsterdam focusing on curricula in transgender voice and communication for students and practicing clinicians (Papp et al., 2016).

In October 2017, ASHA's SIG 10, *Perspectives on Issues in Higher Education*, focused on curriculum in transgender voice and communication. The articles included in this issue described university programs in transgender voice and communication (Kayajian & Pickering, 2017; Oates & Dacakis, 2017; Stewart & Kling, 2017), clinical instruction (Helou, 2017), resonance (Hirsch, 2017), counseling (Adler, 2017), WPATH's clinical guidelines (Davies, 2017), and the application of personal narratives to describe the importance of voice and communication training (Booz, Dorman, & Walden, 2017). Finally, with the increase in clinical programs in transgender voice and communication modification around the world, social media has been used increasingly to promote clinical services, advocacy, and networking. Media coverage has also grown, providing a vehicle to support the public's understanding of the role of voice and communication training for people who are gender diverse.

Based on the growing clinical research, literature, and resources in transgender voice and communication, voice and resonance are viewed as foundational areas of emphasis when working with transgender women (Adler & Pickering, 2015). Other aspects of communication should be addressed depending on individual needs. In regard to voice and resonance, maintaining/improving vocal health (see Chapter 8) should be implemented prior to considering the following goals:

- Elevate fundamental frequency
- Modify use of inflections
- Consider increased breathiness
- Improve projection
- Elevate formant frequencies
- Facilitate forward resonance

Recently, literature focusing on trans men has emerged, building on the previous information provided in the first two editions of this book (Adler, Hirsch, & Mordaunt, 2006, 2012). The expanding information (e.g., Azul, Arnold, & Neuschaefer-Rube, 2018; Block, 2017) provides important, increasingly specific areas of emphasis for assessment and training, as noted in Chapter 9. The literature regarding trans men, like the research supporting training for trans women, states that clinicians should consider client self-reported voice and communication satisfaction as an important component of their service provision.

Client Self-Reported Satisfaction and the TVQ[MtF]

Increasingly, research has focused on transgender clients' self-reported satisfaction of voice and communication. Since client self-perception may not be correlated with acoustic and perceptual change, it becomes an important component to consider in voice and communication modification (Byrne, Dacakis, & Douglas, 2003). In 2008, research by McNeill et al. indicated that a trans woman's happiness with voice was not directly related to f_0, and the way a participant's voice was perceived by listeners did not accurately represent her level of happiness. This study demonstrated the incongruence that can occur between clinician measures of voice and communication, listener perception of voice, and an individual's self-perception of voice and communication.

Around the time that McNeill et al. (2008) published their study, client satisfaction measures were being developed for trans women to assess client self-perception. For example, Pasricha, Dacakis, and Oates (2008) investigated factors that influence communicative satisfaction in the lives of trans women. Their qualitative study provided the basis for the development of the Functional Communication Satisfaction Questionnaire (FCSQ; Pasricha, Dacakis, & Oates, 2008). Just prior, Davies and Goldberg (2006) used the Voice Handicap Index (VHI; Jacobson et al., 1997) as a model to create the Transgender Self Evaluation of Voice Questionnaire (TSEQ). Adler, Hirsch, and Mordaunt (2012) included the TSEQ in an earlier edition of this book.

Hancock et al. (2009) found that the TSEQ was positively correlated to other measures of voice-related quality of life (vQOL), including the VHI, and had strong test-retest reliability. The researchers concluded that the questionnaire was a sensitive instrument that may be useful in measuring trans women's self-perceptions of voice femininity. In 2011, Hancock, Krissinger, and Owen further examined voice-related self-perception and the quality of life of trans women using the TSEQ. Results indicated that vQOL

improved as voice was rated "more feminine" or "likable" by the transgender participants; however, this relationship was not significant when listeners rated the transgender speaker's vocal femininity and likability. These results point out the importance of client self-perception measures as part of a comprehensive examination of transgender voice and communication (see Chapter 7 for information on assessing the voice of transgender and gender non-binary speakers).

Addressing client self-reported voice and communication satisfaction is consistent with the World Health Organization's International Classification of Functioning (WHO-ICF; WHO, 2013), a framework for understanding the impact of a disorder or difference on an individual in the real world. Hancock (2017) discussed transgender voice and communication from a WHO-ICF perspective, highlighting how responses on measures of client self-perception can provide insight on: (a) the impact of body function on quality of life, (b) communication activity and participation, and (c) an individual's environmental and attitudinal contexts. In relation to the WHO-ICF, these factors, in particular a trans person's attitudes about vocal function and the resulting restrictions in life participation, may facilitate or complicate an individual's quality of life; therefore, they need to be considered in assessment and treatment.

As a further step in the development of a valid and reliable client self-reported voice and communication satisfaction measure for trans women, Dacakis et al. (2013) developed the Transsexual Voice Questionnaire (TVQ^MtF). The TVQ^MtF is a 30-item questionnaire that assesses a trans woman's perception of the impact of voice on her daily life. Similar to other client self-perception measures, the TVQ^MtF requires an individual to rate the frequency (1 = never or rarely;

4 = usually or always) with which one of 30 situations occurs (e.g., "I am less outgoing because of my voice," "When I laugh I sound like a man"). Lower scores reflect a lower frequency of adverse voice-related experiences; higher scores suggest that the individual is affected more negatively by her voice. Information on the application of this measure is discussed in Chapter 7.

In their two-part study, Dacakis et al. (2013) first reviewed and modified the content and organization of the TSEQ, applying psychometric content analysis by 2 SLPs and 2 trans females to the results of in-depth interviews with 14 trans women. Once the new tool was prepared, the second part of the study included the administration of the TVQ^MtF to 35 transgender individuals in Australia and Canada. The measure was applied on two occasions, four to six weeks apart, in order to assess internal consistency and test-retest reliability, both of which were determined to be statistically strong. Results of the second part of the study indicated a wide range of difficulties in both (a) vocal functioning, most importantly pitch, and (b) the impact of voice on activity and participation.

In addition to establishing reliability, studies have been completed to determine the validity of the TVQ^MtF. For example, Davies and Johnston (2015) compared the content reflected in the TVQ^MtF with voice-related concerns generated from interviews with five trans women. Initially, the 30 TVQ^MtF questionnaire items were categorized into six themes: effect of voice on social interaction, the effect of voice on emotions, the relationship between voice and gender identity, effort and concentration required to produce voice, physical aspects of voice production, and pitch. The categorized items were then evaluated against thematic interviews with the five participants regarding voice and communi-

cation. Davies and Johnston (2015) found that the content themes from the TVQ^MtF were present in the interviews, and the themes most frequently discussed in the interviews corresponded to items on the TVQ^MtF that were found to be most problematic for trans women.

Dacakis, Oates, and Douglas (2016) investigated the content validity of the TVQ^MtF by comparing client self-perception for 26 trans women who went through gender confirmation surgery and 27 trans women who did not have the surgery. Using known-groups analysis, the researchers found a statistically significant difference between the groups on the TVQ^MtF suggesting that participants who underwent gender confirmation surgery perceived less voice-related difficulties and a decreased impact on their gender identity, consistent with past research that trans females feel more positively about their voice after surgery. However, participants in both groups still reported some impact on their voice-related activity and participation. Collectively, the results supported the construct validity of the TVQ^MtF.

Dacakis, Oates, and Douglas (2017) further assessed the validity and reliability of the TVQ^MtF, this time with a large number of trans women. One hundred fifty-one trans women completed the TVQ^MtF, and the results were subjected to principal components analysis in order to assess construct validity. The analysis uncovered a two-factor structure for the assessment tool. One factor, which accounted for the largest variance, was related to vocal functioning and included items about gender identity (referred to as vocal functioning). The second factor was related to the voice's impact on activity and participation (referred to as social participation). Given this structure, the authors suggest that item-specific responses can be used by clinicians to guide service delivery (Dacakis, Oates, & Douglas, 2017).

In addition to the evidence for construct validity, results from 133 trans women in the study indicated strong internal consistency in their responses (Cronbach's alpha = .97), providing additional evidence for the reliability of the TVQ^MtF.

The studies described above confirm the reliability and validity of the TVQ^MtF as an appropriate client self-perception measure in English. Since its development, the TVQ^MtF has been translated into nine languages according to Davies' website (http://www.shelaghdavies.com/ retrieved on July 18, 2017). Among the translations, test-retest reliability was found to be excellent in studies applying the Portuguese (Santos et al., 2015) and Swedish (Cardell & Ruda, 2014) versions of the TVQ^MtF.

Since Freidenberg's (2002) observation that transgender client satisfaction is sometimes at odds with improvements in acoustic-perceptual features of voice, a number of researchers have advanced our understanding of this important aspect of our clients' lives, leading to the development of a valid and reliable measure for trans women, the TVQ^MtF. Of course, there is more to consider, including further study of the clinical utility of the TVQ^MtF, as well as the self-reported voice and communication satisfaction of trans men (see Azul, Arnold, & Neuschaefer-Rube, 2018) and those who are gender nonconforming.

Pitch-Elevating Surgery for Transgender Speakers

In addition to behavioral methods for modifying voice and communication, surgical procedures have been developed to increase fundamental frequency and its perceptual correlate, pitch. Early surgical procedures were described at approximately the same time that reports of behavioral voice and communication modification emerged (e.g., Kitajima, Tanabe, & Isshiki, 1979; LeJeune, Guice, & Samuels, 1983; Tucker, 1985). Since these early experimental procedures, other surgeries have been described in the literature (e.g., Anderson, 2014; Gross, 1999; Hamdan, 2012; Kanagalingam, Geogalas, & Wood, 2005; Kim, 2016; Kunachak, Prakunhungsit, & Sujjalak, 2000; Mastronikolis, Remacle, & Biagini, 2013; Meister et al., 2017; Orloff, Mann, & Damrose, 2006; Remacle, Matar, Morsomme, Veduyckt, & Lawson, 2011; Thomas & MacMillan, 2013; Wagner, Fugain, Monneron-Girard, Cordier, & Chabolle, 2003; Yang, Palmer, Murray, Meltzer, & Coen, 2002). Van Damme, Cosyns, Deman, Van den Eede, and Van Borsel (2016) completed a systematic review of the efficacy of pitch raising surgery for trans women and reported on 20 studies that met their inclusion criteria: (a) participants were trans women; (b) pre- and post-surgical results were reported; (c) objective and/or subjective measures were included; and (d) surgery was designed to increase pitch. Among the 20 studies reviewed, cricothyroid approximation and anterior glottal web formation were the surgical procedures described most frequently. Results across studies indicated that fundamental frequency was increased as a result of pitch-elevating surgery to levels consistent with normative data on cisfemale speakers. However, voice quality was negatively impacted in some of the studies, particularly by surgeries that facilitate anterior glottal web formation. Most patients who underwent pitch-raising surgery reported being satisfied, but there was no research on long-term results, and none of the studies used a control group or randomization of participants. Interestingly, 13 of the 20 studies mentioned some form of voice therapy before and/or after surgery, but the therapy was not well described.

The cautions discussed in the systematic review (Van Damme et al., 2016) are consistent with those noted by Davies, Papp, and Antoni (2015), who reported limited evidence on the long-term effectiveness and risks of pitch-elevating surgery, something people should be aware of prior to undertaking surgery. Collaboration between the otolaryngologist and SLP is encouraged, consistent with practice in voice disorders. Careful attention to post-surgical measures is recommended, including education before surgery and work with an SLP to ensure appropriate use of voice after surgery. In keeping with this recommendation, a collaborative intervention process involving surgery and behavioral voice training was described in a 12-year retrospective study by Kim (2016).

Kim's study (2016) investigated the results of a surgical procedure called vocal fold shortening and retrodisplacement of the anterior commissure (VFSRAC), performed between 2003 and 2014 on 362 patients, 313 of whom were trans women. Participants had the surgery and took part in post-surgical behavioral intervention referred to as phonatory pattern retraining. VFSRAC is a two-part direct laryngoscopic procedure that includes the de-epithelialization of the anterior one-third of the vocal fold, followed by the placement of sutures to shorten the vocal folds, leaving the posterior two-thirds to vibrate with a higher frequency after healing. A variety of objective and subjective measures were taken pre-operatively and seven days post-operatively, at two months, six months, and one year post-surgery. An SLP performed acoustic, aerodynamic, and perceptual measures and completed phonatory pattern retraining.

After approximately eight weeks, the participants took part in the behavioral voice modification program designed to address a new pattern of phonation, phonatory feedback, and resonance. Activities used during the training regimen included laryngeal relaxation, vocal exercise, and modification of resonance. Results of the study indicated that after surgery and vocal training, the participants demonstrated: (a) a significant increase in fundamental frequency, (b) improvement in voice satisfaction, based on the Voice Handicap Index (VHI), and (c) acoustic measures that approached or were within normal limits. Post-surgical dysphonia occurred but was no longer present after two or three months. Fundamental frequency change occurred over time, and according to Kim (2016) the change was affected by healing and vocal training.

Kim (2016) concluded by saying that surgery alone does not seem to be enough to adequately feminize the voice. The combination of careful pre-surgical assessment, effective surgery, careful post-surgical care, and vocal training supports the development of a female voice for trans women. As noted earlier, the implementation of a collaborative approach between an otolaryngologist and SLP is advised if surgery is going to be undertaken by a transgender speaker (Davies, Papp, & Antoni, 2015). Casado, O'Connor, Angulo, and Adrián (2016) applied this model with 10 trans women who achieved positive acoustic and perceptual results with combined surgery and voice modification.

Like the literature on behavioral voice and communication modification for people who are transgender, the application of pitch-elevating surgery has evolved since the late 1970s. Research has indicated that surgical management of the larynx and vocal folds can increase fundamental frequency; however, the long-term effects of surgery, risk factors, and participant satisfaction continue to be unclear. The combination of surgery and voice modification appears to be promising and may become an effective treatment option for trans women, particularly those who are unable to make significant progress in voice and communication modification alone, or whose age, overall health, or other factors might influence clinical decision making.

Voice and Communication for People Who Are Transgender and Gender Nonconforming: A Current Perspective

At the present time, SLPs have growing evidence to support voice and communication intervention for trans women. The next chapter provides an analysis of this evidence. Clinical resources are also available that can guide effective service delivery in the broader context of transgender health. Increasingly, other gender diverse people, including transgender men and gender nonconforming individuals, are seeking services to understand and modify their voice and communication to match their gender identity, gender expression, and importantly, their sense of self (Azul, 2015, 2016; Azul, Arnold, & Neuschaefer-Rube, 2018; Azul, Nygren, & Sodersten, 2017; Block, 2017; Davies, Papp, & Antoni, 2015; Nygren et al., 2016). We are already seeing increased attention in the literature to voice and communication for trans men (see Chapter 9) and will ultimately need to effectively respond to those who are gender nonconforming, people who do not necessarily seek voice and communication that is consistent with the voice of a cismale or cisfemale.

Providing effective, evidence-based intervention for speakers who are transgender and gender nonconforming requires that clinicians be culturally competent. Kelly and Robinson (2011) cautioned SLPs that members of the LGBTQ community may be hesitant to disclose their membership in the community, even though they think it is important. Furthermore, participants surveyed reported feeling that clinicians may be biased against them because of their membership in the LGBTQ community. These perceptions may affect people who are transgender and gender nonconforming; some may not choose to seek services at all or may find it difficult to develop an effective, collaborative rapport with an SLP.

Hancock and Haskins (2015) suggested that knowledge about the transgender community, transgender health, and voice and communication modification is a place to start when it comes to providing culturally competent services. They surveyed 279 SLPs who reported feeling comfortable working with people who are transgender, although they lacked the clinical knowledge to do so competently. Survey respondents expressed an openness to learn more but felt unprepared to provide services in voice and communication. The majority of participants did not hold any moral concerns about providing intervention to people who are transgender and gender nonbinary, and feelings expressed by participants were largely positive. Interestingly, but not surprisingly, clinicians with less clinical experience (younger individuals) reported greater knowledge of people who are transgender and gender nonconforming, as well as services provided to modify voice and communication.

In her 2015 *Perspectives* article, Hancock (2015) explored cultural competence in the provision of services for transgender and gender nonconforming individuals, suggesting that we continually seek knowledge about the transgender community and transgender health. Increased attention in speech-language pathology curricula during pre-professional preparation, as well as expanded continuing education opportunities, will support improved cultural competence.

Hancock used a case example to illustrate the importance of integrating our clients' overall quality of life into intervention, which allows us to explore communication in the context of the individual's real world and significant communication partners.

As we take a historical view of voice and communication modification for people who are transgender and gender nonconforming, it is interesting to note that the clinical population that first included adult trans women has grown to include adolescents (Hancock & Helenius, 2012) and trans men (Azul, 2015, 2016; Azul, Arnold, & Neuschaefer-Rube, 2018; Azul, Nygren, & Sodersten, 2017; Block, 2017; Davies, Papp, & Antoni, 2015). Additionally, recent transgender choral groups have brought attention to the trans singer (see Chapter 14).

Ultimately, clinical research and service delivery models will need to attend more closely to these and other emerging client groups and be sensitive to other points along the expanding gender identity continuum. These experiences will likely lead to different ways of thinking about and implementing services in transgender and gender diverse voice and communication. It is clear that voice and communication services are expanding and include surgical procedures that modify the vocal folds and voice. At the present time, voice and communication intervention provided by a speech-language pathologist is increasingly supported by research, and is being implemented in the context of a dramatic cultural shift in how we perceive gender, gender identity, and gender expression.

References

Adler, R. (2015). Voice and communication for the transgender/transsexual client: Presenting the WPATH Standing Committee on Voice and Communication. *SIG 3 Perspectives on Voice and Voice Disorders, 25*(1), 32–36.

Adler, R. K. (2017). The SLP as counselor for the transgender client. *SIG 10 Perspectives in Higher Education, 20*(2), 92–101.

Adler, R. K., Hirsch, S., & Mordaunt, M. (Eds.). (2006). *Voice and communication therapy for the transgender/transsexual individual: A comprehensive clinical guide*. San Diego, CA: Plural Publications.

Adler, R. K., Hirsch, S., & Mordaunt, M. (Eds.). (2012). *Voice and communication therapy for the transgender/transsexual client: A comprehensive clinical guide* (2nd ed.). San Diego, CA: Plural Publications.

Adler, R., & Pickering, J. (2015, November). *Supporting the modification of voice and resonance with speakers who are transgender*. Presented at 2015 ASHA Annual Convention, Denver, CO.

Anderson, J. (2014). Pitch elevation in transgendered patients: Anterior glottis web formation assisted by temporary injection augmentation. *Journal of Voice, 28*(6), 816–821.

Andrews, M. L. (1999). *Manual of voice treatment: Pediatrics through geriatrics* (2nd ed.). San Diego, CA: Singular.

Antoni, C. (2015). Service delivery and the challenges of providing service to people who are transgender. *SIG 3 Perspectives on Voice and Voice Disorders, 25*(2), 59–65.

Aronson, A. E. (1990). *Clinical voice disorders: An interdisciplinary approach* (3rd ed.). New York, NY: Thieme.

Azul, D. (2015). On the varied and complex factors affecting gender diverse people's vocal situations: Implications for clinical practice. *SIG 3 Perspectives on Voice and Voice Disorders, 25*(2), 75–86.

Azul, D. (2016). Transmasculine people's vocal situations: A critical review of gender related discourses and empirical data. *International Journal of Language and Communication Disorders, 50*(1), 31–47.

Azul, D., Arnold, A., & Neuschaefer-Rube, C. (2018). Do transmasculine speakers present with gender-related voice problems? Insights from a participant-centered mixed-methods study. *Journal of Speech Language Hearing Research, 61*(1), 25–39.

Azul, D., Nygren, U., & Sodersten, M. (2017). Transmasculine people's voice function: A review of the currently available evidence. *Journal of Voice, 31*(2), 261.e9–261.e23.

Block, C. (2017). Making a case for transmasculine voice and communication training. *Perspectives of the ASHA Special Interest Groups SIG 3, 2*(1), 33–41.

Boone, D. R., McFarlane, S. C. and Von Berg, S. L. (2005). *The voice and voice therapy*. Boston, MA: Allyn and Bacon.

Booz, J., Dorman, K, & Walden, P. (2017). First-person narratives by transgender individuals on voice and communication. *SIG 10 Perspectives in Higher Education, 20*(2), 60–63.

Bralley, R. C., Bull, G. L., Gore, C. H., & Edgerton, M. T. (1978). Evaluation of vocal pitch in male transsexuals. *Journal of Communication Disorders, 11*(5), 443–449.

Byrne, L. A., Dacakis, G., & Douglas, J. M. (2003). Self-perceptions of pragmatic communication abilities in male-to-female transsexuals. *Advances in Speech-Language Pathology, 5*(1), 15–25.

Casado, J. C., O'Connor, C., Angulo M. S., & Adrián J. A. (2016). Wendler glottoscopy and voice therapy in male-to-female transsexuals: Results in pre and post-surgery assessment. *Acta Otorrinolaringologica Espanola, 67*(2), 83–92.

Cardell, F., & Ruda, M. (2014). *Reliability evaluation of the Swedish version of the transsexual voice questionnaire (TVQ^{MtF})*. Unpublished master's thesis.

Challoner, J. (1986). The voice of the transsexual. In M. Fawcus (Ed.), *Voice disorders and their management* (pp. 224–239). London, UK: Croom Helm.

Coleman, E., Bockting, M., Botzer, P., DeCuypere, G., Feldman, J. Fraser, L., . . . Zucker, K., (2012). Standards of Care for the Health of Transsexual, Transgender, and Gender-Nonconforming People, Version 7. *International Journal of Transgenderism, 13*(4), 165–232.

Dacakis, G. (2000). Long-term maintenance of fundamental frequency increases in male-to female transsexuals. *Journal of Voice, 14*(4), 549–556.

Dacakis, G. (2008, October). *Speech pathology for transsexual women: An Australian perspective*. Unpublished manuscript, La Trobe University, Victoria, Australia.

Dacakis, G., Davies, S., Oates, J., Douglas, J., & Johnston, J. (2013). Development and preliminary evaluation of the transsexual voice questionnaire for male-to-female transsexuals. *Journal of Voice, 3*(27), 312–320.

Dacakis, G., Oates, J., & Douglas, J. (2016). Exploring the validity of the Transsexual Voice Questionnaire (male-to-female): Do TVQ^{MtF} scores differentiate between MtF women who have had gender reassignment surgery and those who have not? *International Journal of Transgenderism, 17*(3-4), 124–130.

Dacakis, G., Oates, J., & Douglas, J. (2017). Further evidence of the construct validity of the transsexual voice questionnaire (TVQ MtF). *Journal of Voice, 31*(2), 142–148.

Davies, S. (2015). A brief overview of the WPATH companion document on voice and communication. *SIG 3 Perspectives on Voice and Voice Disorders, 25*(2), 66–74.

Davies, S. (2017). The evidence behind the practice: A review of WPATH suggested guidelines in transgender voice and communication. *SIG 10 Perspectives in Higher Education, 20*(2), 64–73.

Davies, S., & Goldberg, J. M. (2006). Clinical aspects of transgender speech feminization and masculinization. *International Journal of Transgenderism, 9*(3-4), 167–196.

Davies, S., & Johnston, J. R. (2015). Exploring the validity of the Transsexual Voice Questionnaire for male-to-female transsexuals. *Canadian Journal of Speech-Language Pathology and Audiology, 39*(1), 40–51.

Davies, S., Papp, V., & Antoni, C. (2015). Voice and communication change for gender nonconforming individuals: Giving voice to the person inside. *International Journal of Transgenderism, 16*(3), 117–159.

Freidenberg, C. B. (2002). Working with male-to-female transgendered clients: Clinical considerations. *Contemporary Issues in Communication Science and Disorders, 29*(1), 43–58.

Gallena, S. J. K., Stickels, B., & Stickels, E. (2017). Gender perception after raising vowel fundamental and formant frequencies: Considerations for oral resonance research. *Journal of Voice*. [Epub ahead of print] doi: 10.1016/j.jvoice .2017.06.023.

Gelfer, M. P. (1999). Voice treatment for the male-to-female transgendered client. *American Journal of Speech-Language Pathology, 8*(3), 201–208.

Gelfer, M. P., & Bennet, Q. E. (2013). Speaking fundamental frequency and vowel formant frequencies: Effects on perception of gender. *Journal of Voice, 27*(5), 556–66.

Gelfer, M. P., & Mikos, V. A. (2005). The relative contributions of speaking fundamental frequency and format frequencies to gender identification based on isolated vowels. *Journal of Voice, 19*(4), 544–554.

Gelfer, M. P., & Schofield, K. J. (2000). Comparison of acoustic and perceptual measures of voice in MtF transsexuals perceived as female versus those perceived as males. *Journal of Voice, 14*(1), 22–33.

Gelfer, M. P., & Tice, R. M. (2013). Perceptual and acoustic outcomes of voice therapy for male-to-female transgender individuals immediately after therapy and 15 months later. *Journal of Voice, 27*(3), 335–347.

Gelfer, M. P., & Van Dong, B. R. (2013). A preliminary study on the use of vocal function exercises to improve voice in male-to-female transgender clients. *Journal of Voice, 27*(3), 321–334.

Gorham-Rowan, M., & Morris, R. (2006). Aerodynamic analysis of male to-female transgender voice. *Journal of Voice, 20*(2), 251–262.

Gross, M. (1999). Pitch-raising surgery in male-to-female transsexuals. *Journal of Voice, 13*(2), 246–250.

Hamdan, A. (2012). Cricothyroid approximation using silastic sheath: A new approach. *Middle East Journal Anesthesiology, 21*(6), 909–912.

Hancock, A. B. (2015). The role of cultural competence in serving transgender populations. *SIG 3 Perspectives on Voice and Voice Disorders, 25*(1), 37–42.

Hancock, A. B. (2017). An ICF Perspective on voice-related quality of life of American transgender women. *Journal of Voice, 31*(1), 115.e1–115.e8.

Hancock, A. B., Colton, L., & Douglas, F. (2014). Intonation and gender perception: Applications for transgender speakers. *Journal of Voice, 28*(2), 357–366.

Hancock, A. B., & Garabedian, L. (2013). Transgender voice and communication treatment: A retrospective chart review of 25 cases. *International Journal of Communication Disorders, 48*(1), 54–65.

Hancock, A. B., & Haskin, G. (2015). Speech-language pathologists' knowledge and attitudes regarding lesbian, gay, bisexual, transgender and queer (LGBTQ) populations. *American Journal of Speech Language Pathology, 24*(2), 139–149.

Hancock, A. B., & Helenius, L. (2012). Adolescent male-to-female transgender voice and communication therapy. *Journal of Communication Disorders, 45*(5), 313–324.

Hancock, A. B., Krissinger, J., & Owen, K. (2011). Voice perceptions and quality of life of transgender people. *Journal of Voice, 25*(5), 553–558.

Hancock, A., Owen, K., Siegfriedt, L., & Brundage, S. (2009, June). *Relationship between self-perception, listener perception, and acoustic measures of femininity in transgender voice assessment.* Paper presented at WPATH 2009 XXI Biennial Symposium, Oslo, Norway.

Hancock, A. B., Stutts, H. W., & Bass, A. (2015). Perceptions of gender and femininity based on language: Implications for transgender communication therapy. *Journal of Language and Speech, 58*(3), 315–333.

Hardy, T. L. D., Boliek, C. A., Wells, K., Dearden, C., Zalmanowitz, C., & Deardan, J. R. (2016). Pretreatment acoustic predictors of gender, femininity, and naturalness ratings in individuals with male-to-female gender identity. *American Journal of Speech Language Pathology, 25*(2), 125–137.

Helou, L. (2017). Crafting the dialogue: Meta-therapy in transgender voice and communication training. *SIG 10 Perspectives in Higher Education, 20*(2), 83–91.

Hirsch, S. (2017). Combining voice, speech science and art approaches to resonance challenges in transgender voice and communication training. *SIG 10 Perspectives in Higher Education, 20*(2), 74–82.

Holmberg, E. B., Oates, J., Dacakis, G., & Grant, C. (2010). Phonetograms, aerodynamic measurements, self-evaluations, and auditory perceptual ratings of male-to-female transsexual voice. *Journal of Voice, 24*(5), 511–522.

Irwig, M. S., Childs, C., & Hancock, A. B. (2017). Effects of testosterone on the transgender male voice. *Andrology, 5*(1), 107–112.

Jacobson, B. H., Johnson, A., Grywalski, C., Silbergleit, A., Jacobson, G., Benninger, M. S., & Newman, C. W. (1997). The Voice Handicap Index (VHI): Development and validation. *American Journal of Speech-Language Pathology, 6*(3), 66–70.

Kalra, C. (1977). Perceptions of female and male speech. *Language and Speech, 20*(2), 151–161.

Kanagalingam, J., Georgalas, C., & Wood, G. R. (2005). Cricothyroid approximation and subluxation in 21 male-to-female transsexuals. *Laryngoscope. 115*(4), 611–618.

Kapsner-Smith, M. R., Hunter, E. J., Kikham, K., Cox, K., & Titze, I. R. (2015). A randomized controlled trial of two semi-occluded vocal tract voice therapy protocols. *Journal of Speech Language Hearing Research, 58*(3), 535–549.

Kayajian, D., & Pickering, J. (2017). Connecting clinic and classroom to enhance group transgender voice and communication training in a college environment. *SIG 10 Perspectives in Higher Education, 20*(2), 116–122.

Kelly, J., & Robinson G. C. (2011). Disclosure of membership in the lesbian, gay, bisexual, and transgender community by individuals with communication impairments: A preliminary Web-based survey. *American Journal of Speech-Language Pathology, 20*(2), 86–94.

Kim, H. (2016). A new conceptual approach for voice feminization: 12 years of experience. *Laryngoscope, 126*(2), 1–7

King, R. S., Brown, G. R., & McCrea, C. R. (2012). Voice parameters that result in identification or misidentification of biological gender in male-to-female transgender veterans. *International Journal of Transgenderism, 13*(3), 117–130.

Kitajima K., Tanabe M., & Isshiki N. (1979). Cricothyroid distance and vocal pitch. Experimental surgical study to elevate the vocal pitch. *Annals of Otology, Rhinology, and Laryngology, 88*(1), 52–55.

Kunachak, S., Prakunhungsit S., & Sujjalak K. (2000). Thyroid cartilage and vocal fold reduction: A new phonosurgical method for male-to-female transsexuals. *Annals of Otology, Rhinology, and Laryngology, 109*(11), 1082–1086.

LeJeune, F. E., Guice, C. E., & Samuels, P. M. (1983). Early experiences with vocal ligament tightening. *Annals of Otology, Rhinology, and Laryngology, 92*(5), 475–477.

Leung, Y., Oates, J, & Chan, S. P. (2018). Voice, articulation, and prosody contribute to listener perceptions of speaker gender: A systematic review and meta-analysis. *Journal of Speech, Language, Hearing Research, 61*(2), 266–297.

Mastronikolis, N. S., Remacle, M., & Biagini, M. (2013). Wendler glottoplasty: An effective pitch raising surgery in male-to-female transsexuals. *Journal of Voice, 27*(4), 516–522.

McNeill, E. J., Wilson, J. A., Clark, S., & Deakin, J. (2008). Perception of voice in the transgender client. *Journal of Voice, 22*(6), 727–733.

Meister, J., Hagen, R., Shehata-Dielter, W., Kuhn, H., Kraus, F., & Kleinsasser, N. (2017). Pitch elevation in male-to-female transgender persons—the Würzburg approach. *Journal of Voice, 31*(2), 244.e7–244.e15.

Mount, K. H., & Salmon, S. J. (1988). Changing the vocal characteristics of a postoperative transsexual patient: A longitudinal study. *Journal of Communication Disorders, 21*(3), 229–238.

Nygren, U., Nordenskjold, A., Arver, S., & Sodersten, M. (2016). Effects on voice fundamental frequency and satisfaction with voice in trans men during testosterone treatment. *Journal of Voice, 30*(6): 766.e23–766.e34.

Oates, J. M., & Dacakis, G. (1983). Speech pathology considerations in the management of transsexualism—a review. *British Journal of Disorders of Communication, 18*(3), 139–151.

Oates, J. M., & Dacakis, G. (1997). Voice change in transsexuals. *Venereology—the Interdisciplinary International Journal of Sexual Health, 10*(3), 178–187.

Oates, J., & Dacakis, G. (2015). Transgender voice and communication: Research evidence underpinning voice intervention for male-to-female transsexual women. *SIG 3 Perspectives on Voice and Voice Disorders, 25*(2), 48–58.

Oates J. M., & Dacakis, G. (2017). Inclusion of transgender voice and communication training in a university clinic. *SIG 10 Perspectives in Higher Education, 20*(2), 109–115.

Orloff, L. A., Mann, A. P., & Damrose, J. F. (2006). Laser-assisted voice adjustment (LAVA) in transsexuals. *Laryngoscope, 116*(4), 655–660.

Palmer, D., Dietsch, A., & Searl, J. (2012). Endoscopic and stroboscopic presentation of the larynx in male-to-female transsexual persons. *Journal of Voice, 26*(1), 117–126.

Papp, V., Dacakis, G., Oates, J., Lobegeiger de Rodriquez, S., Pickering, J., Kayajian, D., . . . Davies, S. (June, 2016). *Global approaches to a transgender-specific curriculum for speech-language clinicians.* Paper presented at WPATH 2016 XXIV Biennial Symposium, Amsterdam, the Netherlands.

Pasricha, N., Dacakis, G., & Oates, J. (2008). Communicative satisfaction of male-to-female transsexuals. *Logopedics Phoniatrics Vocology, 33*(1), 25–34.

Pickering, J. (2015). Transgender voice and communication: Introduction and international context. *SIG 3, Perspectives on Voice and Voice Disorders, 25*(1), 25–31.

Remacle, M., Matar, N., Morsomme, D., Veduyckt, I., & Lawson, G. (2011). Glottoplasty for male-to-female transsexualism: Voice results. *Journal of Voice, 25*(1), 120–123.

Santos, H. H., Aguilar, A. G., Baeck, H. E., & Van Borsel, J. (2015). Translation and preliminary evaluation of the Brazilian Portuguese version of the Transgender Voice Questionnaire for male-to-female transsexuals. *CoDAS, 27*(1), 89–96.

Schwartz, B., & LaSalle, L. (2008). *Language choice and gender perceptions: Implications for male-to-female voice therapy.* Paper presented at the

2008 American Speech-Language-Hearing Association Convention, Chicago, IL.

Shelagh Davies (n.d.). Transsexual voice questionnaire (TVQ male to female). Retrieved from: http://www.shelaghdavies.com/questionnaire/questionnaire.html.

Skuk, V., & Schwinberger, S. (2014). Influences of fundamental frequency, formant frequencies, aperiodicity, and spectrum level on the perception of voice gender. *Journal of Speech Language and Hearing Research, 57*(1), 285–296.

Söderpalm, E., Larsson, A., & Almquist, S. A. (2004). Evaluation of a consecutive group of transsexual individuals referred for vocal intervention in the west of Sweden. *Logopedics Phoniatrics Vocology, 29*(1), 18–30.

Södersten, M., Nygren, U., Hertegård, S., & Dhejne, C. (2015). Interdisciplinary program in Sweden related to transgender voice. *SIG 3 Perspectives on voice and voice disorders, 25*(2), 87–97.

Stemple, J.C., Glaze, L., & Gerderman, B. (1995). *Clinical voice pathology: Theory and management* (2nd ed.). San Diego, CA: Plural.

Stemple, J. C., Glaze L., & Klaben, B. (2010). *Clinical voice pathology: Theory and management* (4th ed.). San Diego, CA: Plural.

Stewart, C. F., & Kling, I. F. (2017). University practicum for transgender voice modification: A motor learning perspective. *SIG 10 Perspectives in Higher Education, 20*(2), 102–108.

Thomas, J. P., & MacMillan, C. (2013). Feminization laryngoplasty: Assessment of surgical pitch elevation. *European Archives of Oto-Rhino-Laryngology, 270*(10), 2695–2700.

Tucker, H. M. (1985). Anterior commissure laryngoplasty for adjustment of vocal fold tension. *Annals of Otology, Rhinology, and Laryngology, 94*(6), 547–549.

Van Borsel, J., De Cuypere, G., Rubens, R., & Destaerke, B. (2000). Voice problems in female-to-male transsexuals. *International Journal of Language and Communication Disorders, 35*(3), 427–442.

Van Borsel, J., De Cuypere, G., & Van den Berghe, H. (2001). Physical appearance and voice in male-to-female transsexuals. *Journal of Voice, 15*(4), 570–575.

Van Borsel, J., & De Maesschalck, D. (2008). Speech rate in males, females, and male-to-female transsexuals. *Clinical Linguistics and Phonetics, 22*(9), 679–685.

Van Borsel, J., de Pot, K., & De Cuypere, G. (2009). Voice and physical appearance in female-to-male transsexuals. *Journal of Voice, 23*(4), 494–497.

Van Borsel, J., Janssens, J., & De Bodt, M. (2009). Breathiness as a feminine voice characteristic: A perceptual approach. *Journal of Voice, 23*(3), 291–294.

Van Damme, S., Cosyns, M., Deman, S., Van den Eede, Z., & Van Borsel, J. (2016). The Effectiveness of pitch-raising surgery in male-to-female transsexuals: A systematic review. *Journal of Voice, 31*(2), 244.e1–244.e5.

Verdolini-Marston, K., Burke, M. K., Lessac, A., Glaze, L., & Caldwell, E. (1995). Preliminary study of two methods of treatment for laryngeal nodules. *Journal of Voice, 9*(1), 74–85.

Wagner, I., Fugain, C., Monneron-Girard, L., Cordier, B., & Chabolle, F. (2003). Pitch-raising surgery in fourteen male-to-female transsexuals. *Laryngoscope, 113*(17), 1157–1165.

Wolfe, V. I., Ratusnik, D. L., Smith, F. H., & Northrop, G. (1990). Intonation and fundamental frequency in male-to-female transsexuals. *Journal of Speech and Hearing Disorders, 55*(1), 43–50.

WHO-ICF. (2013). *A practical manual for using the International Classification of Functioning, Disability, and Health: ICF.* Geneva, Switzerland: World Health Organization.

WPATH: World Professional Association of Transgender Health. (2017). Retrieved from: http://www.wpath.org.

Yang, C. Y., Palmer, A. D., Murray, K. D., Meltzer, T., & Coen, J. I. (2002). Cricothyroid approximation to elevate vocal pitch in male-to-female transsexuals: Results of surgery. *Annals of Otology, Rhinology, and Laryngology, 111*(6), 477–485.

6

Evidence-Based Practice in Voice Training for Trans Women

Jennifer M. Oates

Introduction

The aim of this chapter is to place the literature on voice training for adult trans women in the context of evidence-based practice and to consider future research developments that could improve the evidence base for voice training with this client group. For these women, achieving gender-congruent voice characteristics is frequently critical to their psychosocial and financial well-being, personal safety, and quality of life (Byrne, 2007; Hancock, Krissinger, & Owen, 2011; Oates & Dacakis, 2015). The term "trans women" is used here to refer to those women who were assigned male at birth, who experience gender dysphoria or gender incongruence, and who meet the criteria for the International Classification of Diseases (ICD-10) (World Health Organization, 1992) diagnosis of transsexualism. The terms "transgender" and "cisgender" are also used in this chapter, the former referring to people whose gender differs from their sex assigned at birth and the latter to individuals whose gender aligns with their birth-assigned sex.

The first part of this chapter provides a summary of the historical development of voice training for trans women and a framework for the application of evidence-based practice principles to voice training. The second section of this chapter outlines and evaluates the available evidence for voice training with trans women. The final section considers future research developments that would ensure that clinical practice in this field is underpinned by best evidence.

The Historical Development of Voice Training for Trans Women

In the middle of the twentieth century, voice and communication clinicians developed a key role in the management of people with a wide range of voice problems (Oates, 2004), and by the 1970s their management approaches were supported by a scientific approach. Voice was conceptualized as a multidimensional phenomenon that could be measured through auditory-perceptual, acoustic, and physiological means, the mechanisms of causation for different voice problems were better understood, and clearer rationales for therapeutic intervention were developed (Baken, 1998).

It was in the late 1970s that the role of speech-language pathologists in the management of trans women first became recognized. One of the earliest references to the role of these clinicians in voice training for these clients occurred in 1977 when Kalra presented a paper that described her therapeutic approach and voice outcomes for one client at the American Speech-Language-Hearing Association (ASHA) convention in Chicago (Kalra, 1977). The first journal report on voice training for a trans woman was published the following year (Bralley, Bull, Gore, & Edgerton, 1978). Both of these single case reports focused on therapeutic methods for modification of the nonsegmental speech markers of average fundamental frequency and fundamental frequency range.

In 1983 the first general framework for voice training with trans women was published (see Oates & Dacakis, 1983). This framework recommended that voice training be directed to changing fundamental frequency characteristics, but the authors also suggested that additional voice features such as prosody, intensity, voice quality, and resonance required intervention if training was to be maximally effective in assisting these clients to develop communication skills consistent with their desired gender. A small number of single case reports (Bralley et al., 1978; Challoner, 2000; Kalra, 1977; Mount & Salmon, 1988) and the general approach proposed by Oates and Dacakis remained the primary source of guidance for clinicians working with trans women for the next decade.

Single case reports on voice training for trans women continued to be published throughout the 1980s and 1990s (see, for example, Hooper, 1985; Kaye, Bortz, & Tuomi, 1993), and during this time and in the early 2000s, general textbooks on voice disorders also began to include short sections

on this topic (e.g., Andrews, 1999; Aronson, 1990; Battin, 1983; Boone & McFarlane, 2000; Challoner, 2000; Colton & Casper, 1996; Mathieson, 2001; Morrison & Rammage, 1994; Stemple, Glaze, & Gerdeman, 1995). Reports of systematic research on the outcomes of voice training were rare (e.g., Günzburger, 1989, 1993; Spencer, 1988). Unfortunately, this remains the situation into the twenty-first century, where only a handful of data-based research papers have been published (e.g., Carew, Dacakis, & Oates, 2007; Dacakis, 2000; Gelfer & Tice, 2013; Gelfer & Van Dong, 2013; Hancock & Garabedian, 2013; Mészáros et al., 2005; Söderpalm, Larsson, & Almquist, 2004). Readers are also referred to Chapter 5 of this volume, where Pickering and Greene provide a more detailed historical perspective and review of the literature on transgender voice and communication from the 1970s to the present time.

A Framework for the Application of Evidence-Based Practice in Voice Training with Trans Women

If clinicians are to practice effectively in providing voice training for trans women, they need to develop relevant clinical questions and then search for and obtain access to evidence that supports their practice. This evidence includes information on the voice features that are most strongly associated with speaker gender identification, voice features that are associated with successful gender transition, and the effectiveness of voice training methods. Clinicians need to be able to evaluate or critically appraise this information so that they can then apply the results to clinical practice with trans women. This process of structuring clinical questions, searching the literature for evidence, evaluating the strength of that evidence, and using the evidence in client care is known as evidence-based practice.

Evidence-based practice originated in the field of medicine, where the most frequently cited definition was proposed by Sackett and his colleagues, who wrote: "Evidence based medicine is the conscientious, explicit and judicious use of current best evidence in making decisions about the care of individual patients" (Sackett, Richardson, & Rosenberg, 1997, p. 2). This definition of evidence-based medicine has since been applied to health care in general and to many non-medical health care disciplines, such as speech-language pathology (Reilly, 2004a). Speech-language pathology is a relatively young discipline, and there are substantial gaps in our knowledge about the effectiveness of management approaches that are used in everyday practice. This is particularly the case in the area of voice training for trans women. Nevertheless, the application of evidence-based practice principles to the management of these clients has the potential to enhance clinical practice, to reduce variability in practice, and to improve the cost-effectiveness of intervention. Professional associations for speech-language pathologists such as the American Speech-Language-Hearing Association and Speech Pathology Australia provide extensive online resources and databases to assist clinicians to implement evidence-based practice (see, for example, https://www.asha.org/Research/EBP/; https://www.asha.org/Education.aspx#Evidence-Maps; http://speechbite.com/ebp/).

The focus of the next section of this chapter is the critical appraisal of the available evidence underpinning voice training practice for trans women. To facilitate this appraisal process, an evidence hierarchy has been adopted. Evidence hierarchies provide a framework for assessing the level

of evidence obtained about a clinical question. The level of evidence is usually defined as the extent to which the research design used to collect the evidence has minimized bias (NHMRC, 2009). There are many published hierarchies in the literature for evaluating the level of the evidence, but most hierarchies range from the highest level of evidence (e.g., systematic review of several randomized controlled trials) to the lowest level of evidence (e.g., expert opinion). The evidence hierarchy adopted here is the updated hierarchy of the Joanna Briggs Institute (JBI) (https://joannabriggs. org/assets/docs/approach/JBI-Levels-of -evidence_2014.pdf). This hierarchy was selected because, while the evidence levels are based on the relatively complex system developed by the University of Oxford Centre for Evidence-Based Medicine (http://www .cebm.net/), they are less complex and relatively straightforward to apply to a clinical field where the evidence is limited. The JBI Levels of Evidence for effectiveness are presented in Table 6–1 below.

In addition to the levels of evidence, it is important to evaluate the quality, statistical precision, and relevance of the evidence (NHMRC, 2009). *Quality* denotes the strategies used by the investigators to reduce bias in both the design and methods of the research (e.g., the adequacy of control groups; the adequacy of the methods used to measure outcomes). *Statistical precision* requires evaluation as to whether the outcomes of the study are accurate or due to chance. *Relevance* requires an evaluation of the extent to which the research findings can be applied in a range of clinical environments and to different clients. Taken together, the level, quality, statistical precision, and relevance of the evidence can be said to indicate the overall strength of that evidence. For the purposes of this evaluation of the quality, statistical precision, and relevance of

Table 6–1. Joanna Briggs Institute Levels of Evidence

Level of Evidence	Treatment Effectiveness
1 Experimental Designs	1.a Systematic review of randomized controlled trials (RCTs) 1.b Systematic review of RCTs and other study designs 1.c RCT 1.d Pseudo-RCT
2 Quasi-experimental Designs	2.a Systematic review of quasi-experimental studies 2.b Systematic review of quasi-experimental studies and other lower study designs 2.c Quasi-experimental prospectively controlled study 2.d Pre-test/post-test or retrospective control group study
3 Observational—Analytic Designs	3.a Systematic review of comparable cohort studies 3.b Systematic review of comparable cohort studies and other lower study designs 3.c Cohort study with control group 3.d Case-controlled study 3.e Observational study without control group
4 Observational—Descriptive Studies	4.a Systematic review of descriptive studies 4.b Cross-sectional study 4.c Case series 4.d Case study
5 Expert Opinion	5.a Systematic review of expert opinion 5.b Expert consensus 5.c Single expert opinion

Source: Courtesy of the Joanna Briggs Institute.

the evidence for the effectiveness of voice training for trans women, the JBI Critical Appraisal tools (Joanna Briggs Institute, 2016) and general principles of validity and reliability in clinical research design (Portney & Watkins, 2015) served as guides.

The Evidence Base for Voice Training for Trans Women

Although there is relatively widespread acknowledgment that communication training for trans women may require a focus on speech sound articulation, vocabulary, pragmatic behaviors, conversational topics and style, and non-verbal communication, vocal behaviors are the most frequent target of communication intervention for this client group (de Bruin, Coerts, & Greven, 2000; Davies, Papp, & Antoni, 2015; Gelfer, 1999; Neumann & Welzel, 2004; Oates & Dacakis, 1997, 2015; Van Borsel, De Cuypere, & Van den Berghe, 2001). This emphasis on voice change arises from research findings demonstrating that voice features such as average fundamental frequency, fundamental frequency range and variability, average intensity, formant frequencies, and other spectral characteristics differ between cis-female and cismale speakers and that these voice characteristics are critical to listener perceptions of gender. Readers are referred to Freidenberg (2002), Oates and Dacakis (1997, 2015), and Pickering and Baker (2012), as well as Chapter 5 of this volume for reviews of published research on these voice markers of speaker gender.

A focus on voice change in trans women is also supported by research that has examined voice differences between trans women and cisgender controls, between trans women when using their "female" versus their "male" voice, and between trans women perceived as women versus those perceived as men (e.g., Gelfer & Schofield, 2000; Günzburger, 1989, 1993, 1995; King, Brown, & McCrea, 2012; Mikos & Gelfer, 2000, 2001; Spencer, 1988; Wolfe, Ratusnik, Smith, & Northrop, 1990). These studies have shown that average fundamental frequency and intensity, upper and lower limits of the fundamental frequency range, and formant frequencies are voice markers of speaker gender in trans women. Further, these studies have demonstrated that transgender voices identified as female are characterized by less extensive downward intonational shifts, a greater proportion of upward shifts, and fewer level intonation patterns. The relative salience of these voice features, however, is not clear. Gelfer and Schofield (2000), for example, found that, while trans women using higher average fundamental frequencies were more likely to be identified as women, some trans women who used average fundamental frequencies within the accepted normal range for women were still perceived as men. In contrast, Spencer (1988) found that fundamental frequency correlated highly with ratings of speaker gender and that trans women with an average fundamental

frequency of 160 Hz or higher were likely to be perceived as women.

Additional evidence supporting a primary focus on voice change comes from studies of the self-perceptions of trans women. Byrne, Dacakis, and Douglas (2003), for example, demonstrated through a qualitative investigation of perceptions of communicative satisfaction among 21 trans women that the strongest contributor to communicative satisfaction was satisfaction with voice. Similarly, Pasricha, Dacakis, and Oates (2007) concluded from their qualitative study of 12 trans women that the voice was of primary concern and that it was the "feature of their communication with which they were least satisfied" (p. 30). These women also reported that the main aspect of their communication that prevented them from "passing" as women was their voice.

A range of general guides for voice training (e.g., Adler, Hirsch & Mordaunt, 2006, 2012; Battin, 1983; de Bruin et al., 2000; Cavalli & Morris, 1998; Challoner, 2000; Davies et al., 2015; Davies & Goldberg, 2006; Descloux et al., 2012; Freidenberg, 2002; Gelfer, 1999; Gold, 1999; King, Lindestedt, Jensen, & Law, 1999; Mills & Stoneham, 2017; Wiltshire, 1995), literature reviews (e.g., Oates & Dacakis, 1983, 1986, 1997), case reports (e.g., Kalra, 1977; Mount & Salmon, 1988; Vasconcellos & Gusmão, 2001), and studies of the outcomes of voice training (e.g., Carew et al., 2007; Dacakis, 2000; Hancock & Garabedian, 2013; Söderpalm et al., 2004) have outlined recommendations for voice training procedures for trans women. The most common targets for voice training are "to increase fundamental frequency to at least 155 Hz, increase formant frequencies, decrease intensity and vocal effort slightly, increase breathiness slightly, and alter intonation patterns so that the use of level and downward tones are reduced, upward tones are increased, and the overall number of intonation shifts is increased" (Oates & Dacakis, 1997, p. 181). Other frequently cited targets of voice training include minimizing *chest* resonance, encouraging anterior oral resonance and *head* resonance, increasing pitch range and flexibility, and feminizing vocalized pauses, coughing, throat clearing, and laughing (Carew et al., 2007; Dacakis, 2002; Davies et al., 2015; Davies & Goldberg, 2006; de Bruin et al., 2000; Freidenberg, 2002; Hirsch & Gelfer, 2012; Mount & Salmon, 1988; Oates & Dacakis, 1997; Pickering, 2015).

There is, therefore, a reasonable volume of published information on voice training for trans women. Two critical questions remain to be answered, however. How strong is the evidence that voice training for these clients is successful and to what extent can clinicians confidently select specific voice training methods that lead to successful outcomes? Answering these questions requires a critical appraisal of the published literature within the framework of the evidence hierarchy outlined earlier in this chapter.

The available literature on voice training for trans women was gathered from the reference lists of original articles and textbooks, searches of relevant electronic databases (MEDLINE, PsycInfo, EMBASE, and CINAHL), and hand-searching through the general textbooks on voice problems and voice therapy. A total of 29 articles on voice training in trans women published between 1977 and mid-2017 were uncovered. Of those 29 articles, 5 are reviews of the literature, 11 are general guides derived from the authors' clinical experience and/or review of the literature, 6 are case reports, and only 7 are reports of systematic research. In addition, 10 voice texts that include information on voice training for trans women were located. Texts include, at best, reviews of the literature (e.g., Aronson & Bless, 2009;

Challoner, 2000; Mathieson, 2001; Rammage et al., 2001; Stemple, Glaze, & Klaben, 2010), and several provide mainly general guides to voice training based on clinical experience and anecdotal evidence (e.g., Andrews, 1999; Aronson & Bless, 2009; Battin, 1983; Boone, McFarlane, Von Berg, & Zraick, 2009; Colton, Casper, & Leonard, 2006; Mills & Stoneham, 2017).

The JBI evidence hierarchy adopted here places systematic reviews of randomized controlled trials, randomized controlled trials (RCTs), and pseudo-RCTs at the top of the hierarchy (Level 1, Experimental Designs). Although literature reviews concerned with voice training for trans women are available (e.g., Davies et al., 2015; Oates & Dacakis, 1983, 1986, 1997, 2015; Pickering & Baker, 2012), these are a long way short of being systematic reviews and there are no published RCTs or pseudo-RCTs in the field of voice training for these clients.

There are only three published studies of the effectiveness of voice training for this population at the next level down the hierarchy (Level 2, Quasi-experimental Designs). The prospectively controlled study (Level 2.c) reported by Mészáros et al. (2005) investigated auditory-perceptual and acoustic voice characteristics, maximum phonation time, and self-rated communicative impairment for three trans women before and after an average of 9.6 months of voice training. These results were compared with the same measures for two trans women who did not undergo voice training. Voice training focused on increasing fundamental frequency (f_0), improving diaphragmatic-abdominal breath support, reducing laryngeal muscle tension, feminizing intonation patterns, and increasing *head* resonance. Although no statistical analyses were reported, this study showed that following intervention, the habitual f_0 of the clients who underwent voice training increased into the female range, their vocal intensity range increased, and their self-ratings of communicative impairment improved from severe limitations to no limitations in everyday communication. The habitual f_0 of the clients who did not have voice training increased, but to a lesser degree than for the trained participants, and there were no other clear improvements in the remaining voice features or ratings of communicative impairment.

Gelfer and her colleagues also conducted two prospectively controlled studies (Level 2.c) to evaluate the effectiveness of voice therapy for trans women. The control participants in these studies, however, were height- and age-matched cisgender men and women rather than trans women. Gelfer and Tice (2013) analyzed college students' auditory-perceptual judgments of speaker gender and both masculinity and femininity, and acoustic measures of speaking fundamental frequency (SFF) (mean, maximum, and minimum f_0) and frequencies of the first three formants on a variety of speech samples in five trans women prior to 8 weeks of twice-weekly voice therapy, immediately on termination of therapy, and then 15 months later. The same measures were made on one occasion for the voices of five control men and five control women. Voice therapy focused on increasing average pitch and pitch range and oral resonance, voice quality, intonation, and speech naturalness. Before therapy, only 2% of the trans women's voice samples were judged to be female, whereas immediately after therapy this had increased to 51%. A second group of listeners rated speaker gender before therapy and at long-term follow-up. These findings were less positive, with 33% of trans women's voice samples being perceived as female in the long-term. The authors concluded that improve-

ments in gender identification achieved after therapy were only partially maintained in the long term. However, the authors advised caution because of the large individual differences in gender ratings at each of the three time points and because different raters made the judgments of gender at the short- and long-term time points. A series of analyses of variance (ANOVAs) conducted on the listener ratings of masculinity and femininity of the trans women's voices indicated that these women were rated as both more feminine and less masculine immediately after voice therapy and in the long term but that, again, there was substantial individual variability in the gains made.

Findings for the acoustic measures made by Gelfer and Tice (2013) showed similar patterns. In general, SFF, the upper and lower limits of SFF, and formant frequencies increased immediately after therapy, and although they decreased in the longer term, they remained higher than immediately before therapy and mostly fell between the values for the cisgender female and male controls. Once again, interindividual variability was substantial and the results varied depending on the type of speech sample (e.g., isolated vowels versus connected speech).

Gelfer and Van Dong (2013) used a similar research design, intervention techniques, and voice measures to those of Gelfer and Tice (2013), but did not incorporate long-term follow-up measures. However, these researchers added Stemple's Vocal Function Exercises (VFEs) (Gelfer & Van Dong, 2013) to their voice intervention program, and in this case, the duration of intervention was considerably shorter (12 sessions over 6 weeks). Although the three trans women who participated in this study thought that VFEs were a valuable aspect of voice training, they felt that VFE alone would be an inadequate intervention method. Gelfer and Van Dong concluded that the addition of VFE did not enhance the effectiveness of voice intervention, but this conclusion was based only on their finding that voice outcomes associated with their intervention program were similar to those of other studies that did not include VFE.

Although the findings reported by Mészáros et al. (2005), Gelfer and Tice (2013), and Gelfer and Van Dong (2013) appear to support the effectiveness of voice training for trans women, an examination of the strength of the evidence provided demonstrates that the effectiveness of vocal intervention has been established to only a limited degree. Even though the level of evidence is at Level 2 on the JBI evidence hierarchy, the very small number of participants and the lack of consideration of confidence intervals or effect sizes reduce the strength of the evidence provided by these three studies. In addition, the study conducted by Mészáros et al. is limited by the possibility of systematic selection bias in the non-random assignment of the trans women to the treatment and no-treatment groups, absence of ratings of masculinity/femininity of voice, and the lack of statistical analyses and long-term follow-up measures. The studies conducted by Gelfer and Tice and Gelfer and Van Dong are limited by the wide individual variability in voice features before and after voice training, the inclusion of only cisgender control participants (that is, these researchers did not compare voice characteristics between trans women who underwent voice training and those who received no intervention), and the absence of self-ratings of voice-related communication impairment. Further, the conclusion of Gelfer and Van Dong that incorporating VFE into voice training did not enhance voice outcomes must be accepted with caution

because this conclusion was not formally tested through their research design.

At the next level down the hierarchy (Level 3, Observational—Analytic Designs), there are no studies. At Level 4 (Observational—Descriptive Studies), there are only five studies. Carew et al. (2007), Dacakis (2000), Hancock and Garabedian (2013), and Söderpalm et al. (2004) reported the findings of case series without control groups; their studies are categorized at a lower level of the evidence hierarchy (Level 4.c) than the studies reported by Gelfer and Van Dong (2013), Gelfer and Tice (2013), and Mészáros et al. (2005). The single case study reported by Mount and Salmon (1988) (Level 4.d) is the only one of the six case reports yielded through this literature search that can be considered as systematic research.

Carew et al. (2007) reported pre- and post-training formant frequencies (*F1, F2, and F3*) for /a/, /i/, and /ʊ/; mean f_0 in connected speech; auditory-perceptual ratings of masculinity/femininity in connected speech; self-ratings of masculinity/femininity; and satisfaction with voice for 10 trans women. The participants were provided with five sessions of structured voice training targeting two aspects of oral resonance: lip spreading and forward tongue carriage. Training sessions were scheduled at weekly intervals and each session was 45 minutes in duration. Carew et al. demonstrated that, following training, *F3* values increased for all three vowels, *F1 and F2* increased for at least one of the three vowels, and mean f_0 increased. The findings for listener ratings of masculinity/femininity were mixed, but the majority of participants' voices were perceived to sound more feminine after training. The participants' self-ratings demonstrated that they believed that they sounded more feminine after intervention and that their satisfaction with their voices also increased. In addition to the finding that oral resonance training was associated with positive changes in all voice outcome measures, the finding that mean f_0 increased is particularly valuable. Because f_0 increased even though training did not specifically target pitch change, it may be that clinicians can use techniques that are less likely to induce vocal misuse (e.g., oral resonance training) than are traditional methods for achieving increased f_0.

The study reported by Carew et al. (2007) is characterized by several positive methodological features. The number of participants was larger than many previous studies; a wider range of acoustic, auditory-perceptual, and self-rating measures of voice were reported; the voice training program was clearly described and delivered by the same clinician for all participants; and statistical analyses were appropriate for the research aims and the study design. Unfortunately, however, the evidence for the effectiveness of intervention provided through this study is limited. There was no control or comparison group, confidence limits and effect sizes were not reported, and no medium- or long-term follow-up voice measures were made. Furthermore, the low inter-rater reliability of the listener ratings requires that the findings for the auditory-perceptual judgments be accepted with caution.

Dacakis (2000) measured f_0 for 10 trans women before voice training commenced, at discharge from training, and subsequently between 1 and 8.9 years after discharge. Self-ratings of satisfaction with voice and pitch were also obtained at the time of discharge from voice training and at follow-up. The clients' ratings of satisfaction with their voices were obtained retrospectively for the discharge time point. Voice training focused primarily on increasing f_0, and the intervention techniques were reported to be similar across all participants. Dacakis demonstrated that average f_0 for the group increased significantly from pre-treatment to discharge and from pre-treatment to follow-up but that f_0 reduced significantly between discharge and follow-up. That is, while the increases in f_0 achieved after training were not fully maintained, the participants continued to use a higher f_0 at follow-up than they did prior to voice training. Satisfaction ratings were high at both discharge from training and at follow-up. Dacakis also examined the relationships between the number of treatment sessions and f_0 at discharge and between the number of treatment sessions and maintenance of f_0 increases. While the correlation between the number of training sessions and f_0 at discharge was not significant, there was a moderately strong association between the number of sessions and the maintenance of f_0 increases.

The research reported by Dacakis (2000) demonstrates several strengths relative to other publications in this field. Her research included a larger number of trans women than most earlier studies, a relatively long follow-up period was incorporated, both instrumental and self-reported voice measures were used, appropriate statistical analyses were undertaken, and the study examined a possible predictor of voice outcomes (i.e., number of training sessions). Again, however, consideration of the strength of the evidence provided demonstrates that the effectiveness of vocal intervention has been established to only a limited degree. Unfortunately, the relatively low level of evidence (Level 4.c), the lack of a control group, inclusion of only one instrumental voice measure (f_0), no auditory-perceptual measures, lack of reporting of confidence limits or effect sizes, and the possibility of bias arising from the retrospective measure of satisfaction with voice at discharge from training, restrict the degree to which the findings from this study can be applied with confidence to clinical practice.

Hancock and Garabedian (2013) reported on a retrospective chart review of 25 trans women who were discharged from voice feminization training at a university speech and hearing clinic over a five-year period from 2006 to 2010. Duration of intervention varied between 2 and 77 sessions for these trans women. Increasing mean f_0, forward resonance, relaxation, and intonation were the most frequent goals of voice training. Intervention also aimed to reduce the use of phonotraumatic behaviors and improve breath control for approximately half of the participants. Mean f_0 on sustained /a/, a reading passage, and a monologue, semitone (ST) range and the lower and upper limits of f_0 on ascending and descending glissandos, and intensity on sustained /a/ were measured before and after intervention. Although auditory-perceptual ratings were made for some clients and some completed self-report questionnaires on their voice-related quality of life, the large amount of missing data meant that these data could not be reported or analyzed statistically. Repeated-measures ANOVAs, however, were able to be conducted for the f_0 and intensity data. Mean f_0 on all speech samples increased significantly between initial assessment and discharge from intervention. On average, trans women in this study gained 6 ST on the sustained vowel and 5 ST on reading and monologue between initial assessment and discharge. No significant changes on the remaining acoustic variables were detected.

Although the sample size of trans women for the study reported by Hancock and Garabedian (2013) was larger than that of most other treatment studies for this population and while the significant increases in f_0 after intervention are

promising, the retrospective nature of the study, lack of a control group, large amount of missing data, wide variability in number of intervention sessions, and the limited number and type of voice outcome measures reduce the strength of evidence provided through this study.

Söderpalm et al. (2004) reported on a consecutive case series of 22 trans women (3 trans men were also included in their study). Measures of habitual and "preferred" f_0 (mean, range, and variability) were made at baseline and then at varying time points during training and at follow-up. Self-reported ratings of masculinity/femininity were also made by the clients at baseline and at follow-up, and 13 of the participants answered questions addressing various aspects of voice-related quality of life and compliance with vocal exercises at follow-up interviews. Of the 22 trans women who provided baseline data, 17 underwent voice training ranging in duration from one month to more than four years. Voice training comprised vocal hygiene exercises (e.g., relaxation and breath control for phonation), as well as specific pitch-raising exercises and anterior articulation training. Intervention followed the theories of the *Accent Method* of voice training, but training was "broadened and individualized to meet the needs of the transgendered patient" (Söderpalm et al., 2004, p. 20).

Söderpalm et al. (2004) demonstrated that for this series of trans women, fundamental frequencies increased significantly following intervention. At the follow-up interviews, most of the clients reported that they no longer experienced vocal fatigue, hoarseness, and sore throats. There were no major changes in self-ratings of masculinity/femininity after voice training. The findings of this study are difficult to discern, however, because there was a large amount of missing data, not all voice measures were made at baseline as well as follow-up, only limited statistical analyses were reported, effect sizes and confidence intervals were not reported, and not all follow-up questions were answered by all of the trans women. The strength of the evidence provided by Söderpalm et al. is weakened further by the lack of a control group, the variations in voice training procedures across participants, and the limited number of voice outcomes that were measured. As was the case for the studies reported by Carew et al. (2007), Dacakis (2000), and Hancock and Garabedian (2013), the effectiveness of voice training has been established to only a limited degree.

The case study (Level 4.d) reported by Mount and Salmon (1988) is also placed at this level on the evidence hierarchy. Mount and Salmon reported f_0 and formant frequency data for one trans woman at the time of initial assessment, discharge from voice training, and five years after discharge. A comprehensive description of the voice training procedures is provided. These authors concluded that f_0 and the frequency of the second formant increased to levels that would be expected for female speakers after training and that these increases were maintained at follow-up. In addition, Mount and Salmon reported that the client was perceived as a woman over the telephone at the five-year follow-up. Unfortunately, this study did not include a baseline control period, no auditory-perceptual voice measures were made, and no statistical analyses were reported. The strength of the evidence provided is therefore weak.

Conclusions

There is no escaping the general conclusion that the evidence for the effectiveness of voice training in general for trans women

is weak. Of the 29 publications uncovered through this literature search, only 8 (28%) can be considered to yield evidence that is stronger than single case report or expert opinion. Of these 8 publications, however, 3 provide moderately strong evidence for the effectiveness of voice training for trans women. These 3 papers (Mészáros et al., 2005; Gelfer & Tice, 2013; Gelfer & Van Dong, 2013) all report on quasi-experimental prospectively controlled studies that are placed at Level 2 on the JBI evidence hierarchy. The findings of these studies provide promising evidence for the effectiveness of voice training, but their conclusions must be accepted with caution because of design and method limitations, including the very small number of participants, non-random assignment to treatment and control groups, and the absence of long-term follow-up measures.

Not only is the evidence for the effectiveness of voice training generally weak, but no studies have demonstrated the relative effectiveness of specific intervention methods or the relative effectiveness of targeting particular voice features. Nearly all publications reviewed for this chapter reported on the use of similar voice intervention approaches through either quasi-experimental or observational case series designs. However, there are no reports of studies that compare the effectiveness of two or more specific treatment methods, and few reports that provide evidence as to whether targeting a particular voice characteristic or combination of voice characteristics leads to superior outcomes. Several authors recommend that effective voice intervention should target resonance characteristics, intonation, intensity, respiratory control, and voice quality in addition to f_0 (e.g., Carew et al., 2007, Davies et al., 2015; Gelfer, 1999; Freidenberg, 2002; Oates & Dacakis, 1983, 1997; Vasconcellos & Gusmão,

2001; Wiltshire, 1995), but treatment effectiveness studies to support such recommendations are not yet available.

The literature on voice training for trans women provides little guidance as to prognostic indicators or predictors of successful intervention. Dacakis (2000) has provided some evidence that there is a positive correlation between the number of training sessions and the maintenance of f_0 increases following training, but this author cautions that there is no clear evidence as to the number of sessions required for successful outcomes. Hancock and Garabedian (2013) demonstrated that although the total number of intervention sessions was not associated with acoustic measures of voice outcome, an increased number of sessions was correlated with greater gains in f_0 in a sustained vowel, reading, and monologue. Other reports provide only anecdotal suggestions as to who will benefit most from voice training. Gelfer (1999), for example, suggests that the trans woman who is living full-time in the female role will have a strong need to develop a voice consistent with her gender and will, therefore, make the most rapid gains in learning to use female voice characteristics. The assumption underlying this conclusion is that such trans women will be more motivated to practice and comply with training regimes. Similarly, Gold (1999) states that clients who live full-time as women are most likely to succeed in acquiring female voice patterns. Gold also suggests that clients who have performance skills or experience and those who are willing to experiment with their voices are most likely to achieve positive outcomes through voice training. Gelfer (1999) indicates that trans women who misuse their voice, smoke, or suffer from upper respiratory tract allergies will be less successful in voice training. Other authors (e.g., Spencer, 1988; Wolfe et al., 1990) indicate that trans

women who begin intervention with average fundamental frequencies close to or within the expected female range will be most successful. In line with this suggestion, Kaye et al. (1993) and Spencer (1988) propose that the size of the clients' vocal folds, larynx, and vocal tract can limit the extent to which they are able to develop female voice features. These suggestions as to prognostic indicators have some face validity, but the evidence base to support these proposals is far from adequate.

Does the conclusion that the evidence base to support voice training for trans women is insufficient and that the effectiveness of voice training with this population has been established to only a limited degree mean that voice and communication clinicians should not offer services to these clients? Should we wait until higher quality effectiveness research has been reported? These are controversial questions (Carding, 2017; Reilly, 2004a), but it is widely acknowledged that evidence-based practice does not provide all of the answers to guide clinical practice, particularly in fields where only limited effectiveness data are available. Proponents of evidence-based practice have frequently stressed that best practice results only when the expertise of the clinician and client circumstances, preferences, and goals are combined with critical appraisal of research evidence (Carding, 2017; NHMRC, 2009; Reilly, 2004b). The strength of evidence available is therefore only one component of clinical decision making.

Clinicians working with trans women can be encouraged by the high levels of satisfaction with voice training among these clients, the relatively strong consensus among experts as to recommended approaches to voice training for trans women, and the relatively strong evidence available as to voice markers of gender (Davies et al., 2015; Oates & Dacakis, 2015; Pickering & Baker, 2012).

In addition, although the strength of the evidence for the effectiveness of voice training is weak, the most common conclusion from effectiveness studies and case reports is that voice training is associated with positive outcomes for many trans women. Clinicians would, therefore, be negligent to decline requests by these clients for voice training, until a stronger evidence base is available.

Meeting the Challenge of Improving the Evidence Base for Voice Training for Trans Women

Although the application of evidence-based practice principles to clinical practice in the general field of voice disorders has influenced the care of clients with voice problems (Carding, 2017; Oates, 2004), this is not yet true for the specialty area of voice training for transgender clients. Until the strength of evidence provided by intervention studies increases, clinicians cannot be confident that voice training for trans women will be successful or that they have the best evidence on which to select the most effective intervention schedules and methods.

The appraisal of the existing literature on voice training for trans women provided in this chapter provides many pointers to the types of research designs and methods that will improve the evidence base in this field. This area of clinical practice will be advanced dramatically if at least some of the following recommendations are adopted in future research with these clients:

1. Randomized controlled studies, quasi-experimental studies, and single case experimental designs are conducted (i.e., research designs at higher levels of evidence that minimize bias and that can provide data for future systematic reviews and meta-analyses)

2. The effectiveness of specific voice intervention techniques rather than of only broad voice training programs are investigated

3. The comparative effectiveness of alternative voice training methods and of targeting specific parameters of voice (e.g., pitch, resonance, voice quality, intonation) are evaluated

4. Longer follow-up periods are incorporated into intervention studies

5. Intervention methods and training schedules (i.e., duration, dosage, and intensity of training) are described clearly and comprehensively so that replication is possible and the application of the research findings to clinical practice is facilitated

6. Multiple voice measures with established validity and reliability are investigated; auditory-perceptual ratings, instrumental measures, and self-report of impairment, activity and participation restriction, psychosocial well-being, and satisfaction with intervention should all be considered

7. Appropriate statistical analyses are conducted and effect sizes and confidence intervals are reported for all intervention studies

8. Predictive studies are conducted to establish patient, clinician, and intervention factors that are associated with the best voice training outcomes

In 2000, Carding proposed that the most appropriate way to improve the evidence base for voice training in general would be to follow the randomized clinical trial model. Whether this approach to effectiveness research in the field of voice training for trans women will prove to be the gold standard or even feasible is a difficult question to answer. Trans women are not a homogeneous population in terms of their physical, psychological, and social characteristics or with regard to their clinical presentation, motivation, and personal goals (Davies & Goldberg, 2006). This heterogeneity makes scientific control difficult and can limit the feasibility and value of randomized controlled trials. Heterogeneity among these clients may also mean that voice training should be individualized; this may further reduce the suitability of the large-scale randomized clinical trial for effectiveness research with this population. Other research approaches such as quasi-experimental studies with extended pre-intervention control phases and single-subject experimental designs therefore require consideration if we are to further develop the evidence base for voice training with trans women.

References

Adler, R. K., Hirsch, S., & Mordaunt M. (Eds.). (2006). *Voice and communication therapy for the transgender/transsexual individual: A comprehensive clinical guide*. San Diego, CA: Plural Publications.

Adler, R. K., Hirsch, S., & Mordaunt, M. (Eds.). (2012). *Voice and communication therapy for the transgender/transsexual client: A comprehensive clinical guide* (2nd ed.). San Diego, CA: Plural Publications.

Andrews, M. L. (1999). *Manual of voice treatment. Pediatrics to geriatrics* (2nd ed.). San Diego: Singular.

Aronson, A. E. (1990). *Clinical voice disorders: An interdisciplinary approach* (3rd ed.). New York, NY: Brian C. Decker.

Aronson, A. E., & Bless, D. (2009). *Clinical voice disorders: An interdisciplinary approach* (4th ed.). New York, NY: Thieme.

Baken, R. J. (1998). Foreword. In T. Harris, S. Harris, J. S. Rubin, & D. M. Howard (Eds.), *The voice clinic handbook*. London, UK: Whurr Publishers.

Battin, R. R. (1983). Treatment of the transsexual voice. In W. H. Perkins (Ed.), *Voice disorders* (pp. 63–66). New York, NY: Thieme-Stratton Inc.

Boone, D. R., & McFarlane, S. C. (2000). *The voice and voice training* (6th ed.). Boston, MA: Allyn and Bacon.

Boone, D. R., McFarlane, S. C., Von Berg, S. L., & Zraick, R. (2009). *The voice and voice training* (8th ed.). Boston, MA: Allyn and Bacon.

Bralley, R. C., Bull, G. L., Gore, C. H., & Edgerton, M. T. (1978). Evaluation of vocal pitch in male transsexuals. *Journal of Communication Disorders, 11*, 443–449.

de Bruin, M. D., Coerts, M. J., & Greven, A. J. (2000). Speech training in the management of male-to-female transsexuals. *Folia Phoniatrica et Logopaedica, 52*, 220–227.

Byrne L. A. (2007). *My life as a woman: Placing communication within the social context of life for the transsexual woman* [unpublished doctoral dissertation]. Melbourne, Australia: La Trobe University.

Byrne, L. A., Dacakis, G., & Douglas, J. M. (2003). Self-perceptions of pragmatic communication abilities in male-to-female transsexuals. *Advances in Speech Language Pathology, 5*, 15–25.

Carding, P. (2000). *Evaluating voice therapy. Measuring the effectiveness of treatment*. London, UK: Whurr.

Carding, P. (2017). *Evaluating the effectiveness of voice therapy. Functional, organic and neurogenic voice disorders* (2nd ed.) Oxford, UK: Compton Publishing.

Carew, L., Dacakis, G., & Oates, J. (2007). The effectiveness of oral resonance training on the perception of femininity of voice in male-to-female transsexuals. *Journal of Voice, 21*, 591–603.

Cavalli, L., & Morris, M. (1998). Working with transgender patients. *RCSLT Bulletin*, October, pp. 11–13.

Challoner, J. (2000). The voice of the transsexual. In M. Freeman & M. Fawcus (Eds.), *Voice disorders and their management* (3rd ed.) (pp. 245–267). London, UK: Whurr Publishers.

Colton, R., & Casper, J. K. (1996). *Understanding voice problems. A physiological perspective for diagnosis and treatment* (2nd ed.). Baltimore, MD: Williams and Wilkins.

Colton, R., Casper, J. K., & Leonard, R. (2006). *Understanding voice problems. A physiological perspective for diagnosis and treatment* (3rd ed.). Baltimore, MD: Lippincott Williams and Wilkins.

Dacakis, G. (2000). Long-term maintenance of fundamental frequency increases in male-to-female transsexuals. *Journal of Voice, 14*, 549–556.

Dacakis, G. (2002). The role of voice training in male-to-female transsexuals. *Current Opinion in Otolaryngology and Head and Neck Surgery, 10,* 173–177.

Davies, S., & Goldberg, J. M. (2006). Clinical aspects of transgender speech feminization and masculinization. *International Journal of Transgenderism, 9,* 167–196.

Davies, S., Papp, V. G., & Antoni, C. (2015). Voice and communication change for gender nonconforming individuals: Giving voice to the person inside. *International Journal of Transgenderism, 16,* 117–159.

Descloux, P., Isoard-Nectoux, S., Matoso, B., Matthieu-Bordeau, L., Schneider, F., & Scweizer, V. (2012). Transsexualité: accompagnement logopédique sur la 'voix' de las transformation. *Revue de Laryngologie Otologie Rhinologie, 133,* 41–44.

Freidenberg, C. B. (2002). Working with male-to-female transgendered clients: Clinical considerations. *Contemporary Issues in Communication Science and Disorders, 29,* 43–58.

Gelfer, M. P. (1999). Voice treatment for the male-to-female transgendered client. *American Journal of Speech-Language Pathology, 8,* 201–208.

Gelfer, M. P., & Schofield, K. J. (2000). Comparison of acoustic and perceptual measures of voice in male-to-female transsexuals perceived as female versus those perceived as male. *Journal of Voice, 14,* 22–33.

Gelfer, M. P., & Tice, R. M. (2013). Perceptual and acoustic outcomes of voice therapy for male-to-female transgender individuals immediately after therapy and 15 months later. *Journal of Voice, 27,* 335–347.

Gelfer, M. P., & Van Dong, B. R. (2013). A preliminary study on the use of vocal function exercises to improve voice in male-to-female transgender clients. *Journal of Voice, 27,* 321–334.

Gold, L. (1999). Voice training for the transsexual. *VASTA Newsletter, 13,* 10–15.

Günzburger, D. (1989). Voice adaptation by transsexuals. *Clinical Linguistics and Phonetics, 3,* 163–172.

Günzburger, D. (1993). An acoustic analysis and some perceptual data concerning voice change in male-female trans-sexuals. *European Journal of Disorders of Communication, 28,* 13–21.

Günzburger, D. (1995). Acoustic and perceptual implications of the transsexual voice. *Archives of Sexual Behavior, 24,* 339–348.

Hancock, A. B., & Garabedian, L. M. (2013). Transgender voice and communication treatment: A retrospective chart review of 25 cases. *International Journal of Language and Communication Disorders, 48,* 54–65.

Hancock, A. B., Krissinger, J., & Owen, K. (2011). Voice perceptions and quality of life of transgender people. *Journal of Voice, 25,* 553–558.

Hancock, A., Owen, K., Siegfriedt, L., & Brundage, S. (2009, June). *Relationship between self-perception, listener perception, and acoustic measures of femininity in transgender voice assessment.* Paper presented at WPATH 2009 XXI Biennial Symposium, Oslo, Norway.

Hirsch, S., & Gelfer, M. P. (2012). Resonance. In R. Adler, S. Hirsch, & M. Mordaunt (Eds.), *Voice and communication training for the transgender/transsexual client. A comprehensive guide* (2nd ed., Chap. 10). San Diego, CA: Plural Publishing.

Hooper, C. R. (1985). Changing the speech and language of the male to female transsexual client: A case study. *Journal of the Kansas Speech-Language-Hearing Association, 25,* 1–6.

Joanna Briggs Institute (2014). *New JBI Levels of Evidence.* https://joannabriggs.org/assets/docs/approach/JBI-Levels-of-evidence_2014.pdf.

Joanna Briggs Institute (2016). *The Joanna Briggs Institute Reviewers' Manual: 2016 edition.* Australia: Joanna Briggs Institute.

Kalra, M. A. (1977). *Voice training with a transsexual.* Paper presented at the American Speech and Hearing Association Convention, Chicago, IL.

Kaye, J., Bortz, M. A., & Tuomi, S. K. (1993). Evaluation of the effectiveness of voice training with a male-to-female transsexual subject. *Scandinavian Journal of Logopedics and Phoniatrics, 18,* 105–109.

King, J. B., Lindstedt, D. E., Jensen, M., & Law, M. (1999). Transgendered voice: Considerations in case history management. *Logopedics Phoniatrics Vocology, 24,* 14–18.

King, R. S., Brown, G. R., & McCrea, C. R. (2012). Voice parameters that result in identification or misidentification of biological gender in male-to-female transgender veterans. *International Journal of Transgenderism, 13*(3), 117–130.

Mathieson, L. (2001). *Greene and Mathieson's The voice and its disorders* (6th ed.). London, UK: Whurr Publishers.

Mészáros, K., Vitéz, L. C., Szabolcs, I., Góth, M., Kovács, L., Görömbei, Z., & Hacki, T. (2005).

Efficacy of conservative voice treatment in male-to-female transsexuals. *Folia Phoniatrica et Logopaedica, 57*, 111–118.

Mikos, V. A., & Gelfer, M. P. (2000, April). Significant voice change: The male-to-female transgendered individual. *Proceedings of the Student Scientific Research Symposium* (pp. 29–32). University of Wisconsin School of Allied Health Professionals.

Mikos, V. A., & Gelfer, M. P. (2001, November). *The relative contribution of speaking fundamental frequency and formant frequencies to gender identification of biological males, biological females, and male-to-female transgendered individuals based on isolated vowels.* Paper presented at the Convention of the American Speech-Language-Hearing Association, New Orleans, LA.

Mills, M., & Stoneham, G. (2017). *The voice book for trans and non-binary people. A practical guide to creating and sustaining authentic voice and communication.* London, UK: Jessica Kingsley Publishers.

Morrison, M., & Rammage, L. (1994). *The management of voice disorders.* New York, NY: Chapman and Hall.

Mount, K. H., & Salmon, S. J. (1988). Changing the vocal characteristics of a postoperative transsexual patient: A longitudinal study. *Journal of Communication Disorders, 21*, 229–238.

NHMRC (National Health and Medical Research Council) (2009). *NHMRC levels of evidence and grades for recommendations for developers of guidelines.* Canberra: Australian Government.

Neumann, K., & Welzel, C. (2004). The importance of the voice in male-to-female transsexualism. *Journal of Voice, 18*, 153–167.

Oates, J. (2004). The evidence base for the management of individuals with voice disorders. In S. Reilly, J. Douglas, & J. Oates (Eds.). *Evidence-based practice in speech pathology* (pp. 110–139). London, UK: Whurr Publishers.

Oates, J. M., & Dacakis, G. (1983). Speech pathology considerations in the management of transsexualism—a review. *British Journal of Disorders of Communication, 18*, 139–151.

Oates, J. M., & Dacakis, G. (1986). Voice, speech and language considerations in the management of male-to-female transsexualism. In W. A. W. Walters & M. W. Ross (Eds.), *Transsexualism and sex reassignment* (pp. 82–91). Melbourne, Australia: Oxford University Press.

Oates, J., & Dacakis, G. (1997). Voice change in transsexuals. *Venereology. The Interdisciplinary, International Journal of Sexual Health, 10*, 178–187.

Oates, J., & Dacakis, G. (2015). Transgender voice and communication: Research evidence underpinning voice intervention for male-to-female transsexual women. *Perspectives on Voice and Voice Disorders, 25*, 48–58.

Oxford Centre for Evidence-Based Medicine (2009). *Oxford Centre for Evidence-Based Medicine—Levels of Evidence March 2009,* viewed July 5, 2011, http://www.cebm.net/

Pasricha, N., Dacakis, G., & Oates, J. (2007). Communicative satisfaction of male-to-female transsexuals. *Logopedics Phoniatrics Vocology, 33*, 25–34.

Pickering, J. (2015). Transgender voice and communication: Introduction and international context. *Perspectives on Voice and Voice Disorders, 25*, 25–31.

Pickering, J., & Baker, L. (2012). Voice and communication intervention for individuals in the transgender community: An historical perspective and review of the literature. In R. Adler, S. Hirsch, & M. Mordaunt (Eds.), *Voice and communication training for the transgender/transsexual client. A comprehensive guide* (2nd ed., Chap. 1). San Diego, CA: Plural Publishing.

Portney, L. G., & Watkins, M. P. (2015). *Foundations of clinical research: Applications to practice* (3rd ed.). Philadelphia, PA: F. A. Davis Company.

Rammage, L., Morrison, M., & Nicholl, H. (2001). *Management of the voice and its disorders* (2nd ed.). Vancouver, BC, Canada: Singular Thomson Learning.

Reilly, S. (2004a). The move to evidence-based practice within speech pathology. In S. Reilly, J. Douglas, & J. Oates (Eds.). *Evidence based practice in speech pathology* (pp 3–17). London, UK: Whurr Publishers.

Reilly, S. (2004b). What constitutes evidence? In S. Reilly, J. Douglas, & J. Oates (Eds.), *Evidence-based practice in speech pathology* (pp. 18–34). London, UK: Whurr Publishers.

Sackett, D. L., Richardson, W. S., & Rosenberg, W. M. C. (Eds.). (1997). *Evidence-based medicine.* London, UK: Churchill Livingston.

Söderpalm, E., Larsson, A., & Almquist, S. (2004). Evaluation of a consecutive group of transsexual individuals referred for vocal intervention in the west of Sweden. *Logopedics Phoniatrics Vocology, 29*, 18–30.

Spencer, L. E. (1988). Speech characteristics of male-to-female transsexuals: A perceptual and acoustic study. *Folia Phoniatrica, 40,* 31–42.

Stemple, J. C., Glaze, L. E., & Gerdeman, B. (1995). *Clinical voice pathology. Theory and management* (2nd ed.). San Diego, CA: Singular Publishing Group.

Stemple, J. C., Glaze, L. E., & Klaben, B. (2010). *Clinical voice pathology. Theory and management* (4th ed.). San Diego, CA: Plural Publishing.

Van Borsel, J., De Cuypere, G., & Van den Berghe, H. (2001). Physical appearance and voice in male-to-female transsexuals. *Journal of Voice, 15,* 570–575.

Vasconcellos, L., & Gusmão, R.J. (2001). Phonoaudiological training in male transsexuals: Report of three cases. *Brazilian Journal of Otorhinolaryngology, 67,* 114–118.

Wiltshire, A. (1995). Not by pitch alone: A view of transsexual vocal rehabilitation. *National Student Speech-Language-Hearing Association Journal, 22,* 53–57.

Wolfe, V. I., Ratusnik, D. L., Smith, F. H., & Northrop, G. (1990). Intonation and fundamental frequency in male-to-female transsexuals. *Journal of Speech and Hearing Disorders, 55,* 43–50.

World Health Organization (1992). *The ICD-10 International Statistical Classification of Diseases and Related Health Problems.* 10th Revision (2016 version). Geneva, Switzerland: Author.

7

Considerations for Intake and Assessment

Georgia Dacakis

Assessment and Goal Setting for Trans and Gender Diverse Individuals

Assessment of trans women, trans men, gender non-binary, and gender diverse individuals provides its own unique set of challenges and rewards. However, it is important that the speech-language clinician be aware that the technical and therapeutic skills and knowledge required to assess the voice and communication of these individuals are not dissimilar to those required to assess a range of everyday communication disorders unrelated to gender identity. The significant difference lies in the imperative for the clinician to achieve cultural competency (Hancock, 2015) and to gain a thorough understanding of the medical and psychosocial factors associated with the individual's transition from living as their birth-assigned gender to living as their self-identified gender. Poor cultural competency and the lack of understanding of the transition process have the potential to significantly negatively impact the client, the client/clinician relationship, and the outcomes of voice and communication (VAC) training.

This chapter proposes the necessary preparation that a clinician requires when embarking on a first-time contact with trans and gender diverse individuals. The author provides an overview of assessment for these individuals followed by considerations for establishing client-centered goals. Readers seeking information relating to specific assessment techniques, training goals, and procedures for targeting verbal and nonverbal communication characteristics will find this information addressed in later chapters of this book. Because of the paucity of research and clinical reports pertaining to assessment of trans men and gender non-binary and gender diverse individuals, the information provided is derived largely from reports and research involving trans women. The information outlined in this chapter, however, provides guidance for those working with trans and gender diverse individuals who seek an authentic expression of their gender.

Preparing to Work with Trans and Gender Diverse Clients

While gender diversity may be valued in certain cultures (Bockting & Cesaretti, 2001;

Bolin, 2004; Coleman et al., 2012; Coleman, Colgan, & Gooren, 1992; Kalra, 2012;), negative societal responses toward gender non-conformity predominate globally, and the stigma attached to trans and gender diverse individuals frequently results in substantial psychosocial, physical, and financial consequences (Budge et al., 2012; Clements-Nolle, Marx, & Katz, 2006; Pitts, Couch, Mulcare, Croy, & Mitchell, 2009; Whittle, Turner, Combs, & Rhodes, 2008). For those individuals who are not visual conformers, that is, who are identified as gender non-conforming by strangers in casual situations based on how they look and sound, the risk of adverse consequences is higher than for those who are visual conformers (Byrne, 2007; Grant et al., 2011). Due to these adverse societal responses, this client population must have faith that the clinician fully understands their condition and respects their gender position.

Freidenberg (2002) makes a valuable contribution when she proposes that published trans and gender diverse autobiographies provide "compelling and informative" clinical resource material to increase one's understanding of the experience of trans and gender diverse individuals. The Internet and social media now also provide speech-language clinicians with unprecedented access to material that reflects the lived experiences of trans and gender diverse individuals. To ensure and maintain credibility with the client, the clinician must also be familiar with the requirements of any Gender Dysphoria Program that the client may be enrolled in. While not all trans and gender diverse individuals choose a medically assisted transition, accessing the Standards of Care (SOC) for the Health of Transsexual, Transgender and Gender Non-Conforming Individuals Version 7 (Coleman et al., 2012) will provide the clinician with an understanding of the psychiatric, psychological, medical, and

surgical undertakings that a client may be negotiating. The clinician must be culturally sensitive to trans and gender diverse issues (Davies & Goldberg, 2006a; Hancock, 2015); and at minimum must employ correct gender-status terminology to ensure that the client is not inadvertently offended, as would most likely be the case if a trans woman were to be referred to as a transvestite by an ill-informed clinician.

Davies and Goldberg (2006a) recommend as a prerequisite for working with trans and gender diverse clients that a speech-language clinician attain a minimum of two years of experience in the assessment and treatment of adult speech and voice disorders. They, along with Freidenberg (2002), Gelfer (1999), and Hancock (2015), also emphasize the importance of clinicians possessing knowledge of the trans and gender diverse experience and, in particular, an understanding of the transformative process that clients will undergo on their journey toward achieving comfort and an authentic expression of their gender identity. In addition to the minimum two years' expertise noted above, prior to a first-time assessment of a trans or gender diverse client, clinicians should comply with the recommendations outlined in SOC v7 (Coleman et al., 2012, pp. 197–198). These include:

1. *Specialized training and competence in the assessment and development of communication skills in transsexual, transgender, and gender-nonconforming clients.*

2. *A basic understanding of transgender health, including hormonal and surgical treatments for feminization/masculinization and trans-specific psychosocial issues as outlined in the SOC, and familiarity with basic sensitivity protocols such as the use of preferred gender pronoun and name (Canadian*

Association of Speech-Language Pathologists and Audiologists; Royal College of Speech and Language Therapists, United Kingdom; Speech Pathology Australia).

3. *Continuing education in the assessment and development of communication skills in transsexual, transgender, and gender nonconforming clients. This may include attendance at professional meetings, workshops, or seminars; participation in research related to gender-identity issues; independent study; or mentoring from an experienced, certified clinician.*

Freidenberg (2002), de Bruin, Coerts, and Greven (2000) and King, Lindstedt, Jensen, and Law (1999) acknowledge that clinicians may experience hesitancies in working with trans and gender diverse individuals. The authors variously cite religious, moral, and psychological reasons as well as generalized feelings of unease and uncertainty as the cause of these hesitations. The clinician treating these clients must be aware of the possibilities for tacit discrimination and must ensure that the client is given "full regard" and is treated with the courtesy and respect provided to every client who attends a speech-language clinic (King et al., 1999). The clinician who believes that his or her treatment provision may be compromised by personal beliefs or discomfort in treating this population should refer the client to another clinician.

When to Assess?

There are few published guidelines or protocols surrounding the timing of referral of trans and gender diverse clients for VAC assessment. In speech-language facilities that accept self-referrals, individuals will likely be accepted for assessment when a request is made. Protocols exist, however,

for services associated with gender clinics. In Sweden, for example, all trans men and trans women are referred for voice assessment once a diagnosis of gender dysphoria has been confirmed (Södersten, Nygren, Hertegård, & Dhejne, 2015; see Chapter 1 of this volume). De Bruin et al. (2000) recommend that all trans women attending a gender clinic be referred, as a matter of course, approximately three months after the commencement of hormone therapy, while trans men be referred only if they have a specific concern. Although trans men are usually only referred for assessment if there is an expressed communication difficulty, a growing number of research reports indicate that voice change in trans men is not totally "unproblematic" and recommend voice assessment of these individuals (Azul, Nygren, Södersten, & Neuschaefer-Rube, 2016; Nygren, Nordenskjöld, Arver, & Södersten, 2016; Scheidt, Kob, Willmes, & Neuschaefer-Rube, 2004; Van Borsel, De Cuypere, Rubens, & Destaerke, 2000).

Voice assessment for the purpose of providing trans and genderdiverse individuals with advice regarding the VAC training process can be undertaken at any stage. However, because of testosterone-induced voice change in trans men and the findings that in trans women the impact of a gender-incongruent voice changes with a myriad of fluctuating personal and social factors, assessment for the purposes of determining VAC training goals must be undertaken in close proximity to the commencement of the training to ensure appropriateness of training goals and to facilitate successful outcomes. Examples of the personal and social factors associated with the impact of voice on trans women include the length of time since they have transitioned to living in their self-identified gender (Byrne, 2007; Dacakis, Davies, Oates, Douglas, & Johnston, 2013; Holmberg, Oates, Dacakis, & Grant,

2010), their social network, the extent of acceptance by colleagues and close others, and the nature of the communication situation (Byrne, 2007; Pasricha, Dacakis, & Oates, 2008). These factors may also apply to trans men and gender diverse individuals. Consequently, for all populations where intervention does not commence soon after the initial assessment, it is imperative that the client be reassessed prior to the commencement of VAC training.

Referral to an Ear, Nose, and Throat Specialist

It is generally accepted as good clinical practice that clients who are referred to a speech-language clinician for assessment and management of a voice disorder are referred to an ear, nose, and throat (ENT) specialist or otolaryngologist for a laryngeal examination prior to being seen. However, although trans and gender diverse clients usually require voice modification, they do not usually have a "voice disorder" per se (Stemple, Glaze, & Klaben, 2000, p. 139). Söderpalm, Larsson, and Almquist (2004) provide support for this assumption. Their study, which reported the findings of stroboscopic examinations of 22 transgender individuals referred for phoniatric examination between 1991 and 2002, found "no laryngeal pathology except for a minor sulcus on one vocal cord in one patient" (p. 21).

Freidenberg (2002) indicates that the clinical setting influences whether or not a trans or gender diverse client undergoes laryngeal examination prior to attending the VAC assessment. For example, in speech-language clinics attached to a hospital-based Gender Dysphoria Program, all clients may be examined by an ENT using laryngeal endoscopy with stroboscopic light to eliminate vocal pathology and confirm normal vocal

cord functioning. In addition, at these clinics, the presence of any other ear, nose, or throat complaints are investigated. In contrast, speech-language clinicians in private practice or a clinical facility not attached to an ENT department may assess the cost/benefit of this intervention according to the individual client. The decision to refer a client for ENT assessment is determined by: a close examination of the client's voice use; perceptual and acoustic analyses of vocal characteristics; and the identification (from the case history interview) of upper respiratory tract infections, hearing loss, or other relevant medical conditions. Any suspicion of a voice disorder or adverse changes in vocal characteristics following the implementation of voice training should result in a referral to the ENT.

While visual examination of the larynx using indirect laryngoscopy with the patient phonating on /i/ will reveal vocal fold approximation and any gross pathology, it is preferable that the function of the larynx be examined endoscopically to observe vocal fold function during pitch change and check for the presence of ventricular fold and anterior-posterior constriction. There is a risk that increased laryngeal muscle tension and constriction may be more prevalent in trans and gender diverse individuals who attempt to increase the pitch of their voice without professional guidance (Palmer, Dietsch, & Searl, 2012).

The Assessment

Comprehensive assessment of trans and gender diverse individuals draws on the speech-language clinician's extensive knowledge of voice and communication. Clinicians will potentially assess all verbal and nonverbal components of the clients' communication. As noted above, the assessment process may require referring clients to ENT specialists. It will certainly require collecting both voice and speech samples, undertaking detailed case history interviews, and gathering the individuals' self-perceptions of their vocal functioning and the impact of their voice on their everyday lives.

Voice Sample

An integral component of the assessment of the voice and communication characteristics of trans and gender diverse individuals involves obtaining an audio-recorded sample of the individual's voice and speech. These samples are used for acoustic analysis of the individual's vocal characteristics and screening for articulation precision and language use. Ideally the sample would be recorded in a sound-treated room with a high quality digital recorder (e.g., Marantz Solid PMD671 Flash recorder) and a pre-polarized dual-diaphragm condenser, head-mounted microphone (e.g., AKG C477 WR). The sample would be analyzed using a computer software program such as Multispeech, Model 3700 (KayPentax). Affordable options are, however, available for clinicians in smaller practices where client numbers do not support an expensive recording and acoustical analysis suite. In the absence of a sound-treated room, the voice can be recorded in a quiet room with ambient noise <50 dB (Dejonckere et al., 2001) and analyzed using a free-to-download program such as PRAAT (www.praat.org) or Wavesurfer (http://www.speech.kth.se/wavesurfer/man.html).

A standard voice sample will include:

- Four-second sustained /a/. Most stable of three attempts for analysis of voice quality: Jitter, shimmer, and noise-to-harmonic ratio.
- Sustained /a/, /i/, and /u/. Analysis of resonance: F1, F2, and F3.

- Reading sample, e.g., The Rainbow Passage* (Fairbanks, 1960). Analysis of fundamental frequency: mean, modal, SD, minimum, maximum, and range in semitones (ST).
- Monologue sample* at comfortable pitch and loudness. Analysis of intonation: f_0 SD and frequency of upward and downward intonation patterns.
- /i:/ at comfortable loudness on ascending and descending glissandos. Analysis of maximum phonation range in ST.
- Maximum prolongation of /i/, /a/, and /u/. Analysis of maximum phonation time.

*Also to examine for articulation precision and language

Case History

The traditional case history assists in the overall differential diagnosis of a communication disorder. Causal and maintaining factors are isolated, the severity of the disorder is ascertained, and the client's motivation is examined—with the clinician aware that information provided by the client during the interview will change according to altered circumstances. For trans and gender diverse clients, the potential for frequently changing case history information is high. For example, information gathered from a trans man living and working full-time while still presenting as female will bear little resemblance to case history information obtained when he has transitioned to full-time presenting as male. The clinician must be attuned to the potential for the client's emotional, social, psychological, and financial status to alter significantly and, consequently, impact on self-perceptions of communication, motivation, and ability to comply with speech-language intervention. This change dynamic requires the preparedness of the clinician to review case history information on a regular basis.

Identifying Information

From the outset, the clinician must establish the name and pronoun by which the client wishes to be referred. Although some clinicians may find it a challenge to address a client dressed as a male by a female name, it is a simple courtesy to call a client by their preferred name (Brown & Rounsley, 1996; Davies & Goldberg, 2006a; Hancock, 2015). As indicated above for a good working relationship to be established, the trans or gender diverse client must detect full support from the clinician. The clinician must also establish whether the name identified for use within the clinic is the preferred name to be used in all extra-clinical situations. For those clients who are in the process of transitioning from one binary gender presentation to another, there may be periods when they will use both the male and female versions of their name. To ensure clients' confidentiality, it is necessary that both the clinician and reception staff are fully acquainted with the name(s) used by clients in the differing aspects of their lives. Although client files must be identified by the client's legal name, postal documents and telephone calls can be addressed using the client's preferred name (with the requisite pronoun inserted into telephone conversations) so that client confidentiality is not inadvertently breached.

Again, for those transitioning from one binary gender to another, it is useful to establish the duration of time (expressed as a percentage) that the client lives concurrently in each gender, the circumstances determining the gender presentation of each situation and whether or not there is a clear delineation between gender presentations. For example, does the client only present as

male while engaged in employment activities? This information will indicate clients' opportunities to transfer new communication characteristics from the confines of the clinic room to everyday living situations and will give the clinician valuable insight into the stresses experienced by clients as they attempt to balance their double lives.

Referral

Trans and gender diverse clients may be referred to a speech-language clinician from a variety of sources. Some clinics require a referral from a general medical practitioner, while others require a referral from a mental health counselor or treating psychiatrist. There are still others that are comfortable with a self-referral. Establishing the referral source and reason for referral provides an indication of the client's perception of both their communication needs and their motivation. The client who self-identifies a communication difficulty and subsequently seeks help from a clinician is usually insightful and highly motivated. A client who is referred by a member of a Gender Dysphoria Program may be as equally motivated as the self-referral or, on the other hand, may be attending VAC training, believing it will facilitate their access to gender reassignment surgery (GRS).

Medical Information

Traditionally, when gathering medical information, the clinician will strive to ascertain the presence of any condition that may have an impact on the client's ability to achieve the goals of intervention. The majority of trans and gender diverse clients referred to speech-language clinicians require voice modification, thus case history questions related to the voicing mechanism are specifically targeted. In this respect, questions posed to trans and gender diverse clients are no different than those asked when taking a voice case history from cisgender individuals presenting with voice concerns unrelated to gender. Identification of respiratory disease is important because respiration provides the power source of phonation. Relevant questions will include: Does the client suffer upper respiratory tract infections, asthma, frequent colds, or allergies? Does the client suffer laryngopharyngeal reflux or a thyroid condition? Has the client ever had surgery (including cosmetic surgery) or trauma to the head/neck/chest regions? Information regarding the presence of any neurologic disorders or hearing loss will be equally important to the client's prognosis. As with all clients requiring voice modification, cigarette smoking and/or recreational drug taking places trans and gender diverse clients at risk for voice quality disturbances. A more than moderate intake of alcohol not only may affect the mucous membrane of the vocal folds, but will also make it difficult for the speaker to monitor and adjust gender-inappropriate communication. For example, it may be more difficult to maintain a gender-appropriate pitch while under the influence of alcohol (de Bruin, Coerts, & Greven, 2000).

The clinician should establish a complete list of the client's current medications that includes the condition for which the medication is prescribed as well as any side effects described by the client. The significant medication trans and gender diverse individuals may be taking will be cross sex hormones (see Chapter 4). It is also not uncommon, given the life-changing experience of seeking to live in one's authentic gender and the frequency of negative societal responses to gender non-conformity, for trans and gender diverse individuals to experience high rates of anxiety, depression, and suicidal ideation (Hyde et al., 2013; Pitts

et al., 2009) and to therefore be prescribed antidepressants. Information must be gathered on any prescribed antidepressants and their impact on therapy, in terms of the efficacy of the prescription in managing the depression and whether or not the client's mental concentration is affected.

If a doctor has not referred the client, it is important to establish the details of the client's treating doctor, and the frequency of the client's appointments. A client who is attending doctor's appointments more frequently than might be expected may be either unwell or experiencing difficulty with the transition process. Additional problems can arise from the client's need to attend frequent and regular appointments with specialists such as psychiatrists, endocrinologists, and laser therapists. This is particularly pertinent in the case of the employed client who has not "come out" at work and whose employer becomes concerned by the extent of their absenteeism. Workplace reaction to absenteeism may affect the timing of the commencement of speech-language intervention and the client's ability to attend regular therapy appointments.

Those individuals diagnosed with gender dysphoria may be under the care of a consulting psychiatrist. It is often the case that psychiatric appointments are scheduled several months apart, whereas clients undergoing VAC training usually attend on a weekly basis. Given the contrasting frequency of the appointments, it is not uncommon that a client/clinician relationship is established such that it is the speech-language clinician rather than the psychiatrist to whom the client is inclined to reveal any emotional discomfort arising from the transition process. Freidenberg (2002) advises that in order to pre-empt a client's emotional state intervening with the progress of VAC training, from the outset the clinician should request the client's permission to contact the treating psychiatrist if required. In cases where a client is unwilling to agree to this, the clinician may counsel the client to speak with his or her psychiatrist or refer the client to another qualified professional.

Psychosocial Aspects

In everyday clinical practice, the speech-language clinician encounters clients ranging from infancy to old age. Most of these cisgender clients, irrespective of age and diagnosis, will enjoy unqualified approval and support from family, friends, and, where appropriate, employers in their attempts to modify their voice or communication. In this respect, trans and gender diverse clients often stand alone and isolated. For example, rarely are the attempts by a birth-assigned male (trans woman) to acquire the communication characteristics of a female supported or approved by all those who know her. In instances where support does become available, it is rarely present for the duration of the transition process. Case history questions should establish which of the client's nominated contacts are supportive of their need to modify communication characteristics: Who is available to say to the client, "Yes, you are doing the right thing. I support you" or "Sure, you can practice your new voice with me."

Emotional and psychological state can have a significant impact on the client's ability to concentrate on the clinical task at hand and, therefore, on the ability to transfer learned skills into everyday communication situations. Information gained in this section of the case history will help clinicians gauge how clients are dealing with the transition process and how they are coping emotionally and psychologically. Simple, direct questions will best reveal this information. As noted above, trans and gender diverse clients may suffer not only social rejection but also the loss of family, friends, employment, financial assets, and concomitant lifestyle (Budge et al., 2013; Clements-Nolle et al., 2006; Pitts et al., 2009; Whittle et al., 2008). Much will be gained in the clinical interaction if the clinician and the client discuss the possibility of potential loss in the latter's life and how it may affect the client's attendance and compliance with the requirements of the VAC training program. Clients must be proactive in notifying the clinician when situations causing feelings of rejection/depression arise that affect their ability to focus on the program. In these instances, the clinician may assume a counseling role (see Chapter 3). If necessary, the intervention program should be modified accordingly. Indeed, Freidenberg (2002) recommends that when a client is experiencing emotional "upheaval and depression" (p. 47), it may be appropriate to temporarily interrupt the VAC training program. With a new client, it may be necessary to postpone the commencement of clinical intervention.

Social Information

To gain insight into the client's motivation to communicate, the clinician must ask specific questions about the client's social support network and social interactions: "Are you a social person?" "How do you socialize?" "What do you like to do in your spare time?" Clearly, if clients are socially withdrawn (e.g., solely interested in playing computer games in isolation or socializing through computer chat rooms that do not require verbal communication), there are far fewer opportunities for them to practice new communication skills than if they have an active verbally driven social network. It is also important that clients are encouraged to talk about their friends, and the extent to which they believe their friends will support the modification of their communication characteristics. Rejection by friends, however, is high in the trans and gender diverse population, and questioning must be treated sensitively. In the study by Grant et al. (2011) 67% of trans women, 51% of trans men, and 61% of transgender respondents reported the loss of close friends as a result of their gender presentation. Generally speaking, it is to be expected that the client who has maintained close social contacts will have more situations to conquer. It is also to be expected that such clients will have more situations in which to practice. However, Pasricha, Dacakis, and Oates (2008) report that loving and supportive friends can provide a safe haven for trans women where they do not have to "pass," and, therefore in these situations, do not worry about maintaining gender modified communication.

Family and Close or Significant Others

The reactions of family members to the trans and gender diverse individual's "coming out" range from outright rejection (including verbal and physical abuse) through to qualified acceptance (Freidenberg, 2002). It is therefore important to identify the significant people in the client's life and to ascertain the extent to which they support the individual's transition to presenting in their self-identified gender. This support may contribute to positive outcomes of the VAC training by providing practice opportunities; however, the absence of this support will certainly have a negative impact on individuals' emotional and psychological well-being and, in turn, their ability to focus on achieving their goals. Questions regarding support of family will require a measure of sensitivity, as many clients suffer great loss of family and close other support, and questions may evoke an emotional response.

It may come as a surprise to the clinician working with trans and gender diverse clients for the first time to discover that many of these individuals have been (or are still) married, and have children. For trans women (and likely for trans men), attempts in adolescence and young adulthood to prove that they "belonged" to their birth-assigned gender or to overcompensate for feelings of belonging to the opposite gender often resulted in these individuals committing to conventional marriage (Gagne & Tewksbury, 1999). It may be that a trans woman, for example, still lives with her wife and their children who may or may not support her attempts to modify her voice and communication. In the case of trans women, the author's experience is that there are few clients who are able to practice feminized communication characteristics with a wife, ex-wife, their children, or their own parents. Indeed, there often exists an unspoken understanding that they will refrain from using feminized speech in the family home. It is not uncommon for family members to announce that they prefer clients to speak in their "real" voice, or even for clients themselves to choose to use their "old" voice so as not to "upset" their family and close others.

Clinicians must pay particular attention to a client whose case history reveals significant rejection by family. The loss of the safe haven provided by family support is associated with increased suicidal ideation and suicide rates within the trans and gender diverse population. Grant et al. (2011) reported that 32% of trans and gender diverse adults who had family support attempted suicide, while the figure was 51% for those whose family had rejected them. The finding of Bauer and Scheim (2015) that 57% of trans individuals aged between 16 and 24 years without parental support for their gender identity attempted suicide in the year prior to the study, compared with a rate of 4% for individuals who reported strong parental support, is testament to the gravity of loss for this population.

Employment

The rate of unemployment in trans and gender diverse populations is significantly higher than that of the general population. A study of European countries reported 39% employment (full-time and part-time combined) for trans women (Whittle et al., 2008). This figure is lower than employment rates for Ireland (McNeil, Bailey, Ellis, & Regan, 2013), Canada (Ontario) (Bauer & Scheim, 2015), and Australia (Hyde et al., 2014), who all reported employment rates around 50%. In a study by Grant et al. (2011) of an American transgender population, 47% of the respondents experienced being fired, not hired, or denied promotion because of their gender identity. In the same study, 90% of the participants reported harassment and mistreatment at work. In view of these damning statistics, the clinician must determine the extent of awareness and acceptance levels in the workplace environment as regards the client's self-identified gender. In workplaces where the employer and colleagues are accepting of the client's transgender status, greater opportunities for practice are available and less anxiety will surround the transfer of newly learned voice and communication characteristics to the workplace. Conversely, where the client plans to but has not "come out" in the workplace, information regarding timing of transition and the communication load attached to the employment position will help identify realistic and safe opportunities for transferring voice and communication characteristics to the workplace.

Voice

The perceived imperative for voice modification by trans and gender diverse individuals seeking the services of speech-language clinicians necessitates a detailed investigation of the client's voice. Case history questions will identify past and current voice problems unrelated to gender identity, concerns about voice in the context of gender identity, previous attempts to re-gender the voice and the results of such attempts, expectations of the voice and communication program and the client's reliance on voice for communication. This information will expose the extent of the client's concerns and the importance of appropriate voice usage as a motivational factor.

Although trans and gender diverse individuals seek the services of speech-language clinicians for training of a physiologically healthy larynx, it cannot be assumed that the client has not already experienced, or is not experiencing, an underlying voice problem unrelated to gender identity. The clinician should ask: "Do you think you have a voice problem unrelated to wanting a voice to match your gender identity?" "Do you ever lose your voice?" "Does the quality/sound of your voice change of its own accord?" "Does your throat feel sore after you have spoken for a long time?" "Have you been treated by a speech-language clinician or an ENT in the past?" The clinician will also determine whether the client is engaging in vocal abuse or misuse behaviors or is at risk of a voice disorder (see Chapter 8). The client is observed for obvious signs of vocal abuse (e.g., throat clearing) and is asked case history questions relating to their voice use patterns. Does the client misuse their voice by using extreme laryngeal tension in attempts to change vocal pitch? Does the client abuse their voice in situations unrelated to attempts to achieve a gender congruent voice? Often, a simple case history question such as, "Do you need to raise your voice over background noise or force it in any way?" will point to instances of vocal abuse; however, it is also useful to compile a comprehensive list of the client's speaking situations and discuss how the client uses their voice in each situation. This communication diary will help the clinician identify actual or potential vocal abuse situations not immediately obvious to the client. The clinician can also access the diary to establish a hierarchy of situations in which the client can practice (transfer) their newly acquired communication characteristics.

Within the context of their gender identity, trans and gender diverse individuals commonly describe their perceived voice concern as related to voice pitch. Not infrequently, they will have a vocal image in mind as a target voice and some will have attempted themselves to modify their voice using programs developed by speech-language clinicians or resources produced by trans individuals. Because of the potential for vocal misuse resulting from the absence of feedback when using these resources, it is important to ask the client questions that establish the nature of any past or ongoing attempts to change voice characteristics. These questions can include: "Do you have a specific vocal image in mind?" "Have you attempted to achieve this vocal image?" "Have you tried to increase vocal pitch?" "What resources did you use to aid these attempts?" "How successful were these attempts?" "Did these attempts to change your voice result in your voice tiring easily or the quality of your voice changing?" It may be that the client has achieved, without VAC training, the maximum that can be achieved. Alternatively, it may be that a successful increase in pre-training pitch, with no accompanying signs of tension, indicates that the client has the potential for further increases in pitch or will readily respond to training aimed at modifying other aspects of voice not originally considered by the client (e.g., increasing intonation variability). Having identified any changes in voice characteristics since the individual's decision to modify their voice, the clinician faces the somewhat more complex task of establishing situational variability of voice use and how the voice impacts the individual.

Traditionally, symptoms of voice disorders vary according to a number of internal and external factors affecting the client: levels of fatigue and stress; exposure to environmental noise (resulting in compensating louder voice levels); exposure to air conditioning; cheering/yelling at sports and entertainment venues; hydration levels; and sensitivity to listener reactions. It is clinically important to examine these factors and establish whether the individual's voice use varies under these conditions. The variability of the client's voice, and importantly the individual's perception of voice as a concern, will result from their ability to use gender-congruent voice characteristics under the conditions outlined above, and will be also be significantly determined by the responses of listeners to the individual's self-identified gender. This dynamic phenomenon ensures an exponential list of possible situations in which the extent of voice concern and its impact vary. The full scope of these impacts may be best obtained by encouraging clients to keep their ongoing communication diary of speaking situations but will also be accessed through self-report measures.

Client Perspective— Voice and Communication

Objective and acoustic data can provide accurate information regarding the degree to which the communication characteristics of the client differ from those of a person of the same age and build, but a different sex. These data do not, however, necessarily reveal the impact of gender-inappropriate communication characteristics on the client's everyday life. Obtaining clients' perspective of their vocal functioning and the impact of their voice is therefore integral to a comprehensive assessment of voice (Davies, Papp, & Antoni, 2015; Hancock, 2016; Hardy, Boliek, Wells, & Rieger, 2013; Ma & Yiu, 2011). Health frameworks such as the International Classification of Functioning, Disability, and Health (ICF) framework (World Health Organization, 2001) that coalesce the social and medical aspects of a health condition further highlight the importance of incorporating the client's perspective into assessment, and increasingly the ICF is applied to the voice and communication characteristics of transsexual individuals (Byrne, 2007; Hancock, 2016; Hardy et al., 2013). Validated self-report voice measures provide the means for the individual's perspective to be captured and incorporated into planning client-centered management, assessing progress, and measuring outcomes of voice training.

A number of self-report measures for the cisgender population provide clinicians with a means of obtaining voice-related quality of life information (Ma & Yiu, 2011). By and large, these self-reports draw on the WHO disablement model. The WHO's original usage of the term *disability* has been replaced by "activity limitation," and *handicap* by "participation restriction." These terms fit nicely within the context of the impact of voice disorders on an individual client, as well as offering an effective means for assessing the effect of gender-incongruent voice on the trans and gender diverse individual. A trans woman may, for example, have a low pitch that is particularly marked

on the telephone where there is an absence of visual clues as to gender. The fact that the client cannot speak with the appropriate pitch means there is an activity limitation. If the client refrains from making telephone calls and deals with her tasks on a face-to-face basis or appoints someone else to take care of the telephoning, then according to the contemporary WHO definition, the client is experiencing participation restriction.

In the absence of a systematically developed and psychometrically validated voice self-report questionnaire for trans and gender diverse individuals, the Voice Handicap Index (VHI) (Jacobson et al., 1997) in particular was used by researchers seeking a measure to ascertain the self-perceptions of trans women regarding their voice (Geneid, Rihkanen, & Kinnari, 2015; Mastronikolis, Remacle, Biagini, Kiagiadaki, & Lawson, 2013; Remacle, Matar, Morsomme, Veduyckt, & Lawson, 2011). While self-report voice measures designed for cisgender adults with a voice disorder contain items that may be relevant to the activity and participation of trans and gender diverse individuals (e.g., *I am less outgoing because of my voice*), none contain items intrinsic to the voice experience of this population, such as the impact of voice on listener perceptions of their gender. It is therefore not surprising that the VHI lacks sensitivity to the voice-related experiences of trans women (Hancock, 2016; Remacle et al., 2011; T'Sjoen et al., 2006;).

In 2005, Canadian speech-language pathologist Shelagh Davies developed the Transgender Self-Evaluation Questionnaire (TSEQ) (Davies & Goldberg, 2006b) for use in her clinical practice. Davies based the TSEQ on the VHI and adapted items informed by her extensive clinical experience working with trans men and trans women; a version was available for each of these populations and she had no plan to psychometrically evaluate the questionnaire (personal communication, June 19, 2005). In 2013, the TSEQ was superseded by the Transsexual Voice Questionnaire ([TVQ^{MtF}] Dacakis et al., 2013), a systematically designed and psychometrically evaluated self-report voice questionnaire for trans women (Dacakis et al., 2013; Dacakis, Oates, & Douglas, 2016, 2017a, 2017b). The 30-item questionnaire (see online resources for Chapter 7 in the section "forms for assessment") was designed to elicit the trans woman's perception of her vocal functioning (e.g., *the pitch of my voice is too low*) and the frequency of adverse voice-related experiences (e.g., *I feel discriminated against because of my voice*). Significantly, the TVQ^{MtF} includes items that reflect the relationship between voice and perceptions of gender (e.g., *It distresses me when I am perceived as a man because of my voice*). The trans woman rates the frequency with which she experiences each situation, event, or perception on a four-point Likert scale with never or rarely (1) at one end and usually/always (4) at the other end. The minimum and maximum scores achievable are 30 and 120, respectively, with a higher score representing more frequent perceptions of negative voice-related experiences.

The significant strength of the TVQ^{MtF} is that the items were informed by the personal experiences of trans women and that it has been shown to be reliable and have strong support for its construct validity (Dacakis et al., 2013, 2016, 2017a, 2017b). Good reliability has also been reported for the Portuguese translation of the TVQ^{MtF} (Santos, Aguiar, Baeck, & Van Borsel, 2015) and the Swedish translation (Cardell & Ruda, 2014). The TVQ^{MtF} has been translated into 12 languages that are available from the author. The questionnaire has, however, only been validated with trans women who have transitioned to living full-time in their self-

identified gender "usually or always" and will therefore be most appropriate for this population. While the authors of the TVQ^{MtF} had originally intended to extend the TVQ for use by trans men, this plan was discontinued when it became apparent that the experiences of trans men were different from those of trans women and therefore a questionnaire for trans men could not easily be developed simply by changing the pronouns on the TVQ^{MtF} and the direction of, for example, pitch change. The TVQ^{MtF} has, however, been modified by others in this way and consequently fails to meet the significant criteria for the development of client self-report questionnaires, i.e., that items are informed by the people for whom they are designed (Branski et al., 2010).

Two additional questionnaires relating to voice and communication have been used with trans women. Firstly, Pasricha, Dacakis, and Oates (2008) developed an evaluative instrument specifically for trans women, the Functional Communication Satisfaction Questionnaire (FCSQ). The FCSQ enables trans women to indicate the level of communication satisfaction experienced in a comprehensive range of life situations, for example, "Speaking to men," "Speaking on the telephone." Respondents are also asked to rate their perceptions of themselves and others toward their gender presentation, for example, *Overall, I am satisfied with my ability to portray myself as female* and *Overall, I feel other people perceive me as female*. Secondly, the La Trobe Communication Questionnaire (LCQ) (Douglas, O'Flaherty, & Snow, 2000) has been administered to trans women to elicit their perceptions regarding their pragmatic abilities and to determine whether the LCQ results predicted communication satisfaction (Byrne, Dacakis, & Douglas, 2003). Examples of questions on the LCQ include: *When talking to others, do you carry on talking about things for too long in the conversation? Do you find it easy to change your speech style according to the situation you are in?* The LCQ provides baseline data on clients' perceptions of their pragmatic skills. Statistical analysis of the LCQ results and measures of communication satisfaction found that the LCQ is also predictive of communication satisfaction in trans women. The LCQ was, however, designed for measuring perceived pragmatic ability in individuals with acquired communication disorders and, therefore, may contain items that are not of particular relevance to the trans and gender diverse population.

As the trans population–specific questionnaires to date address the experiences of trans women, there is an urgent need for reliable and valid measures designed specifically to reflect the experiences of individuals with a range of gender identities.

Client Perspective—Gender Congruence

A recent inclusion by speech-language clinicians in the assessment of the trans and gender diverse population is the Transgender Congruence Scale ([TCS] Kozee, Tylka, & Bauerband, 2012), which measures the extent to which individuals feel "genuine, authentic, and comfortable with their gender identity and external appearance" (Kotzee et al., p. 179). This scale is composed of two underlying factors. *Appearance Congruence* measures the perceptions of transgender individuals in terms of how comfortable and authentic they are with their external appearance/gender presentation. This factor includes items such as: *I am generally comfortable with how others perceive my gender identity when they look at me.* The second factor, *Gender Identity Acceptance*, measures comfort with and acceptance of their self-identified gender. This factor includes items such as: *I am happy that I have the gender identity that I do.* Originally a 25-item questionnaire, the TCS was reduced to 12 items during the psychometric evaluation of the scale. Although the TCS does not have specific items related to voice, given that voice is closely tied to the individual's perception of self-identified gender (Byrne, 2007; Dacakis et al., 2016), it is conceivable that future research using this scale will demonstrate that a positive outcome of VAC training is improved self-perceptions of gender congruence. A comprehensive, culturally sensitive assessment of the individual's voice, their wishes and expectations, and the facilitators and barriers to modification of their voice and communication will provide a sound foundation for establishing client-centered VAC training goals.

Guidelines for Setting Voice and Communication Goals

Setting appropriate client-centered goals for trans and gender diverse individuals results from a respectful collaboration between the speech-language clinician and the gender diverse client. The speech-language clinician brings knowledge about gender differences in voice and communication, characteristics that contribute to listener perceptions of gender, known stereotypical beliefs regarding gendered communication, as well as personal and environmental factors that may act as either facilitators or barriers to making gains in voice and communication training. The clinician also brings the skills to effect change to voice and communication characteristics. This expertise will form the platform of goal setting; however, each client will bring an equally important set of individual circumstances that will ultimately determine the VAC training goals. The client's choice of voice and communication characteristics that feel authentic, situation-specific needs, stage in gender transition, biological constraints, and access to voice and communication training programs will all contribute to the selection of VAC training goals, which will be prioritized to facilitate a client-centered approach and optimum benefit from the speech-language intervention.

Client-Perceived Authenticity of Goals

Modification of speaking pitch is the priority goal for many trans and gender diverse individuals referred to a speech-language clinician. As noted above, it is not uncommon for clients to attend VAC training with a preconceived image of the type of voice they would like to achieve (often based on the voice of a celebrity). However, in recent years, as a result of increased Internet access, many clients understand that pitch is not the only aspect of communication that may be targeted in VAC training. Other aspects of voice that may be modified include pitch range, resonance, intonation, volume, and voice quality. In addition, speech preciseness, vocabulary, and nonverbal behaviors such as gesture and posture are targeted (see Chapters 9, 10, 11, 12). An early goal of VAC training is to determine which of these aspects of communication are relevant, or feel authentic, to the individual client. It is important for the clinician to be aware that the voice and communication characteristics that are perceived as gender congruent from the individual's perspective (i.e., authentic to their gender identity) may not necessarily match the listener's perception of the speaker's communication as gender congruent (i.e., matching the listener's perception of the speaker's gender).

The client's perspective regarding the voice and communication characteristics to be modified can be obtained from the case history information, self-report questionnaires, and facilitated observation of voice and communication in the client's everyday environment. Voice self-report questionnaires such as the TVQ^{MtF} (Dacakis et al., 2013) identify concerns of the trans woman regarding her vocal functioning, for example, *When I speak, the pitch of my voice does not vary enough*. Recent research findings indicate that the trans woman's beliefs about what contributes to her *voice femininity* should also inform goal setting. Dacakis et al. (2017b) reported an association between self-perceptions of voice femininity in trans women and the frequency of their negative voice-related experiences. The higher the trans woman rated her voice femininity, the less frequent were her negative voice-related experiences. A similar study by Hancock, Krissinger, and Owen (2011) shows an inverse relationship between self-ratings of voice femininity and voice-related quality of life. These findings indicate the importance of the trans woman's perception of the femininity of her voice and suggest that when selecting voice training goals for the trans woman, those characteristics she believes increase the femininity of her voice should be prioritized in voice training.

The technique of directed observation whereby the trans woman studies the voice and communication characteristics of others can also help identify client-centered goals. The clinician can provide the client with a list of masculine and feminine verbal and nonverbal communication characteristics that may influence perceptions of gender—for example, speaking pitch and articulation precision, as well as characteristics that are considered stereotypical, such as the use of tag questions such as, "She's very bright, *isn't she?*" The client will be instructed to observe speakers in their everyday lived environments and to familiarize themselves with these characteristics. Clients are then asked to identify the characteristics they feel are most appropriate to their gender identity, social milieu and life circumstance. This refined list will become the client's personal communication checklist. The scenario may arise where the speech-language clinician and the client differ as to whether a specific characteristic should be targeted. For example, the clinician may believe that the presence of an f/th substitution in a trans woman client promotes the perception of the speaker as more masculine. The client, on the other hand, may believe that intervention to correct this articulation error will cause her to sound "posh" and "different" to those in her social and/or work milieu. The specific communication characteristics targeted for intervention will ultimately emerge from a combination of the clinician's knowledge and the client's wishes; however, it is the client who determines which of these characteristics is/are relevant to their gender identity and communication needs.

Situation-Specific Needs

Having identified the voice and communication characteristics to be targeted in VAC training, it is important to confirm with individual clients that they wish to achieve gender-modified communication characteristics consistently across all everyday situations. This may appear an unusual recommendation to speech-language pathologists who will, as a rule, when working with cisgender populations strive for voice or communication modifications to be transferred across all everyday life situations. For the trans and gender diverse population, however, two factors come into play. Firstly, the individual

may identify as a non-binary gender (e.g., gender fluid) and require the ability to use gender-modified voice and communication characteristics with one gender presentation and not another. Secondly, even for individuals who identify on the gender binary scale, satisfaction with their communication and, therefore, their need for gender-modified communication can be situation specific and alter according to the environment or life context in which they find themselves (Byrne, 2007; Pasricha, Dacakis, & Oates, 2008; Dacakis et al., 2013). Pasricha et al. (2008), for example, reported that the impact of voice on trans women varied according to factors such as the level of intimacy with their communicative partner and the desire to be perceived as their self-identified gender within socially specific situations (e.g., being referred to with a male pronoun by a stranger in a social setting resulted in substantial distress); whereas, the use of a male pronoun by a friend did not have this impact. Client communication satisfaction is also positively impacted by the passage of time. A number of authors have reported that trans women report less concern and fewer negative impacts of voice with the passage of time lived in their female identity (Byrne, 2007; Dacakis et al., 2013, ; Holmberg et al., 2010). Finally, trans women who have undergone GRS also report less frequent negative impact of their voice (Byrne, 2007; Dacakis et al., 2016). Byrne (2007) proposed that consolidation of the trans woman's gender identity as female as well as the freedom from the burden of concealing her birth-assigned gender underpins this association. It may be that GRS, by providing a sense of security unavailable prior to surgery, has an impact on the salience of acquiring gender-appropriate communication characteristics, and thus may reduce client motivation.

Simple case history question such as, "Do you want to change your communication in all speaking situations?" will give an initial indication of the client's wishes. Administering questionnaires such as the TVQ^MtF provides a psychometrically validated means of identifying daily living situations in which the individual experiences voice-related impact (e.g., *I avoid speaking in public because of my voice*). Encouraging the client to maintain a communication diary will also enable the clinician to identify the specific situations in which the client is experiencing communication difficulties and desiring voice modification. In the author's experience, clients who express across-the-board dissatisfaction with their communication characteristics are often surprised at the number of situations in which they have no need to alter these characteristics when asked to keep a diary of their communication in their everyday situations. This finding is particularly relevant to clients for whom pitch modification may prove problematic. Indeed, there are many cases where VAC training goals target modification in only certain situations. Take, for example, the trans woman whose gender status is known among her social, familial, and employment circles and who is satisfied with her voice and communication characteristics in these situations, but who is frustrated when referred to as "Sir" on the telephone. In this situation, a single goal of developing strategies to increase listener perceptions of femaleness on the telephone would be appropriate.

Stage of Transition

Historically, the prerequisite for attending VAC training related to gender identity was that the individual attended sessions presenting in their self-identified gender. Despite the fact that this requirement was implemented to facilitate acquisition of gender-

congruent voice through increased opportunities for practice and transfer, it is no longer universally enforced. A requirement that delays the commencement of VAC training for individuals who cannot comply (e.g., those working in their birth-assigned gender and only able to attend sessions during their lunch break) is particularly inappropriate for those whose voice contributes to their gender dysphoria or who are delaying their transition to living socially as their self-identified gender fearing that their voice will be the one characteristic that will betray their birth-assigned gender. The central challenges arising from commencing VAC training with trans or gender diverse individuals who have not informed others of their gender status are: (a) the risk of setting VAC training goals that might unwittingly expose the individual's gender status and (b) the potential for poor outcomes associated with limited opportunities for practicing gender-modified communication.

With a clear understanding of the client's network of supports and situations where they present in their self-identified gender, the client and clinician can agree on goals that parallel the client's stage in transition—goals that may not necessarily require immediate and obvious changes to everyday communication. These goals may include ensuring that the client has optimum respiration support for the anticipated voice modification, a healthy voicing mechanism (vocal hygiene education), an awareness of communication characteristics appropriate to the client's desired gender, and an awareness of the communication characteristics that will be targeted for modification in the long term. Although individuals may not be ready to use gender-modified pitch in their everyday communication, the study by Lee (2011) demonstrated that introducing Vocal Function Exercises (Stemple, Glaze, &

Klaben, 2010) in trans women still presenting as their birth-assigned gender of male had the benefit of increasing within clinic speaking pitch (mean f_0), pitch variability, and f_0 range (ST). These gains provide a useful stepping stone to increasing variability of intonation and pitch inflection at the end of words, and ultimately directly increasing pitch for everyday speaking situations when the client and the clinician agree that the timing is appropriate. As the client progresses through the transition process and reports an ability to incorporate more obvious gender-appropriate characteristics into everyday communication, goals to modify these are introduced.

Biological Constraints

There are no research reports regarding an association between physical characteristics and the ability of trans and gender diverse individuals to modify their voice. Inevitably, however, there will always be a proportion of trans women who will present with a large stature and very low speaking pitch that is difficult to modify. Biological constraints related to the size of the larynx and the vocal folds can prove a difficult barrier to overcome. In these cases, where the client is large in stature, the goals of VAC training will include informational and affective counseling to ensure that the client understands that pitch must be appropriate to stature, and that females of tall stature often have lower-pitched voices. The client can be directed to observe women's voices and take note of this association. Although VAC training for clients with low pitch will, nevertheless, target an increase in pitch, the target will need to be realistic to prevent setting up the client for failure. A number of authors have demonstrated that an increase in pitch is possible (Dacakis, 2000;

Gelfer & Tice, 2013; Hancock & Garabedian, 2013); however, probing tasks should be introduced over several sessions to establish an individualized target pitch; one that may not fall within, or above, the gender ambiguous range of 145–165 Hz. It must be remembered that a percentage of trans women, irrespective of stature, remain satisfied with their communication despite a voice of low pitch (Dacakis, 2000; McNeill, Wilson, Clark, & Deakin, 2008). This observation may be related to the recent findings of reduced concern with voice in trans women with increased time living in the self-identified gender, and in those who have undergone GRS (Byrne, 2007; Dacakis et al., 2013; Holmberg et al., 2010). It may also be that these individuals have taken on sufficient verbal and nonverbal gender-appropriate communication characteristics, other than pitch, to enhance their own perceptions of the femininity of their communication and/or listener perceptions of them as their self-identified gender. It may therefore be particularly important, when working with trans women who find pitch modification problematic, to focus not only on verbal characteristics other than speaking pitch but also on nonverbal aspects of communication and on visual appearance (Hirsch, 2003; Van Borsel, De Cuypere, & Van den Berghe, 2001).

Access to Voice and Communication Training and Transfer

Although there is an increasing number of speech-language clinicians providing face-to-face and online services for trans and gender diverse individuals, access to VAC training is still restricted for many by geographic, financial, and personal considerations. Those trans and gender diverse individuals who have also chosen a medically assisted transition may be committed to regular and frequent visits to medical specialists and are left with little additional time to commit to regular VAC training sessions. Employed clients, in particular, may meet resistance from employers for additional weekly absences to attend sessions, especially where the client has not transitioned at work and the employer remains unaware of the reason for the absenteeism.

In cases where clients have indicated that they are unable to attend regular weekly sessions, clinicians may: (a) investigate the feasibility of supplementing face-to-face sessions with a telehealth option (e.g., via an online instant messenger) and (b) limit the number and focus of goals targeted in each session. For example, in a situation where the clinician and client agree that an increase in pitch constitutes an appropriate goal but the client is able to attend only monthly sessions, it may be prudent to schedule a double session with the focus almost exclusively on pitch and to ensure that the client is provided with comprehensive take-home support material, including, where appropriate, information on suitable apps. This will increase the likelihood of the client practicing the techniques correctly over the ensuing month. When treating "time-poor" clients who are seen infrequently, it is advisable to target non-interventionist VAC training goals, such as increasing the client's awareness of gender differences in verbal and nonverbal communication and determining which of these characteristics are appropriate to the client's environment. These tasks do not require modification of the larynx or articulators, and therefore minimize the risk of voice damage through inappropriate use.

Finally, it is important to develop specific goals that provide the client with a structured approach to the transfer of new communication skills to everyday situations. This is best achieved by employing a hierarchical model of communication situations, ranging from where the client feels "most supported" to "least supported" when using newly acquired voice and communication characteristics. The client is guided to transfer skills in increasing increments of difficulty, which furthers their chances of experiencing success and improves the client's confidence to face more difficult transfer tasks (see Chapter 16 for additional information).

The importance of setting appropriate VAC training goals cannot be underestimated, nor can the potentially damaging consequences of inappropriate goal setting. Goals must be achievable if the client is to maintain motivation and not be put at risk of experiencing a sense of failure. At a time when it is still difficult, and in some places impossible, for trans and gender diverse individuals to have their needs met by public health providers, it is imperative that these limited services be employed effectively. Effective service can only come about in a context of a comprehensive assessment that leads to collaborative goal setting, with the clinician and the client both cognizant of which communication characteristics are appropriate to the client's gender identity, which characteristics are appropriate to the client's individual needs, as well as the extent to which the client wants these characteristics to become part of their individual persona.

References

Azul, D., Nygren, U., Södersten, M., & Neuschaefer-Rube, C. (2016). Transmasculine people's voice function: A review of the currently available evidence. *Journal of Voice*. doi: http://dx.doi.org/10.1016/j.jvoice.2016.05.005

Bauer, G. R., & Scheim, A. I. (2015). *Transgender people in Ontario, Canada: Statistics to inform human rights policy*. London, Ontario: TransPULSE.

Bockting, W. O., & Cesaretti, C. (2001). Spirituality, transgender identity, and coming out. *Journal of Sex Education and Therapy, 26*(4), 291–300.

Bolin, A. (2004). French Polynesia. In R. T. Francoeur & R. J. Noonan (Eds.), *International encyclopedia of sexuality* (pp. 431–449). New York, NY: Continuum.

Branski, R. C., Cukier-Blaj, S., Pusic, A., Cano, S. J., Klassen, A., Mener, D., Patel, S., & Kraus, D. H. (2010). Measuring quality of life in dysphonic patients: A systematic review of content development in patient-reported outcomes measures. *Journal of Voice, 2*(24), 193–198.

Brown, M. L., & Rounsley, C. A. (1996). *True Selves: Understanding transsexualism—for families, friends, coworkers, and helping professionals*. San Francisco, CA: Jossey-Bass Publishers.

Budge, S. L., Katz-Wise, S. L., Tebbe, E. N., Howard, K. A. S., Schneider, C. L., & Rodriguez A. (2012). Transgender emotional and coping processes: Facilitative and avoidant coping throughout gender transitioning. *The Counseling Psychologist, 41*(4), 601–647. doi: 10.1177/0011000011432753

Byrne, L. A. (2007). *My life as a woman: Placing communication within the social context of life for the transsexual woman*. Unpublished PhD thesis, La Trobe University, Melbourne, Australia.

Byrne, L. A., Dacakis, G., & Douglas, J. M. (2003). Self-perceptions of pragmatic communication abilities in male-to-female transsexuals. *Advances in Speech Language Pathology, 5*, 15–25.

Cardell, F., & Ruda M. (2014). Reliability of the Swedish version of Transsexual Voice Questionnaire Male-to-Female (TVQ^MtF) (Unpublished masters thesis). Karolinska Institute, Stockholm, Sweden.

Clements-Nolle, K., Marx, R., & Katz M. (2006). Attempted suicide among transgender persons: The influence of gender-based discrimination and victimization. *Journal of Homosexuality, 51*(3), 53–69.

Coleman, E., Bockting, W., Botzer, M., Cohen-Kettenis, P., De Cuypere, G., Feldman, L., . . . Zucker, K. (2012). Standards of Care for the Health of Transsexual, Transgender, and Gender Non-conforming people, Version 7. *International Journal of Transgenderism, 13*(4), 165–232. doi: 10.1080/15532739.2011.700873

Coleman, E., Colgan, P., & Gooren L. (1992). Male cross-gender behaviour in Myanmar (Burma): A description of the acault. *Archives of Sexual Behaviour, 21*(3), 313–321.

Dacakis, G. (2000). Long-term maintenance of fundamental frequency increases in male-to-female transsexuals. *Journal of Voice, 14*, 549–556.

Dacakis, G., Davies, S., Oates, J. M., Douglas, J. M., & Johnston, J. R. (2013). Development and preliminary evaluation of the Transsexual Voice Questionnaire for male-to-female transsexuals. *Journal of Voice, 27*(3), 312–320.

Dacakis, G., Oates, J. M., & Douglas, J. M. (2016). Exploring the validity of the Transsexual Voice Questionnaire (Male-to-Female): Do TVQ^MtF scores differentiate between MtF women who have had gender reassignment surgery and those who have not? *International Journal of Transgenderism, 17*(3–4), 124–130. doi: 10.1080/15532739.2016.1222922

Dacakis, G., Oates, J. M., & Douglas, J. M. (2017a). Further evidence of the construct validity of the Transsexual Voice Questionnaire (TVQ^MtF) using principle components analysis. *Journal of Voice, 31*(2), 142–148. doi: 10.1016/j.jvoice.2016.07.01

Dacakis, G., Oates, J., & Douglas, J. M. (2017b). Associations between the Transsexual Voice Questionnaire (TVQ^MtF) and self-report of voice femininity and acoustic measures. *International Journal of Language and Communication Disorders*. doi: 10.1111/1460-6984.12319

Davies, S., & Goldberg, J. M. (2006a). Clinical aspects of transgender speech feminization and masculinization. *International Journal of Transgenderism, 9*, 167–196.

Davies, S., & Goldberg J. M. (2006b). Trans care gender transition: Changing speech. Vancouver, British Columbia: Vancouver Coastal Health, Transcend Transgender Support & Education Society, and Canadian Rainbow Health Coalition. Available at: http://transhealth.vch.ca/resources/library/tcpdocs/guidelines-speech.pdf. Accessed March 15, 2011.

Davies, S., Papp, V., & Antoni, C. (2015). Voice and communication change for gender nonconforming individuals: Giving voice to the person inside. *International Journal of Transgenderism, 16*(3), 117–159. doi: 10.1080/15532739.2015.1075931

de Bruin, M. D., Coerts, M. J., & Greven, A. J. (2000). Speech therapy in the management of male-to-female transsexuals. *Folia Phoniatrica et Logopaedica, 52*(5), 220–227.

Dejonckere, P. H., Bradley, B., Clemente, P., Cornut, G., Grevier-Buchman, L., Friedrich, G., . . . Woisard, V. (2001). A basic protocol for functional assessment of voice pathology, especially for investigating the efficacy of (phonosurgical) treatments and evaluating new assessment techniques: Guideline elaborated by the Committee on Phoniatrics of the European Laryngological Society (ELS). *European Archives of Otorhinolaryngology, 258,* 77–82. http://pareonline.net/getvn.asp?v=14&n=20

Douglas, J. M., O'Flaherty, C. A., & Snow, P. C. (2000). Measuring perception of communicative ability: The development and evaluation of the La Trobe Communication Questionnaire. *Aphasiology, 14*(3), 251–268.

Fairbanks, G. E. (1960). *Voice and articulation drillbook* (2nd ed.). New York, NY: Harper.

Freidenberg, C. B. (2002). Working with male-to-female transgendered clients: Clinical considerations. *Contemporary Issues in Communication Science and Disorders, 29,* 43–58.

Gagne, P., & Tewksbury, R. (1999). Conformity pressures and gender resistance among transgendered individuals. *Social Problems, 45*(1), 85–101.

Gelfer, M. P. (1999). Voice treatment for the male-to-female transgendered client. *American Journal of Speech-Language Pathology, 8,* 201–208.

Gelfer, M. P., & Tice, R. M. (2013). Perceptual and acoustic outcomes of voice therapy for male-to-female transgender individuals immediately after therapy and 15 months later. *Journal of Voice, 27*(3), 335–347. doi: 10.1016/j.jvoice.2012.07.009

Geneid, A., Rihkanen, H., & Kinnari, T. J. (2015). Long-term outcome of endoscopic shortening and stiffening of the vocal folds to raise the pitch. *European Archives of Otorhinolaryngology, 272,* 3751–3756.

Grant, J. M., Mottet, L. A., Tanis, J., Harrison, J., Herman, J. L., & Keisling, M. (2011). *Injustice at every turn: A report of the National Transgender Discrimination Survey.* Washington, DC: National Center of Transgender Equality and National Gay and Lesbian Task Force.

Hancock, A. B. (2015). The role of cultural competence in serving transgender populations. *Perspectives on Voice and Voice Disorders, 25,* 37–42.

Hancock, A. B. (2016). An ICF perspective on voice-related quality of life of American transgender women. *Journal of Voice, 31*(1), 115e1–115e8. doi: 10.1016/j.jvoice.2016.03.013

Hancock, A. B., & Garabedian, L. M. (2013). Transgender voice and communication treatment: A retrospective chart review of 25 cases. *International Journal of Language and Communication Disorders, 48*(1), 54–65.

Hancock, A. B., Krissinger, J., & Owen, K. (2011). Voice perceptions and quality of life in transgender people. *Journal of Voice, 25*(5), 553–558.

Hardy, T. L., Boliek, C. A., Wells, K., & Rieger, J. M. (2013). The ICF and male-to-female transsexual communication. *International Journal of Transgenderism, 14*(4), 196–208. doi:10.1080/15532739.2014.890561

Hirsch, S. (2003, November). *Approaches to nonverbal communication in male-to-female voice feminization treatment.* Paper presented at the annual conference of the American Speech-Language-Hearing Association, Chicago, IL.

Holmberg, E. B., Oates, J. M., Dacakis, G., & Grant, C. (2010). Phonetograms, aerodynamic measurements, self-evaluations, and auditory perceptual ratings of male-to-female transsexual voice. *Journal of Voice, 24*(5), 511–522. doi: 10.1016/j.jvoice.2009.02.002

Hyde, Z., Doherty, M., Tilley, P. J., McCaul, K. A., Rooney, R., & Jancey, J. (2013). *The first national trans health mental health study: Summary of results.* School of Public Health, Curtin University, Perth, Australia.

Jacobson, B. H., Johnson, A., Grywalski, C., Silbergleit, A., Jacobson, G., Benninger, M. S., & Newman, C. W. (1997). The Voice Handicap Index (VHI): Development and validation. *American Journal of Speech-Language Pathology, 6*(3), 66–70.

Kalra, G. (2012). Hijras: The unique transgender culture of India. *International Journal of Culture and Mental Health. 5*(2), 121–126.

King, J. B., Lindstedt, D. E., Jensen, M., & Law, M. (1999). Transgendered voice: Considerations in case history management. *Logopedics Phoniatrics Vocology, 24,* 14–18.

Kozee, H. B., Tylka, T. L., & Bauerband, L. A. (2012). Measuring transgender individuals' comfort with gender identity and appearance: Development and validation of the Transgender Congruence Scale. *Psychology of Women Quarterly, 36*(2), 179–196.

Lee, Y-Q. (2011). *The role of Stemple's vocal function exercises in voice feminisation for male-to-female transsexuals.* Unpublished honors thesis, La Trobe University, Melbourne, Australia.

Ma, E. P-M., & Yiu, E. M-L. (2011). *Handbook of voice assessments.* San Diego, CA: Plural.

Mastronikolis, N. S., Remacle, M., Biagini, M., Kiagiadaki, D., & Lawson, G. (2013). Wendler glottoplasty: An effective pitch raising surgery in male-to-female transsexuals. *Journal of Voice, 27*(4), 516–522.

McNeil, E., Bailey, L., Ellis, S., & Regan, M. (2013). *Speaking from the margins: Trans mental health and wellbeing in Ireland.* Transgender Equality Network Ireland. Retrieved from: http://www.teni.ie

Nygren, U., Nordenskjöld, A., Arver, S., & Södersten, M. (2016). Effects of voice fundamental frequency and satisfaction with voice in trans men during testosterone treatment—a longitudinal study. *Journal of Voice, 30*(6), 766.e23–766.e34. doi: 10.1016/j.jvoice.2015.10.016

Palmer, D., Dietsch, A., & Searl, J. (2012). Endoscopic and stroboscopic presentation of the larynx in male-to-female transsexual persons. *Journal of Voice, 26*(1), 117–126.

Pasricha, N., Dacakis, G., & Oates, J. (2008). Communicative satisfaction of male-to-female transsexuals. *Logopedics Phoniatrics Vocology, 33*, 25–34.

Pitts, M., Couch, M., Mulcare, H., Croy, S., & Mitchell, A. (2009). Transgender people in Australia and New Zealand: Health, well-being and access to health services. *Feminism and Psychology, 19*(4), 475–495. doi: 10.1177/0959353509342771

Remacle, M., Matar, N., Morsomme, D., Veduyckt, I., & Lawson, G. (2011). Glottoplasty for male-to-female transsexualism: Voice results. *Journal of Voice, 25*(1), 120–123.

Santos, H. H., Aguiar, A. G., Baeck, H. E., & Van Borsel, J. (2015). Translation and preliminary evaluation of the Brazilian Portuguese version of the Transgender Voice Questionnaire for male-to-female transsexuals. *Communication Disorders and Science, 27*(1), 89–96.

Scheidt, D., Kob, M., Willmes, K., & Neuschaefer-Rube, C. (2004, August). *Do we need voice therapy for female-to-male transgenders?* Paper presented at the 26th World Congress of the International Association of Logopedics and Phoniatrics, Brisbane, Australia.

Söderpalm, E., Larsson, A., & Almquist, S. (2004). Evaluation of a consecutive group of transsexual individuals referred for vocal intervention in the west of Sweden. *Logopedics Phoniatrics Vocology, 29*, 18–30.

Södersten, M., Nygren, U., Hertegård, S., & Dhejne, C. (2015). Interdisciplinary program in Sweden related to transgender voice. *SIG 3 Perspectives on Voice and Voice Disorders, 25*, 87–97. doi: 10.1044/vvd25.2.87

Stemple, J. C., Glaze, L. E., & Klaben, B. G. (2000). *Clinical voice pathology: Theory and management* (3rd ed.). Vancouver, BC: Singular Thomson Learning.

Stemple, J. C., Glaze, L., & Klaben, B. (2010). *Clinical voice pathology: Theory and management* (4th ed.). San Diego, CA: Plural Publishing.

T'Sjoen, G., Moerman, M., Van Borsel, J., Feyen, E., Rubens, R., Monstrey, S., . . . De Cuypere, G. (2006). Impact of voice in transsexuals. *International Journal of Transgenderism, 9*(1), 1–7.

Van Borsel, J., De Cuypere, G., Rubens, R., & Destaerke, B. (2000). Voice problems in female-to-male transsexuals. *International Journal of Language and Communication Disorders, 35*(3), 427–442.

Van Borsel, J., De Cuypere, G., & Van den Berghe, H. (2001). Physical appearance and voice in male-to-female transsexuals. *Journal of Voice, 15*(4), 570–575.

Whittle, S., Turner, L., Combs, R., & Rhodes, S. (2008). *Transgender EuroStudy: Legal survey and focus on the transgender experience of health care.* Brussels, Belgium: International Lesbian and Gay Association Europe.

World Health Organization (2001). *ICF: International Classification of Functioning, Disability and Health.* Geneva, Switzerland: WHO.

8

Vocal Health and Phonotrauma

Richard K. Adler and Christella Antoni

Phonotrauma

Many transmasculine and transfeminine clients come to voice training having already attempted some "self-therapy" through the use of videotapes made by lay people and/or following some YouTube video presentations. From a professional speech-language pathologist (SLP) point of view, it becomes a matter of safety when using techniques that have no evidence base or to use therapy ideas without the guidance of professionals. This is particularly true if the techniques put undue strain or tension on the vocal mechanism which could lead to damage. Due to many aspects of voice and communication training for the transgender and gender non-conforming client, it is imperative that clients do not unknowingly or unsuspectingly cause phonotrauma to their vocal folds and larynx without realizing the dangerous after effects. In a study by Hancock and Garabedian (2013), 25 cases of voice and communication change in transgender clients were reviewed. The authors found that 28% of the subjects presented with a voice disorder that was separate from gender presentation concerns. Therefore, preventing phonotrauma is of the utmost importance when engaging in a voice and communication training program.

The speech-language pathologist/speech clinician is the professional who can safely guide transgender clients to prevent phonotrauma by helping them to eliminate factors that contribute to damage or maladaptive use of the vocal mechanism. It is worth noting that Special Interest Group 3, Voice and Voice Disorders, from the American Speech-Language-Hearing Association endorsed the term *phonotrauma* to describe its use in assessment and therapy. This term replaces former terminology such as vocal abuse and vocal misuse. It becomes more consumer friendly and less invasive, rather than using terms that appear to put all the blame on the patient or client. Therefore, we explain to our clients that the word *phonotrauma* encompasses both misuse of the vocal folds and knowing or unknowing abuse of the vocal folds, and clients usually accept that term and begin to use it.

Weinrich, Gottliebson, and LeBorgne (2016) emphasize the importance of applying good vocal behaviors. They purport that good posture and relaxed muscles are pertinent to good vocal health. "The adage 'sit up straight' is applicable as this position allows for adequate breath support for voice production" (PowerPoint slide 13). It is important to note that Weinrich et al. emphasize that many inoptimal or damaging vocal behaviors are instinctively occurring, but many are collective and happen over time, such as using an inappropriate pitch out of habit. These all may be prevented by using good vocal health practices.

Phonotrauma may result from a number of behaviors. Excessive phonatory effort (Boone et al., 2010; Boone & McFarlane, 1988; Colton, Casper, & Leonard, 2011; Laver, 1980) often causes hyperfunctional dysphonia. From this, many clients display a compensatory muscle tension dysphonia that results from changes in the vocal fold mucosa or vocal fold lesions. Weinrich et al. (2016) further emphasize that many emotional states that a person exhibits and particularly that involve crying, screaming, and even laughing are often displayed by the lay person. Actors/actresses often need to portray characters that are wrought with these emotional behaviors. They emphasize that "vocal naps" should be part of the actor's daily schedule, especially if these behaviors must be performed on a continuous basis during rehearsals or during a live play performance. These may lead to poor vocal hygiene and therefore have an impact on the performer's vocal health (more information on the transgender performer is found in Chapter 15). And in many emotional states, this may result in a primary muscle tension dysphonia in some people.

Many gender diverse individuals are part of choirs and acting ensembles and enjoy portraying a variety of characters. Many of these people must lead meetings at their workplace or coach sports for children or adults, and often find themselves suffering from vocal fatigue, "scratchy throat," or a certain degree of hoarseness due to their lack of knowledge of good vocal health practices. If one couples these with emotional trauma or ever-changing emotional states of being, it makes it difficult for some transgender/non-binary in-

dividuals to maintain sound vocal health habits. This is an example of how phonotrauma sometimes occurs without a conscious knowledge of harming the vocal folds. Weinrich et al. (2016) emphasize that many coaches who scream throughout a game are hoarse by the end, and that learning how to shout in a vocally healthy manner may help reduce vocal damage. This is an important factor for transmasculine or transfeminine (TM/TF) clients, as they have to learn healthy functional vocal behaviors on top of their communication modification challenges. Many TF/TM clients, for example, are surprised to hear that they have to learn healthy techniques for increasing volume.

In her classic reference manual, Andrews (2006) outlined many common causes of vocal fold irritation or injury, and the American Academy of Otolaryngology Head and Neck Surgery (2017) reiterated these causes, including:

1. Generalized laryngeal tension
2. Overcontraction of the posterior cricoarytenoid muscle
3. Excessive elevation of the larynx, i.e., elevating the larynx to raise the fundamental frequency as opposed to spontaneous elevation needed for swallowing. It should be noted here that laryngeal manipulation is often a technique used to help the transfeminine client raise the larynx to help produce an elevated pitch. Because these clients do not constrict the intrinsic laryngeal muscles, they often do not develop extralaryngeal muscle tension. Over-engaging the intrinsic laryngeal muscles creates a risk of hyperfunctional voice output. As SLPs, we work to avoid this as therapy proceeds.
4. Frequent singing with poor technique
5. Endocrine imbalance (hypothyroidism) Bulimia-induced spasms and acidity

6. Smoking, alcohol, and drug use
7. Excessive coughing and throat-clearing
8. Using an inappropriate pitch level: to some this appears to be an issue when working with trans women because it becomes problematic to have a low male pitch. Voice and communication training provides strategies and techniques that increase the pitch of trans women's voices without causing phonotrauma. To avoid laryngeal muscle tension, it is best to review the laryngeal manipulation exercise (Craig, 2016) and have the client note in both a tactile or kinesthetic manner that the larynx can be raised yet not produce an inappropriate pitch level.
9. Inhalation of airborne irritants and allergies (Andrews, 2006, p. 281)

The American Academy of Otolaryngology–Head and Neck Surgery (AAOHNS) suggests that phonotrauma is a problem that affects any person's voice. "Speaking is a physical task that requires coordination of breathing with the use of several muscle groups" (AAOHNS, 2017). It is pointed out that one can use the voice efficiently or inefficiently but that unnecessary prolonged use of a loud voice would lead to vocal difficulties. Furthermore, there is research evidence that indicates that the amount of talking and the volume one uses when talking clearly affect the vocal folds and voice quality, and would lead to phonotrauma (Voice Doctor, 2017). When working with transmasculine and transfeminine clients, it is of great importance that they understand the importance of vocal health and the elimination of phonotrauma as part of their vocal transition.

Other aspects of daily life may contribute to poor vocal health habits, including environmental factors such as chemicals, fumes, secondary smoke, and other chemical irritants that directly affect the vocal folds and the entire vocal tract (Weinrich et al., 2016). Of course, the transgender individual who is working on transfeminine or transmasculine voice changes should try to avoid these environmental factors or even try to avoid working in the presence of these irritants unless adequate ventilation is provided. Any individual who is exposed to environmental factors is in danger of developing a voice disorder and/or poor vocal behaviors, but this is especially true for the transgender individual who has other circumstances that could contribute to vocally abusive behaviors during voice transition and training, such as self-therapy, family conflicts, etc. Counseling clients often helps them to understand these adverse work or social environments (see Chapter 3). We have learned, from experience, that transgender individuals are often exposed to noisy environments in bars, restaurants, and workplaces. Many of our transgender clients who attend vocal training have remained in their jobs during transition. They are teachers, lawyers, factory workers, accountants, real estate agents, line cooks, playground monitors, cafeteria workers, and a wide range of other professions. Like any individuals in these professions, it is important for the clients to understand how these may affect their voice quality and, if they are not properly aware, may lead to phonotrauma.

Weinrich et al. (2016) further emphasize the importance of hydration for general health and well-being (PowerPoint slide 24). We have found that many of our transgender clients are not aware of the importance of hydration to keep the voice healthy and flexible. Weinrich et al. (2016) suggest that "keeping the vocal folds well-hydrated has long been considered an important component of vocal hygiene recommendations" (PowerPoint slide 24). Keeping the folds flexible helps to maintain the right balance of breath support, air pressure, and flow, which will decrease the likelihood of excessive tension of the vocal folds during voice production. Weinrich et al. (2016) emphasize the importance of using external hydration in the form of humidifiers, facial steamers, and vaporizers. Cool mist humidifiers, fans, and ultrasonic high frequency vibrations can create fine mist that keeps the internal vocal apparatus hydrated. Additional information on hydration is included in the next section.

Voice Safety

Hydration

The benefits of good hydration would be especially important to the transgender individual. Weinrich et al. (2016) point out several factors that are important when considering adequate hydration to keep the voice safe during voice training and overall transition.

1. Increasing water intake often helps eliminate the thick, sticky mucus in the larynx which in turn might prevent traumatic throat-clearing.
2. "Sensory effects of drinking water may make individuals feel that voicing is easier" (slide 33).
3. "Swallowing water may be a useful substitute for reducing harmful vocal behaviors such as chronic coughing and throat-clearing" (slide 33).

As with any others, transgender individuals should often check with their medical team if medicines are prescribed: "Specific prescription and over-the-counter medications such as decongestants and allergy medicine result in the release of fluids from body tissues . . . that may affect the vocal folds

although specific research in these areas is currently lacking" (slide 36). It is known that some blood pressure lowering medications and some heart medications such as beta blockers may cause excessive coughing or dry mouth, so patients should consult with their physician or medical team if they are prescribed a blood pressure lowering medicine.

Food Intake and Vocal Care

It is also important to think about what food and drink are included in a client's diet. Cazden (2012) reminds us that "[b]everages, medicine, and common home remedies taken by mouth may contain helpful ingredients" (p. 40), but she further states the following about eating and drinking critically for voice care:

1. Although important, food and drink are only two aspects of voice care.
2. Sip water throughout the day to stay hydrated.
3. The temperature of beverages is not crucial; use what you like best.
4. Caffeine or alcohol do not count toward daily hydration goals.
5. Fresh, watery fruits and vegetables can help you stay hydrated.

Cazden states that "none of these substances directly 'wets' or 'lubricates' the vocal cords." Their benefits are indirect, as the chemicals are processed through digestion" (p. 40). It is important to eat foods that feel and taste good to the client; the "more important principle is to choose foods based on overall health rather than on . . . what might feel good for an instant on your throat" (Cazden, 2012, p. 40).

Cazden (2012) also summarizes some very important thoughts about food and drink intake that a transmasculine and transfeminine client should consider, especially those with high vocal demands and people in a choir or who sing or act professionally:

1. Develop an optimal eating plan for voice care, including understanding preferences, allergies, and budget.
2. Follow general nutrition guidelines.
3. Take reasonable precautions about reflux issues.
4. Stay open minded about dairy intake.

Many transmasculine and transfeminine clients come to the clinic with a diagnosis from their physician labeled "Reflux." When acid backs up from the esophagus and settles near the vocal folds it is often diagnosed as laryngo-pharyngeal reflux (LPR). Often the client complains of a lower pitch and a "rough" voice usually in the form of hoarseness but without a cold, the flu, or other respiratory condition. Cazden (2012) mentions that the "voice can sound low pitched and crackly and it can get tired more easily as the LPR becomes more serious.... [C]hronic cough and breathing difficulties may develop" (p. 43).

The Voice Foundation (2017) explained that reflux laryngitis is caused by a backflow of stomach acid and fluids into the throat and vocal mechanism. It is a potential consequence of LPR and results in irritation and edema of the vocal mechanism. The client will usually complain of excessive throat-clearing, a sensation that "something is caught in the throat," heartburn, or sore throat. A referral to an ENT for LPR is essential here, but the SLP/speech language therapist (SLT) can discuss this problem with the gender diverse client and talk about vocal health and how it relates to reflux in the throat. The medical community is very aware of this condition and usually prescribes medicines after an evaluation to make sure the client is presenting with gastroesophageal reflux disease or LPR and not something more serious. If the patient has not seen a physician for these complaints, the SLP/SLT should refer directly.

Psychosocial Issues and Vocal Health

Psychosocial issues can often play a significant role in causing phonotrauma. Depression, lack of self-confidence, fear, guilt, embarrassment, and anxiety are often the etiological culprits of phonotrauma in gender diverse clients. Andrews (1999) suggested that part of the therapy for vocal misuse [or abuse] would be to "probe psychosocial dynamics that may be precipitating or manipulating factors" (p. 231). As a nurse, Alegria (2011) emphasizes the importance of understanding psychosocial issues that transgender clients have to cope with in order to treat them fairly and to ensure progress. This will be helpful to clients who often present with a "poor vocal quality" due to "hiding" the voice or overly lowering the volume and becoming "too embarrassed" to engage in modification because they would feel silly.

The use of an overly low volume by some trans women is also a potentially limiting factor in voice change. Trans men may initially present with low volume, frequently accompanied by roughness in the vocal tone. Psychosocial factors can play a significant role in low volume and/or constricted voice use patterns in both trans women and trans men. These may include self-consciousness, low confidence, and a wish to hide the voice. Encouraging an appropriate volume and a voice quality that is not too strongly characterized by breathiness or roughness will maximize the potential for healthy and successful voice changes.

Predisposing Factors

A good example of how psychosocial issues affect one's voice comes from Deary and Miller (2011), who considered the role of psychosocial factors in the case of a cisgender client diagnosed with functional dysphonia. Occupational susceptibility and perfectionism were thought to be predisposing factors of this client's voice disorder as well as general fatigue. Phonotrauma often leads to functional dysphonia and it is up to the SLP/SLT to note this during the intake process or at least during the first therapy session, so that proper outside referrals can be made when needed. These predisposing factors must be dealt with in order to make progress with voice transition.

Providing a Safe Environment to Reduce Phonotrauma

The clinician is concerned with providing a safe environment for the transmasculine and transfeminine client in voice training and during times outside of the therapy environment when the client is on his/her own and the clinician is not there for support. By empowering the client to assist in goal and objective planning, the clinician is affording him/her an opportunity to delve into the various aspects of voice that are important to that individual. Goals and objectives, including those for counseling, will likely be followed when the client has some say in them. This is crucial in the case of TM/TF clients. Helping the client to gain confidence in formulating some of the counseling goals is essential to progress. Helms-Estabrooks and Albert (2004) wrote about counseling for clients with aphasia and their families, but their premise is very valid for the gender diverse client.

They stated that therapy must have face validity for the client and his/her family. The transgender client has a right to know that the elimination of phonotrauma is a critical component of his/her voice and communication treatment plan. The vocal health program will help the client reach functional goals and complete transition in the areas of voice and communication.

Flasher and Fogle (2004) suggested that the clinician's job is not to *cure* the negative emotions and psychosocial issues faced by a client, but rather the clinician may help to identify emotional states and situations that might interfere with voice and communication progress. When working with a gender diverse client, it is often valuable to consult with the psychologist or psychiatrist on the case and integrate the psychotherapy with the vocal health program and voice/speech counseling goals for optimum progress and safety. For further information on the effects of counseling on psychosocial issues as well as the positive aspects of counseling for the transgender individual, see Chapters 2 and 3.

Throat-Clearing

Most gender diverse clients, like other clients with voice disorders, are unaware of the phonotrauma that occurs from throat-clearing. This often happens when a transmasculine or transfeminine client tries to position the larynx for pitch change, or when allergies, cold, and excessive mucus are present. Safe throat-clearing, although not immediately satisfying and slower to achieve in a gratifying way, can be taught as a precautionary measure. In addition, it will help alleviate the "burning" feeling or the "fatigued tight" feeling that is left in the throat after many continuous episodes of traditional,

Table 8–1. Safe Throat-Clearing

1. Client closes his/her mouth.
2. Client is instructed to gather and swallow saliva one time.
3. Client is then instructed to "clear" the throat with the usual laryngeal and pharyngeal movements used for swallowing but without using the vocal cords. Repeat five times.
4. Client is then told to immediately swallow.
5. Client repeats above steps three or four times.
6. Client is again reminded of the benefit of safe throat-clearing.

aggressive clearing. Applying a technique that helps the client use an extra swallow or an additional sip of water is very helpful to the client who might be seeking ways to avoid a harsh throat-clearing episode.

Stemple (2000) offers some suggestions about safe throat-clearing and emphasizes the speech-language clinician's role in teaching non-abusive behaviors that will guide the client into using safe throat-clearing methods. "Holistic voice therapy programs integrate all of the voice subsystems—respiration, phonation, and resonance—into the rehabilitation of the voice disorder" (p. 33). Holistic programs usually include an overall review of functions such as throat-clearing, coughing, and laughing to make sure the client does not incorporate phonotraumatic behaviors while doing these automatic vocal behaviors. Most transgender/gender diverse clients who have been seen in a clinic are often surprised to learn just how many times they actually clear their throats within an hour and are especially astounded to learn just how many phonotraumatic behaviors occur during this time. Teaching the gender diverse client to perform safe throat-clearing is essential for an effective vocal hygiene program. Table 8–1 illustrates a safe throat-clearing protocol.

Safe Coughing

Related to safe throat-clearing is safe coughing (see Table 8–2). The Healthline Newsletter (2017) explains that the University of North Carolina School of Medicine estimated that over 25% of excessive clearing and coughing was due to reflux. These patients often do not have symptoms of heartburn but rather do an inordinate amount of coughing. It is suggested that the client have an upper endoscopy or esophagogastroduodenoscopy (EGD) to determine the best treatment.

Furthermore, the online newsletter SLTinfo (2017) offers a tutorial for clients on how to stop excessive throat-clearing that would lead to safe coughing procedures. It states that clearing the throat can be traumatic to the folds and may cause misuse if this is done over a prolonged period of time. To break this cycle, it is suggested

Table 8–2. Safe Coughing Technique

1. When one feels a cough coming on, inhale a small deep breath through the nose.
2. Instead of coughing very forcefully emitting several glottal attacks, produce a cough that is short in duration, several times in sequence, and produced by approximating the vocal folds approximately one-half to three-quarters of the way closed.
3. Avoid harsh coughing that slams the vocal folds into each other at the point of approximation. It is best to try and cough in the abductor position to avoid irritation (adapt the language here to your client's level of understanding).
4. Use herbal, honey-laden cough lozenges/drops to soothe the throat after coughing or to prevent a cough.
5. After a bout of coughing, drink at least one cup of warm or hot (not iced) herbal tea with a scant teaspoon of honey or agave (no sugar or lemon). This will soothe the mucous membranes of the pharynx and relax the muscles that were just used for coughing (especially forceful coughing).

that the patient take a sip of water, firmly swallow, and then use a dry cough on the /h/ sound followed by another sip of water. This should help relieve the lump sensation in the throat and lead to more safe coughing when needed.

If a client presents with a history of excessive talking or throat-clearing or coughing, it is essential to have that client understand the concept of voice conservation. "Vocal Conservation practices typically range from absolute vocal abstinence to whisper or minimal use of a quiet (breathy) voice . . . which involves lightly adducted vocal folds" (Titze & Verdolini-Abbott, 2012, p. 211). Titze and Verdolini-Abbott (2012) further emphasize that "voice conservation makes imminent sense in cases of serious trauma from phonation or other causes. . . . [F]urther injury should be avoided" (p. 211). They go on to say that the "traditional approach to the management of phonotrauma or other laryngeal injury has been voice conservation" (p. 211). Therefore, it is essential that vocal health practices be instituted when working with a gender diverse client to prevent unnecessary phonotrauma.

Addressing Optimal Vocal Behaviors

When dealing with a client who exhibits phonotrauma, it is critical to be alert to the causative factors or at least the client's attitude toward the phonotraumatic behavior. The first thing to introduce is the concept that this behavior will change. The client needs to hear that the clinician is there to help. First the client has to identify and acknowledge the behavior(s) that is/are causing the phonotrauma to happen. The clinician can then describe the effects this has on one's voice, and how the clinician will empower the client to work on vocal

parameters to do some self-teaching and therefore change the behavior. Drawing up a hierarchy of specific occurrences and scenarios where phonotraumatic behaviors occur would be helpful in confronting the abusive behaviors. Finally, the clinician would be there to help the client learn to modify his/her vocally phonotraumatic behavior (Stemple, Glaze, & Klaben, 2000). Ultimately, it is the role of the SLT/SLP to work with the client to help achieve a modified voice that is produced effectively and safely or at least in a manner that does not cause phonotrauma and to practice vocal behaviors that reduce or eliminate phonotrauma.

It is helpful to set up a complete and detailed vocal health program for the client. Many instructions or precautionary methods may be included in such a program, and the clinician may pick and choose those items that would be the most helpful for a client. The following vocal health program parameters should be considered from an ethical and practical viewpoint. Make sure that each step used is written in laymen's terms in a style easily understood by non-professionals.

1. Utilize progressive relaxation—this works for many clients, especially when there is suspected or diagnosed muscle tension. So, this may be indicated for some clients where stress or overt body and laryngeal tension is a feature of their vocal usage.
2. Employ abdominal breathing for inhalation and exhalation.
3. Utilize easy onset of speech; reduce harsh attack when initiating speech. Do not hold one's breath when speaking; make sure one inhales before speaking, and do not just speak on residual airflow.
4. Employ a stop smoking strategy or at least limit smoking as much as possible; try to avoid secondhand smoke.

5. <u>Decrease</u> caffeine usage—as a diuretic, caffeine may be a drying agent to the mucous membranes of the pharynx and surrounding laryngeal tissues; this includes pop or sodas, coffee, regular tea, and chocolate. Herbal or green teas are recommended as a substitute for high caffeine drinks.

6. <u>Decrease</u> use of acidic citrus juices such as orange, grapefruit, pineapple, and lemon. Citrus juice contains a great deal of acid, and for some people, it is harmful to the laryngeal tissue, especially with a diagnosis of reflux. The following fluids are recommended: water, herbal or green teas, and diluted fruit juices. One can purchase "low acid" orange juice in the local grocery store.

7. <u>Keep</u> well hydrated: 64 ounces (1.5 to 2 liters) of water to include the water in teas and diluted juices. Fruit juices count toward the daily recommended fluid intake. Juices such as apple, grape, and cranberry or a combination of cranberry with another juice are often chosen, but the individual should realize that many of these juices have a great deal of sugar, so that must be considered. Diluting juices with water is a good way of reducing sugar, acidity, and caloric content. Avoid juices containing Aspartame or Saccharin, as these are chemically made in a lab and there is a lack of clear evidence of their effects on the human body.

8. <u>Avoid</u> spicy foods if there is a concern or diagnosis of reflux because they may be irritants to the throat tissue. Moderation is the key word here. If a client has acid reflux, his/her physician should be consulted, and orders followed.

9. <u>Limit</u> alcoholic beverages at least during the transition period for voice and communication training; resume in moderation after discussing with the speech-language clinician and client's personal physician.

10. <u>Be aware</u> that decongestants and antihistamines may dry out the laryngeal and pharyngeal mucosa. Try to include more water intake when taking this type of medication.

11. <u>Limit</u> coughing; aim to use a safe coughing technique when this is not possible (see Table 8–2).

12. <u>Limit</u> throat-clearing when possible (see Table 8–1).

13. <u>Avoid</u> whispering—this can be more detrimental to the laryngeal area than talking, since the vocal folds work harder and have a tendency to be overused during a whisper. Remember, Colton et al. (2011) stated that "there is not yet sufficient evidence available to state unequivocally that whispering is not harmful . . . but it may be helpful for some clients with some caveats" (p. 357).

14. <u>Employ</u> good general fitness and get adequate sleep and rest, both of which support breathing and voice production.

15. <u>Avoid</u> shouting and talking over loud noises (music, airplanes, television, parties, bars, clubs, etc.).

16. <u>Do not</u> strain the voice (do not force words; use of some vocal exercises are helpful). Professional guidance is recommended when embarking on voice modification. Vocal warm-ups are a good source to help the client with easy onset of voice production (see Chapter 14). It is imperative for the SLP/SLT to teach the client about the importance of good voicing techniques, including safe voice projection using breath support at the main source of power. This will also help to alleviate some of the strenuous behaviors on the vocal folds such as speaking on residual air, holding one's breath when speaking, and taking a very short, choppy breath when initiating voicing/speaking.

17. Build in some vocal rest periods during the day, especially if the client is a professional voice user; the average person could use some vocal rest as a means to relax the vocal cords and larynx.

18. Be aware of dust or pet allergies that may affect breathing and could irritate nasal passages and throat tissue. In some cases, it will be necessary to rid the home of animal dander and hairs.

19. Consider some type of amplification at work if a client needs to project his/her voice frequently.

20. Apply good posture, which promotes a good voice: maintain a 90/90 degree sitting posture and head up at a 90-degree angle when speaking to ease the tension in the laryngeal area.

21. When needed, wear a mask when around toxic chemicals, fluids, or other harmful agents in the home or workplace.

Transmasculine and transfeminine clients will greatly benefit from a vocal health program made up of several of the above suggestions. For some clients, counseling sessions by the clinician would be most beneficial to reinforce the seriousness of the hygiene program. Clients could involve their spouse, significant other, children, and co-workers to help reinforce the program on an everyday basis.

It is imperative to include goals and objectives in a client's treatment plan that address phonotrauma and better vocal health. It may be necessary to include a 15-minute segment of each session to address psychosocial issues and other behaviors that would affect whether a vocal health program is being followed. To reiterate, it is important for the SLP/SLT to teach the client about the importance of good voicing techniques, including safe voice projection using breath support as the main source of speaking power. This will also help to alleviate some of the strenuous behaviors on the vocal folds, such as speaking on residual air, holding one's breath when speaking, and taking a very short, choppy breath when initiating speaking.

Vocal Quality Considerations

Apart from the vocal health aspects that contribute to healthy and safe voicing, the issue of initial voice quality is also an important consideration. Dysphonia may be evident in the client's voice at the start of training, and traditional voice advice and exercises to reduce this will be required at the early stage of intervention and training. Hancock and Garabedian (2013) reviewed 25 cases of voice and communication change in transgender clients. The authors found that 28% of the participants presented with a voice disorder that was separate from gender presentation concerns.

For trans women, common vocal presentation in the early stage of treatment may include a breathy and/or strained voice quality. Typically, the dysphonic elements of voicing are due to the client's own attempts to modify her voice without professional guidance or due to clients following suggestions made by other transgender individuals via the internet. Softer onsets and articulation can be a valid goal for some trans women. However, it is advisable to address excessive breathiness at the start of the voice therapy process to ensure safe voice modification. An overly breathy voice quality will contribute to laryngeal dryness, vocal fatigue, and laryngeal strain. In addition, it will limit the client's ability to safely project the voice, since the vocal folds will not adduct adequately.

A Word About Setting Goals

As noted previously, vocal health goals should be part of the treatment plan for a transmasculine or transfeminine client. Clients often

Table 8–3. Goals within the Context of Vocal Health

1. Client will write one entry per day into a journal describing vocal use and/or misuse from the activities of the day.
2. Client will follow, practice, and demonstrate safe throat-clearing techniques without cues or prompts from the clinician and in 90% of all throat-clearing episodes in one session as measured by the clinician.
3. Client will follow, practice, and demonstrate safe coughing techniques without cues or prompts from the clinician and during 80% of all coughing episodes as measured by the clinician and client.
4. Client will write a daily entry into the voice journal illustrating the increasing and habitual use of safe throat-clearing and coughing techniques.
5. During a 1-minute segment of a voice therapy session, the client will be able to name [identify] two emotions or psychosocial issues that affect the voice, work, social situations, school, or family without prompting from the clinician.
6. With minimum cues or prompts from the clinician, the client will be able to describe two ways or techniques that could be used to deal with a psychosocial issue that affects the voice, work, school, or family.
7. With moderate cueing or prompting from the clinician, the client will be able to describe and demonstrate how two techniques could be applied to decrease the effects on the voice, family, school, or work of his/her specific psychosocial issues.
8. The client, with moderate to maximum cues and prompts from the clinician, will be able to write and describe a rank-ordered hierarchy of situations where he/she is "read" due to inadequate voice transition. (The client, with clinical guidance, notes any feelings that might have come from vocal misuse as a result of being read.)
9. The client, with minimum to moderate cues and prompts from the clinician, will be able to name and describe two ways to improve/eliminate each "being read" event.

need goals that deal with safe throat-clearing, safe coughing, psychosocial issues, and counseling/emotional issues (see Tables 8-1 and 8-2 for tips on safe throat-clearing and safe coughing). Transmasculine and transfeminine clients should be especially cognizant of safe throat-clearing and safe coughing to preserve their voices. Examples of goals for the above vocal health parameters are illustrated in Table 8-3.

Psychosocial Factors Affecting Voice Transition

When working with the TM/TF client, psychosocial dynamics can be intertwined as causative factors not only in phonotrauma but also in the transition process. Therefore, it makes it more critical for the clinician

working with a transmasculine or transfeminine client to not only probe psychosocial issues, but include "speech or voice counseling" to address these issues during therapy (see Chapter 3). Andrews (2006) stated emphatically that "patients who are not comfortable seeking counseling may frequently feel more comfortable consulting a speech pathologist because it is less threatening to them" (p. 547). Holland and Nelson (2014) agree that "counseling is necessary to support decisions and behaviors that optimize quality of life" (p. 1). They also stated that appropriate counseling will increase optimal progress for clients. This holds true for voice clients in general but for clients coming in for voice and communication training as well.

Occasionally a dilemma arises because some clinicians are not confident when it comes to including counseling principals in their treatment plans. But as Andrews (2006) so eloquently stated, "speech pathologists are well trained and most do in fact work on the enhancement of self-esteem, social interactions, and increased self-determination for their patients" (p. 546). This only further substantiates the need to incorporate counseling techniques in therapy plans for the TM/TF client. "The speech pathologist's ability to help patients integrate new insights about their feelings and relationships into their communicative strategies is significant" (Andrews, 2006, p. 546). Rao (1997) suggested that clinicians deal with their clients' emotions as they arise in therapy. A TM/TF client may be undergoing hormonal treatment during the time voice and communication therapy is begun. These clients might express sadness, loss, anger, euphoria, and many other emotions during a therapy visit, and the clinician should be

able to incorporate counseling into the treatment session (Rao, 1997).

Mental health professionals, such as social workers, counselors, and psychologists, are very well trained to help their clients understand the dynamic psychosocial relationship of a voice problem or the need for vocal change; it is part of the transition process (see Chapter 2 for a description of this important role). However, the SLP/SLT's roles are to establish and habituate (generalize) safe and appropriate vocal behaviors. In this way, the combination of "speech and voice" counseling and voice and communication training for the TM/TF client sets up a working dichotomy for safe voice transition and the elimination of phonotraumatic behaviors.

Holland and Nelson (2014) stated, "[C]ounseling for communication disorders has a different theoretical perspective. This approach requires essentially abandoning a

Table 8–4. Psychological Issues in TF/TM Transition and Voice Disorders (also see Chapter 3)

Issue	TF/TM Client's Experience	Client is at risk for:
A. Fear	Loss of job; loss of family; loss of friends; self-respect; loss of marriage	Muscle tension dysphonia
		Conversion dysphonia or aphonia
		Chronic cough/damage to the laryngeal tissue
		Other psychogenic voice disorders
B. Guilt	Family strife, family is not accepting; rejection by the children or spouse	Muscle tension dysphonia; chronic clearing of the throat
C. Rage/anger	At God; at family; at the "system," and at the children; anger at him or herself	Severe phonotrauma; poor fundamental frequency ratings; obtrusive yelling or screaming
D. Denial	"I just have a cold," "My voice always gets this way," "I can still work, no problem"	Vocal nodules/polyps; excessive throat clearing; poor singing fundamental frequency range
E. Depression/anxiety	"I just can't do this job anymore," "I am totally afraid to speak"	Voice deteriorates; social isolation; lack of motivation to speak or talk; less social—loses friends; voice seems always fatigued

treatment model based on what is *wrong* with people. . . . [I]instead the emphasis is what is *right* with them and how to . . . deal with adversities that have befallen them" (p. 3). This idea fits directly into the model of TM/TF voice and communication as a voice difference and not a voice disorder. The SLP is in a perfect position to counsel clients who need to overcome their fears and doubts about voice transitioning. Holland and Nelson further stated many ideas of how we, as SLPs or SLTs, can capitalize on the positive nature of voice change, focusing on difference rather than disorder, much like counselors or life coaches address the theme of wellness and positive psychology.

Many clients who come for either voice feminization or masculinization as part of their transition to their gender identity, or for purposes of a voice disorder (perhaps from phonotrauma), have several psychosocial factors that have a direct bearing on the formation of the voice disorder. Several of these factors have an equal bearing on the progress of voice transition or the elimination of the voice disorder. These data have been observed and recorded by the chapter authors for over 25 years of working with TM/TF clients. Table 8–4 outlines the psychosocial issues that are critical to address in therapy sessions with the transmasculine or transfeminine client.

Conclusion

It is important to remember that there is no best or better vocal health program that a transgender client should follow. Most importantly, the client needs to understand that the voice can be at risk for phonotrauma even if unintentionally, and that following a vocal health program is essential. Monitoring the client's progress will be enhanced by the client keeping a journal, which would be a part of the vocal health program. Most clients realize early on in their journal writing and in their vocal health program how essential cooperation is to success. The clinician can be the key figure in facilitating this cooperation.

References

Alegria, C. A. (2011). Transgender identity and health care: Implications for psychosocial and physical evaluation. *Journal of the American Association of Nurse Practitioners, 23,* 175–182.

American Academy of Otolaryngology–Head and Neck Cancer (2017). Retrieved June 29, 2017 from http://www.entnet.org/content/common -problems-can-affect-your-voice

American Academy of Otolaryngology–Head and Neck Surgery (2017). Retrieved July 26 from http://www.entnet.org/content/common -problems-can-affect-your-voice

American Speech-Language-Hearing Association (2016). *Scope of practice in speech-language pathology.* Rockville, MD, Author. Retrieved July 1, 2017 from http://www.asha.org/policy /SP2016-00343/#Framework

Andrews, M. (1999). *Manual of voice treatment: Pediatrics through geriatrics* (2nd ed.). San Diego, CA: Singular Publishing Group.

Andrews, M. (2006). *Manual of voice treatment: Pediatrics through geriatrics* (3rd ed.). Clifton Park, NY: Thomas Delmar Learning.

Aronson, A. E. (1990a). *Clinical voice disorders: An interdisciplinary approach* (3rd ed.). New York, NY: Thieme.

Aronson, A. E. (1990b). Importance of the psychological interview in the diagnosis and treatment of "functional" voice disorders. *Journal of Voice,* 4(4), 287–289.

Boone, D., McFarlane, S., Von Berg, S. & Zraick, R. (2010). *The voice and voice therapy* (8th ed.), Boston, MA: Allyn & Bacon.

Cazden, J. (2012). *Everyday voice care: The lifestyle guide for singers and talkers*. Milwaukee, WI: Hal Leonard Books.

Colton, R. H., Casper, J. K., & Leonard, R. (2011). *Understanding voice problems: A physiological perspective for diagnosis and treatment* (4th ed.). Baltimore, MD: Wolters Kluwer/Lippincott Williams, and Wilkins.

Craig, J. (2016). *Digital manipulation and laryngeal massage*. Retrieved December 21, 2017 from https://prezi.com/cntnf1qgstku/digital-manipulation-and-laryngeal-massage

Deary, V., & Miller, T. (2011). Reconsidering the role of psychosocial factors in functional aphonia. Retrieved June 30, 2017 online from PubMed. doi: 10.1097/MOO.0b013e328346494d

Flasher, L., & Fogle, P. (2004). *Counseling skills for speech-language pathologists and audiologists*. New York, NY: Delmar Learning.

Healthline Newsletter. (2017). Retrieved June 30, 2017 from http://www.healthline.com/health/gerd/coughing#overview1

Helm-Estabrooks, N., & Albert, M. (2004). *Manual of aphasia therapy* (2nd ed.). Austin, TX: Pro-Ed.

Holland, A. L., & Nelson, R. L. (2014). *Counseling in communication disorders: A wellness perspective* (2nd ed.). San Diego, CA: Plural Publishing Co.

Muller, D. (1999). Managing psychosocial adjustment of aphasia. *Seminars in Speech and Language, 20*, 85–92.

Rao, P. (1997). Adult neurogenic communication disorders. In T. A. Crowe (Ed.), *Applications of counseling in speech-language pathology and audiology*. Baltimore, MD: Williams and Wilkins.

SLTinfo (Speech and Language Therapy Information) (2017). Retrieved June 30, 2017 from http://www.sltinfo.com/stop-throat-clearing/

Stemple, J. C. (2000). *Voice therapy: Clinical studies* (2nd ed.). Clifton Park, N.Y.: Thomson Delmar Learning.

Stemple, J. C., Glaze, L. E., & Klaben, B. G. (2000). *Clinical voice pathology: Theory and management* (3rd ed.). San Diego, CA: Singular Thomson Learning.

Titze, I., & Verdolini-Abbott, K. (2012). *Vocology: The science and practice of voice habilitation*. Salt Lake City, UT: National Center for Voice and Speech.

Voice Foundation (2017). Retrieved from http://voicefoundation.org/health-science/voice-disorders/voice-disorders/reflux-laryngitis/ June 28, 2017.

Weinrich, B. D., Gottliebson, R. O., & LeBorgne, W. D. (2016). *Vocal hygiene: Maintaining a sound voice* (2nd ed.). CD/DVD. San Diego, CA: Plural Publishing.

9

Transmasculine Voice and Communication

Christie Block, Viktória G. Papp, and Richard K. Adler

Introduction

Transgender voice and communication training is an increasingly expanding service that up to now has been focused mainly on the needs of the transfeminine client. For transmasculine individuals, it has been commonly assumed that voice and communication training is not warranted, because testosterone administration, which many undergo for gender dysphoria, is often sufficient for masculine voice and communication presentation (Adler, Constansis, & Van Borsel, 2012; Block, 2017; Van Borsel, De Cuypere, Rubens, & Destaerke, 2000). Because of this assumption, there have been relatively minimal research studies, writings, and clinician trainings in this area (Azul, 2015; Azul, Nygren, Sodersten, & Neuschaefer-Rube, 2017). Ultimately, access to care for transmasculine individuals has been even more limited than it is for transfeminine people (Block, 2017). However, the need is there. Some transmasculine people do not choose testosterone administration, and when they do, pitch lowering can be insufficient. Furthermore, even when pitch lowering is sufficient, other masculine voice and communication patterns may not

be. What's more is that transmasculine people can experience dysphonia for various reasons.

The purpose of this chapter is to illuminate what is known about the voice and communication needs of the transmasculine community and share ideas for best practices in service to it. It is based on the authors' combined clinical and research experience as well as input from transmasculine-identified consultants and experts in trans health, voice, gender, and linguistics.

First, a careful analysis of research on testosterone and various aspects of voice and communication will reveal the complex nature of gendered and transmasculine experiences. What is the role of the clinician in that context? A comprehensive summary of diagnostic and therapeutic issues will then be discussed in terms of how to approach a transmasculine client from start to finish. In addition, samples of exercises and case studies will follow. While the clinical information will often be presented in a Standard American English context and may be familiar to some readers, a recurring call for sensitivity to transgender myths, gender stereotypes, and cultural assumptions will be apparent.

The material in this chapter is intended to address the needs of any person assigned female at birth who wishes to increase the masculine aspects of voice and communication, wherever that may be on the gender spectrum. Though some individuals in the community may use other terms, this discussion, for the sake of simplicity, will employ the terms "transmasculine" and "he" to refer to anyone who falls into this category. The terms "non-binary" and "genderqueer," in the context of this chapter, will refer to a subcategory of individuals who wish to increase masculine aspects of voice and communication, but to a lesser extent, not in all contexts, and/or in a less identifiably stereotypical way. Pronoun reference to the clinician will be in the form of singular "they." While one chapter can barely do justice to such a broad topic, it will provide a thorough overview of the critical issues facing this community in the hopes to boost the reader's interest and confidence in providing transmasculine people with the help they deserve.

Review of the Literature

Though the existing body of research on transmasculine speakers is limited in scope, design, and breadth, it is rich enough to serve as a critically useful developing account of transmasculine experiences and needs. It illuminates both the similarities and differences between transmasculine and transfeminine issues. Given the small body of work, a particularly careful interpretation of what does exist is required to understand why there is a pressing need for increased access to care. The following paragraphs will provide an overview and analysis of what is currently known and not known about transmasculine speakers. First, cisgender and transmasculine pitch, including the effects of testosterone on the human larynx, will be covered, followed by a discussion of pitch-lowering surgery, resonance, non-voice communication variables, breathing, dysphonia, and vocal satisfaction.

The Effects of Physiology and Culture on Cisgender Pitch

A wide range of differences characterize the human voice around the globe. By and large, cis men's speaking fundamental frequency (F0), the main acoustic correlate of pitch, is lower than cis women's, and in many Western cultures it is about half of (or about an octave lower than) cis women's (Titze, 2000). For example, Baken and Orlikoff's (2000) literature review reports the F0 of cis men aged 21 to 59 to be between 107 and 129 hertz (~A2–C3) compared with that of cis women aged 21 to 54, which was between 189 and 224 hertz (~F#3–A3). The majority of gendered voice differences emerge physiologically at puberty when higher testosterone levels cause cis men's vocal folds and vocal tracts to grow faster than overall body growth (Fitch & Giedd, 1999; Lee, Potamianos, & Narayanan, 1999; Vorperian et al., 2005, 2009). The physiological changes in cis women are not comparable in extent. But it is important to ask: Do all differences emerge as a direct result of testosterone?

Research evidence indicates that while F0 is influenced by a speaker's physiology to an extent, it is strongly shaped by sociocultural factors as well. Consider countries where language is shared: English is spoken in the Irish Republic, New Zealand, and South Africa, and Portuguese is the official language of Brazil, Portugal, and Angola. Yet, the acoustic targets of the voicing source, such as mean F0 or the standard deviation of F0, can be as different across the dialects as the targets of the vocal tract resonances. Knowing how hard it can be to understand someone speaking a distant dialect of one's own language, it is easy to appreciate how perceptually salient those differences in the vocal tract resonances can be.

The acoustic targets for mean F0, as well as its standard deviation and probability distribution in general, are also subject to change over time. Table 9–1 presents an example from a very well-documented area, namely, how young speakers' mean reading F0 has changed in the United States over time. The table documents the F0 of cis women and men between 18 and 30 years of age when reading the Rainbow Passage (Fairbanks, 1960). Interestingly, it shows pitch lowering over time in both cis men and women in North American and Australian English, and the dialects of the very same language do not have the same target over time. There is no evidence from medical science or imaging studies suggesting that the human larynx has grown over the past century, so it must be assumed that the behavioral use of the laryngeal structures is changing, and not the laryngeal structures themselves. In practical terms, this means that it is important to keep updated on current information.

Other than a few studies explicitly investigating the effects of ethnic background on speech and voice features (for example, Hudson & Holbrook, 1981, 1982; Szakay, 2006), there is rarely a mention of this variable. This omission might create the impression that clinicians can assume the same target values for coexisting ethnicities. This assumption, however, is well refuted in the literature that did in fact compare across ethnicities, from as early as the 1980s, as shown in Table 9–2. The difference in the F0 between Caucasian American and African American cis women is 2 semitones, and between Māori New Zealanders and New Zealanders of European descent (Pākehā) is nearly 3 semitones, which are both perceptually salient distances.

Besides pitch change over time and dialectal pitch differences, between-language differences are very easy to find around the globe. Table 9–3 shows the extreme ends of mean F0 for cis men.

The difference between cis men's mean F0 in British English (100 Hz) versus Urdu (186 Hz) is 10.7 semitones—which is almost a full octave. To place these values into a relevant context, in many European languages, middle-aged cis women are expected to speak around the same mean F0 targets that were observed for cis men speaking Wù and Shanghai Chinese, and Urdu. Needless to say, these large differences in F0 illustrate that the language spoken is relevant when considering pitch expectations for trans men.

In addition to language-based differences, bilingual, mobile, and contextual identities need to be considered. The literature shows inconsistency across various language pairs (for example, German-French, English-Spanish, etc.) regarding the difference between a bilingual speaker's two F0 means. For an overview, see Dorreen (2017). One thing is clear, however: a bilingual speaker is likely to have more than one target when it comes to F0 (be it mean, standard deviation of the mean, or probability distribution), and these targets may not be simply the targets of the monolingual speakers of the language pair in question. These within-language and between-language differences clearly indicate that social, linguistic, ethnic, and time-related factors are relevant when considering pitch. There is no one F0 value that applies globally but rather there are ranges.

So far we have considered the F0. In addition, the conversational minimum and maximum pitch values, as well as measures expressing the variability of the intonational

Table 9–1. Mean Reading F0 (in Hz) of Cisgender Caucasian Speakers Between the Ages of 18 and 30

Dialect	Year	Female	Male	Source
US English	1924	318	152	Weaver (1924)
	1934	242	129	Murray and Tiffin (1934)
	1941	213–224		Snidecor (1951)
	1953	200		Linke (1953, 1973)
	1966	208		Michel, Hollien, and Moore (1966)
	1967	204		Hanley and Snidecor (1967)
	1969	212		Hollien and Paul (1969)
	1970	217	117	J. L. Fitch and Holbrook (1970)
	1972	224		Hollien and Shipp (1972)
	1978	197	120	Lass and Brown (1978)
	1981	217	117	A. I. Hudson and Holbrook (1981)
	1981	197	110	Benjamin (1981)
	1982	193	110	A. I. Hudson and Holbrook (1982)
	1990	206	113	J. L. Fitch (1990)
	1991	192	118	Brown, Morris, Hollien, and Howell (1991)
	1992	202		Yamazawa and Hollien (1992)
	1993	207	123	Awan (1993)
	1993	206	126	Brown, Morris, Hicks, and Howell (1993); Morris, Brown, Hicks, and Howell (1995)
	1993	206		Garofolo et al. (1993)
	1997	198	114	Hollien, Hollien, and de Jong (1997)
	2005	215		Zraick, Birdwell, and Smith-Olinde (2005)
	2011	191		Schiwitz (2011)
Canadian	1981	224		Stoicheff (1981)
	1990	199	115	Britto and Doyle (1990)
Australian	1936	233	141	Cowan (1936)
	1945	229		de Pinto and Hollien (1982)
	1982	204		Hollien, Tolhurst, and McGlone (1982)
	1992	203	123	Gilmore, Guidera, Hutchins, and van Steenbrugge (1992)
	1993	206		Pemberton, McCormack, and Russell (1998)

melody, are also gendered differently across languages. Generally, cis men and women both exhibit a variety of pitch ranges and intonation patterns, like other speech and language parameters, depending on context. This runs counter to what can be commonly assumed as masculine monotone intonation versus feminine emotional pitch variability in all situations. Even when conducted and considered in context, some studies, in fact, incorrectly interpret pitch ranges to be narrower for cis men and wider

Table 9–2. Mean Reading F0 (in Hz) of Cisgender Speakers in the US and New Zealand by Ethnolect

Ethnolect	Female	Male	Source
US English, Caucasians	217	117	A. I. Hudson and Holbrook (1981)
US English, African Americans	193	110	A. I. Hudson and Holbrook (1981)
Difference in ST	2	1	
Māori New Zealanders	–	128	Szakay (2006)
Pākehā New Zealanders	–	109	Szakay (2006)
Difference in ST		2.8	

Table 9–3. Mean F0 of Cis Men Across Languages

Language	F0 (Hz)	Source
British English	100–106	Nolan, McDougall, de Jong, and Hudson (2006); Hudson, de Jong, McDougall, Harrison, and Nolan(2007)
Taiwanese	110	Chen (2007)
German	110–120	Jessen (2009)
Swedish	121	Lindh (2006)
Persian	122	Izadi, Mohseni, Daneshi, and Sandughdar (2012)
Korean	133	Moon, Chung, Park, and Kim (2012)
Brazilian Portuguese	135	Pegoraro-Krook and Castro (1994)
Punjabi	165	French, Saxena, Harrison, and Künzel (1998)
Wù Chinese	170	Rose (1991)
Urdu	186	French et al. (1998)

for cis women. Moore and Glasberg (1983) and Henton (1989) illustrate this with the results from their own investigations and a recalculation of hertz values from earlier studies. Using semitones rather than hertz to measure pitch range, because it is more perceptually salient, they found there to be no significant difference in pitch range between cis men and women in the studies. Likewise, Rose (1991) used semitone measurements and found no significant difference in mean F0 or the standard deviation between genders in his work on the Wù and Shanghai dialects of Chinese. Furthermore, Simpson (2009) reviewed Herbst's (1964) early, large-scale study in German in which data from over a thousand German speakers showed that, when calculated in semitones, cis men actually have a slightly larger pitch range than cis women. Therefore, though cis men can exhibit a narrower pitch range, this is not the case in all contexts and has sometimes been misinterpreted.

The Effects of Testosterone on Transmasculine Pitch

Not all transmasculine and non-binary speakers may want or be able to afford access to and use of exogenous testosterone, and exogenous testosterone is not the sole path to masculinizing the voice. In this section, however, the current state of research on testosterone is summarized to help clinicians understand the effects and risks that the transmasculine client may be facing.

There is relatively little data (at the writing of this chapter, around 100 speakers) on the changes exogenous testosterone brings about in transmasculine speakers. This is despite the marked increase over the past two decades in both the number of studies on the transmasculine and masculinizing voicing source and the number of speakers on which these studies base their results. According to this limited pool of data, long-term testosterone intake results in significantly lowered F0 in the vast majority of, but not all, speakers (Cosyns et al., 2014; Deuster, Matulat, et al., 2016; Irwig, Childs, & Hancock, 2017; Nygren, Nordenskjöld, Arver, & Södersten, 2016; Papp, 2011; Van Borsel, de Cuypere, Rubens, & Destaerke, 2000; Zimman, 2012).

Magnitude and Speed of Pitch Changes

The magnitude of the lowering is usually calculated in hertz and semitones, and sometimes further evaluated by comparing transmasculine speakers with cismasculine speakers as a reference population. Keeping in mind that not all trans men aim for cis men's vocal targets, the above studies found that the majority of transmasculine speakers' mean reading or speaking pitch reaches cismasculine values by the end of the first year on testosterone and sometimes by the nine-month mark (Deuster, Matulat, et al., 2016), or even by the six-month mark (Irwig et al., 2017). As for how much lowering one can expect, the sources documented 3–11 semitone changes in the mean F0 in the first year, with the majority showing a 6–8 semitone lowering in their mean fundamental. Based on the data available at the time of the writing of this chapter, it is not possible to predict the amount of pitch lowering an individual can expect from testosterone. In general, speakers who had relatively low pitch pre-testosterone (by cisfeminine standards) can expect a smaller amount of change than those who had average or high pitch at the outset.

Besides the expected magnitude of the change in F0, the dynamics and rate of the lowering are also affected. The rate of the lowering is only possible to observe and doc-

ument if the speakers are recorded frequently enough, but longitudinal research infrequently samples speakers more than a few times over the first year. Some sources measured speakers before the onset of testosterone therapy and after 12–18 months (Damrose, 2009; Van Borsel et al., 2000); some, every 3 months (Irwig et al., 2017; Nygren et al., 2016); and yet others more frequently (Deuster, Matulat, et al., 2016; Papp, 2011; Zimman, 2012) from the start of the hormone therapy for a year or two. Studies with a frequent enough sampling design conclude that there is no single path that everyone follows and that the lowering is not a linear process. It is usually faster in the first six months than in the second, and it typically continues into the second year, albeit at a greatly diminished speed. Speakers who do not experience any perceivable change in the first three months were observed to still complete the majority of the changes in the first year (Irwig et al., 2017). There is some weak evidence in Papp (2011) that the pitch of transmasculine speakers changes faster after menopause than before, and similarly, speakers might expect some additional lowering post-hysterectomy if the hysterectomy is performed during the first critical year. Even though both of these outcomes are in keeping with the documented lowering effects of menopause on cis women's pitch (e.g., Stoicheff, 1981), much more data are needed.

Pitch Floor

For speakers who do not experience a (perceptually large enough) lowering of the habitual F0 as a function of time on testosterone, Papp (2011) demonstrated that *some* of these speakers are in fact capable of phonating much lower than their habitual F0, in some cases as much as a whole octave (12 semitones). This "buoyancy" of the habitual F0 reveals two things. First, it shows that the physiological effect of testosterone manifests in the lowering (or lowered) pitch floor. Second, it also demonstrates that the F0 does not necessarily stay behaviorally in lockstep with the lowered (or lowering) pitch floor. The diagnostic section of this chapter will further discuss the measurement of the maximum pitch range, including the pitch floor and consideration of the range as a result of testosterone, habitual pitch use, or both.

Pitch Ceiling and Timing of Dysphonia

The pitch ceiling is the highest fundamental that a speaker can reliably scale or glide up to. Identifying this pitch assists in determining the time when the bulk of the changes happen to the voicing source. Typically, as the pitch floor drops away, the pitch ceiling dips with it (Damrose, 2009; Nygren et al., 2016; Papp, 2011; Van Borsel et al., 2000). Depending on the co-timing of these two events, speakers on testosterone may experience a severely narrowed pitch range, voice breaks (akin to cismasculine adolescents' vocal instability), and a sore throat. This is the time when many of them will be asked if they have a cold or if they attended a concert the night before.

Maximum phonation pitch ranges reported in Papp (2011) and Van Borsel et al. (2000), Voice Range Profiles in Nygren et al. (2016), and phonation frequency ranges in Hancock, Childs, and Irwig (2017), however, show that this drop in the pitch ceiling and consequent narrowing of the pitch range manifesting at around months 4–8 is only temporary, and matches closely to cis men's experience with exogenous testosterone (King, Ashby, & Nelson, 2001). By the end of the first year on testosterone, the pitch ceiling tends to return to its original value. On closer examination (see Table 9–4), it

Table 9–4. Mean F0, Maximum Phonation Frequency Range (MPFR), and Change in MPFR by the End of the First Year on Testosterone

Source	N	Mean F0 (in Hz)	MPFR (in ST)	Change in MPFR (in ST)
van Borsel et al. (2000)	2	132–155	25–27	−0.3–0.3
Papp (2011)	8	101–172	30–40	−4–15
Nygren et al. (2016)	36	89–170	39	4.6

turns out that the incremental regaining of the pre-testosterone pitch ceiling, together with the new lowered pitch floor, yields at least an identical or an expanded pitch range compared with pre-testosterone measures (Hancock et al., 2017; Nygren et al., 2016; Papp, 2011; Van Borsel et al., 2000). This is great news for speakers who sing or use their voice professionally.

Reversibility of Pitch Changes

Based on the irreversible quality of androgen-induced changes (e.g., Pattie, Murdoch, Theodoros, & Forbes, 1998), transmasculine speakers are expected to show only downward, irreversible movement of the habitual pitch, even if they stopped taking testosterone. Upward movement is considered impossible on a physiological basis. However, three speakers in Papp (2011) showed a late rise in their mean habitual pitch, showing a small but significant reversal of the pitch lowering around the eight-month mark (referred to as a reverse J-pattern). As the experiences of trans women and cis women with hyperandrogenism so succinctly show (Baker, 1999; Barbieri, Evans, & Kistner, 1982; Boothroyd & Lepre,

1990; Mercaitis, Peaper, & Schwartz, 1985; Newman & Forbes, 1993; Pattie et al., 1998; Wardle, Whitehead, & Mills, 1983), the *physiological* lowering effects of androgens are irreversible. This irreversibility of physiologically lowered pitch means that any observed upward shift is not due to physiological changes, but to individual choices made by transmasculine speakers. It seems that some transmasculine speakers may choose to speak not only markedly higher than their predicted optimal pitch, but consciously or unconsciously opt to systematically shift their pitch within their accessible range. These shifts in pitch are very similar to the language-based F0 tuning exemplified in Table 9–3, changes in pitch for transfeminine voice training, and the transmasculine participants' in Hancock et al. (2017) use of a habitual speaking pitch than observed values of cis men in a comparable cohort. All four phenomena are different manifestations of speakers' substantial agency over their use of the physiologically given laryngeal structures.

The evidence that transmasculine speakers may make choices that counter the physiologically predicted, and often highly desired, effects of testosterone—for habitual pitch and pitch floor (as discussed above)—sheds light not only on the continuum around gender, but also the conscious or unconscious fine-tuning of vocal behavior that speakers employ in order to represent gender.

Phonosurgery

Not all transmasculine people can or want to take testosterone to masculinize their gender expression. Those who have taken testosterone sometimes wish for faster and larger changes to the F0 (e.g., Söderpalm, Larsson, & Almquist, 2004; Van Borsel et al.,

2000). Failure rates of testosterone therapy for satisfactory voice change may also be underestimated, with voice change not occurring as easily, fast, or to the extent hoped for, as in the case of 3 out of 16 clients in Van Borsel et al. (2000), 12 reporting vocal dysfunction or dissatisfaction out of 50 in Nygren et al. (2016), and 3 out of 7 in Hancock et al. (2017). Clients who want to (further) lower their F0 have similar options as cis men experiencing puberphonia (mutational falsetto), that is, they can and usually opt for voice therapy to relocate the F0 to a lower position in an available range (as described later in this chapter), and/or they may consider pitch-lowering surgery.

Isshiki and colleagues (Isshiki, 2000; Isshiki, Taira, & Tanabe, 1983) examined and classified laryngeal framework surgeries used to raise and lower the habitual pitch in cisgender clients. For lowering the F0, they suggested the Isshiki Type III thyroplasty. This procedure shortens the anteroposterior length of the thyroid cartilage by removing a 2-mm piece of it. The shortened cartilage reduces the length and vibratory mass of the vocal folds and thereby decreases the vocal fold tension. As a result, the F0 lowers substantially and instantaneously. If the change is not adequate, then additional cartilage is removed. The European Laryngological Society (ELS) renamed this technique "shortening thyroplasty with lateral approach."

There does not appear to be any peer-reviewed publications on surgical outcomes in the transmasculine population for this procedure. However, studies examining about 70 cis men diagnosed with puberphonia and mutational falsetto report significantly decreased F0 without any statistically significant differences in the pre- and postoperative measures of vocal intensity or instability (jitter and shimmer) (Chowdhury, Saha, Pal, & Chatterjee, 2014; Hoffman et al., 2014; Koçak et al., 2008; Li, Mu, & Yang, 1999; Nakamura, Tsukahara, Watanabe, Komazawa, & Suzuki, 2013; Remacle, Matar, Verduyckt, & Lawson, 2010; Slavit, Maragos, & Lipton, 1990). The same sources also assert that both self-evaluations and vocal quality evaluations significantly improved post-operatively.

Further investigation needs to be done regarding the efficacy of surgery and voice therapy when performed in conjunction. In addition to being recommended as the primary method of voice intervention by the Standards of Care version 7 (SOC7), of the World Professional Association for Transgender Health (WPATH) (Coleman et al., 2012), voice therapy is recommended to be a rehabilitative adjunct to pitch-changing phonosurgery in order to maximize outcomes. This mirrors the gold standard of general phonosurgical procedures for voice disorders.

Resonance

The resonance structure of a voice is responsible for the tone or timbre of the voice, but more importantly, listeners also use it to evaluate speaker age, height, gender, sexual orientation, and other social factors. The resonant structure of a voice is often evaluated acoustically by measuring formant frequencies of sonorants (the high energy harmonics of vowels, glides, liquids, and nasals), the fricative spectrum (aperiodic noise characteristics of fricatives), and the long-term frequency spectrum as a holistic measure, as is discussed at length in the resonance chapter of this book (see Chapter 11).

Gender perception is a rather slippery concept, but there is plenty of research evidence (Coleman, 1976; Gelfer & Mikos, 2005; Klatt & Klatt, 1990; Smith & Patterson,

2005; Titze, 1989, to name just a few seminal papers) suggesting that when people listen to a voice, the psychoacoustic percept of the resonance structure of the voice can easily drown out the gender percept gained from pitch. This phenomenon makes resonance a key attribute for masculine voice.

Cisgender Formant Frequencies

Research on cisgender spoken formant frequencies falls into two broad categories: one addresses the effects of physiology (specifically, height) and the other the effects of language or dialect on the vowel formants.

Fitch and Giedd's work (1999) shows that formant frequencies are more closely spaced in taller speakers, because their spacing is inversely related to the vocal tract length. Since cis men tend to be taller, their vocal tracts are typically longer; indeed, they are longer not only absolutely but even relative to height compared with cis women. If we take two speakers of the same height, one who went through puberty as a cis man, and one who passed puberty as a cis woman, the cis man will have a longer supralaryngeal vocal tract and lower, less dispersed vowel formants. The reason for this difference is the pubertal growth spurt combined with an increase in the volume of the pharynx caused by larynx lowering and mandibular angles opening during puberty (Loth & Henneberg, 2000; Vorperian et al., 2005). The supraglottal vocal tract length differences explain the presence of the differences between the formant frequencies of gendered sonorants. However, that cannot fully explain the magnitude of the acoustic differences found.

In addition, behavioral choices must also be considered, as discussed in the pitch section above. Johnson (2006, 2007) brings compelling evidence for humans overriding physiological predisposition, and actively, if subconsciously, shaping their resonance system. For example, even if two speakers identify as the same gender, are of the same height, and speak the same language (i.e., their physiology would predict near-identical resonance systems), the two speakers are able to agentively shape their respective resonance systems in a manner that reflects other facets of their identity, such as ethnicity or sexuality. As a result, the two systems, physiology and behavior, could be potentially overlapping.

Since body height is strongly correlated with vocal tract dimensions (González, 2004; Jessen, 2007; van Dommelen & Moxness, 1995) and cis men are typically taller than cis women in a particular society, a prediction based solely on physiology would expect the resonance differences between genders to be proportionate to the height differences between genders, across all speech communities and languages. In simpler terms, in regions with large average height differences between cis women and men, large differences in F1, F2, and F3 between cis men and women are commonly expected, and vice versa. However, this has not been consistently found across studies. Johnson's (2006, 2007) surveys compared the mean normalized F1, F2, and F3 production of genders across 26 languages and correlated them with population height information. In order to make his results comparable across languages and vowel inventories, he normalized the differences by expressing them on a psycho-acoustic scale, the Bark scale. This is a process similar to expressing differences in the F0 on the perceptually realistic semitone scale (or less frequently, the equivalent rectangular bandwidth [ERB] scale) instead of the linear hertz scale. On the quasi-logarithmic Bark scale, each Bark unit corresponds to the same perceptual distance (Howard &

Angus, 2017). Speakers in no two languages communicated gender differences the same way in Johnson's (2006, 2007) work. In French speakers, he found that individual formants (i.e., F1, F2, and F3) were gendered differently. Namely, F1 showed virtually no difference between cis women and men, and in F2 there was over 1 Bark difference between cis women and men. Norwegian speakers show 1.4 Bark distance in F2 between cis men and women, while a close cognate language, Danish, shows only 0.2 Bark distance in F2 between cis men and women. New Zealand English speakers showed relatively little difference across all three formants between cis women and men, while Californian English showed about twice the difference between cis women and men for all three formants.

From these results, it can be concluded that the distance between cis men and women in a resonant space is not solely a property of a gender or specific speaker vocal tract lengths as much as a property of the particular language variety itself. To sample from Johnson's (2006, 2007) results again, articulatory behavior will predictably bear much more perceptual weight in Norwegian, Californian English, and Polish than in Hungarian, New Zealand English, and Danish. In keeping with these findings, the clinical section of this chapter will demonstrate how height and resonance behavior are taken into account in assessment and therapy.

Testosterone and Resonance Characteristics

An important question remains: Does testosterone shape the vocal tract's resonances? Based on the expectation that transmasculine speakers will not experience laryngeal lowering or a growth spurt associated with cis men's puberty, the implicit assumption

in the literature is that vocal tract resonances will retain their pre-testosterone
values. However, Papp (2011) found that by
the end of the first year on testosterone, all
participants experienced significantly lowered F1–3 formant values. The directional-
ity of the changes indicated that the vocal
tract grew longer even though the participants themselves did not grow taller. As laryngeal lowering and maxillary expansion
were not measured in these subjects, their
physiologic effect on the formant values in
this study cannot be ruled out, nor can the
effects of behavioral changes in the use of
the articulators.

There is some evidence for additional
physiological mechanisms operating in transmasculine people as a function of time on
testosterone, beside the growth spurt and
descent of the larynx observed in cis men,
which are so far undocumented in populations on exogenous testosterone. Antoszewski et al. (2009) indicated that the size
of transmasculine people's maxillary and
mandibular canines and the first molars
measure between those of cis men and cis
women. There is also morphological evidence in Mackenzie and Wilkinson (2017)
that suggests that about 70% of their sample
of transmasculine participants experienced
the widening in the mid-face and a wider
upper jaw, and about half also experienced
a wider lower jaw after three-plus years of
taking testosterone. Anecdotally, the angle
between the posterior part of the mandible
and the lower border of the ramus tends
to change noticeably during transitioning
on testosterone, creating a more masculine
jawline. Some speakers experience the appearance of an Adam's apple (due to either
cartilage growth or loss of adipose tissue),
which may be accompanied by other laryngeal cartilage shifts, growths, or ossification.
All these phenomena indicate that smaller
bony and cartilaginous structures in and

around the vocal tract may remain sensitive
to androgens comparatively late in life.

In addition to physiologic changes to formants, a behavioral influence can be found.
On closer examination of Papp's (2011) data
on formant changes, participants who were
measured past the first-year mark continued
experiencing significant changes in resonance
characteristics in their second and third
years on testosterone, but these changes
moved in the *opposite direction* from the
first year—in other words, less masculine
resonance rather than more masculine. This
pattern applied to each case study speaker,
for virtually every vowel. This phenomenon
can be akin to the fine-tuning of the mean
F0, as seen in the above section on pitch. As
speakers experience the virilizing effects of
testosterone on their whole bodies, the relative importance of having a very (binary)
masculine voicing source, formant resonances, fricative spectra, etc. may become
somewhat diminished. As a result, speakers
selectively shift some of these variables
from more masculine to less masculine in
a less physiologically predictable way, and
instead use variables to express other facets of their identity (e.g., ethnic origin or
sexuality).

Speech, Language, and Non-Verbal Communication

In addition to pitch, resonance, and intonation, a whole host of linguistic and
communication-related variables have been
examined for their weight in the gender percept. These include, but are not limited to,
articulatory precision, loudness, speech rate,
lexical choices, syntactic constructions, discourse pragmatics, facial expressions, eye
contact, gestures, posture, gait, and body
movement. For a whistle-stop summary of

some of the Anglo-centric patterns, the reader is referred to Davies, Papp, and Antoni (2015). The clinical section of this chapter also makes reference to a number of studies from sociolinguistics, speech-language pathology, and gender studies.

To date, no one has successfully described a globally applicable gendered communicative system as such, likely because these systems are even more community dependent and context dependent than the use of largely pre-determined physiological structures above, like the fundamental and formant frequencies. Given this variability, this chapter aims to avoid an inevitably incomplete review of these variables as well as potentially inappropriate generalization of Anglo-centric facts. This is in keeping with WPATH and European Professional Association for Transgender Health (EPATH) recommendations on language use in publications (Bouman et al., 2017). In service to that, a discussion of these variables in North America will only be covered clinically in context. See the clinical section below.

Breathing and Implications for Dysphonia

Some transmasculine individuals wear chest compression clothing or binders to de-emphasize chest size and create a more masculine chest contour. A large-scale research study with 1800 binding participants by Peitzmeier, Gardner, Weinand, Corbet, and Acevedo (2017) found the following compression methods, in order of usage frequency: (a) commercial binders, (b) sports bras, (c) layered shirts, (d) multiple sports bras, (e) elastic or other bandage, (f) athletic compression wear, (g) neoprene compression wear, (h) duct tape or plastic wrap, and (i) assorted homemade solutions. From the list of 28 health concerns that binders

can plausibly cause or exacerbate, participants indicated experiencing: (a) coughing (17.2%), (b) respiratory infections (3.4%), and (c) shortness of breath (46.6%), with half of the participants experiencing at least one of these concerns. The two binding methods with the largest association with shortness of breath were commercial binders and the duct tape/plastic wrap method.

In addition to these complications, obstructive sleep apnea (OSA) can also develop or worsen from using binders at night and from sustained testosterone use. While the link between testosterone and OSA is not well understood, the correlation is borne out by studies on cis men, post-menopausal cis women (e.g., Shahar et al., 2003), individuals with poly-cystic ovarian syndrome (e.g., Fogel et al., 2001), as well as hypogonadal, elderly, or obese cis men who are administered exogenous testosterone (e.g., Killick et al., 2013). The risk of OSA is greater in individuals who are obese, smoke, or have chronic obstructive pulmonary disease (COPD). If left untreated, OSA may have significant adverse effects on the heart, blood pressure, mood, and productivity, and it may cause headaches and worsen seizure disorders.

Most relevantly, disrupted breathing has a potential negative effect for voice. Because proper pulmonary support is necessary for maintaining subglottal pressure, a person's laryngeal valving efficiency, phonational stability, and intensity all depend on breathing freely (Proctor, 1980).

Despite these problems above, wearing binders is non-negotiable for many non-surgical or pre-surgical transmasculine individuals because of their positive effect on mental health and quality of life. For a comprehensive discussion about how to address binders in therapy, see the clinical section of this chapter.

Vocal Satisfaction, Voice-Related Quality of Life, and Need for Intervention

According to the research literature, there is no vocal satisfaction survey published about pitch lowering surgery. As for the available information on the effects of testosterone, research evidence suggests that this androgen brings about lower levels of depression, anxiety, and stress, and higher levels of social support and health-related quality of life. Testosterone use is associated with improved mental health outcomes in trans men (e.g., Meier, Fitzgerald, Pardo, & Babcock, 2011).

Surveys on the vocal satisfaction of transmasculine individuals revealed a number of significant associations between variables: (a) the significantly improved self-perception of voice during the first three months on testosterone is attributable to the taking of testosterone only (Bultynck et al., 2017), as opposed to physiological changes; (b) voice satisfaction correlates with lower F0 values over one year on testosterone (Nygren et al., 2016); and (c) by the end of the first year on testosterone, voice-related quality of life improved as a function of change in the fundamental frequency expressed in semitones (Deuster, Vincenzo, Szukaj, Zehnhoff-Dinnesen, & Dobel, 2016), rather than as a function of the absolute F0 reached (expressed in hertz). In spite of these quality-of-life changes, Cosyns et al. (2014) and Nygren et al. (2016) document 10% and 24% of their respective participants reporting voice symptoms, such as: (a) insufficient pitch lowering, (b) vocal instability, (c) vocal fatigue, (d) pitch range instability, (e) inauthentic age percept, (f) diminished vocal power, (g) vocal quality, and (h) the subsequent need for voice training or voice therapy. Most of the participants in Van Borsel et al. (2000) wished for a slightly different outcome as a result of testosterone therapy. Complaints included: (a) wanting a "heavier" voice, (b) feeling vocal strain when trying to speak in a lower pitch, and (c) wanting a faster and/ or more pronounced voice change overall. In her linguistically and anthropologically oriented doctoral dissertation work, Papp (2011) documented complaints from transitioning transmasculine individuals about mismatched fundamental-resonance structure (sounding too young) and buoyant habitual pitch that did not lower with the pitch floor. Zimman's (2012) interviews shed light on speakers who experienced less than satisfactory pitch lowering as a function of time on testosterone. For a detailed overview of published evidence up to 2017 on transmasculine vocal dissatisfaction, see Azul, Nygren, Södersten, and Neuschaefer-Rube (2017).

The studies cited in this section are only the tip of the iceberg. Transmasculine needs and problems are clearly underreported in research and at clinics, and the training of clinicians and the information disseminated at conferences prioritize transfeminine needs. For an overview of the magnitude of the need and recommendations to better serve this population, see Block (2017) and the clinical section in this chapter.

Summary of the Research

The material presented above serves to inform the clinician about the experiences and needs of transmasculine individuals as well as available options for masculine voice and prognosis for voice change. Though transmasculine research is often overlooked and sorely inadequate, even compared with transfeminine research, there are some major takeaways that can be significantly useful in a clinical context. Before covering a variety of diagnostic and therapeutic issues in the rest of the chapter, here first is a collection of main research points for easy reference:

- Transmasculine individuals' socio-cultural and linguistic identities strongly shape their view of the gendered voice, desired vocal changes, and satisfaction outcomes. Furthermore, these identities potentially change in the course of a changing presentation.
- Though pitch-lowering from testosterone can be sufficient for many transmasculine individuals, it is not currently possible to predict the magnitude or speed of the pitch changes one can expect from sustained testosterone use. Testosterone, in fact, may "under-deliver" relative to one's expectations or needs. False confidence in the masculinizing powers of testosterone may give speakers little motivation to work on other masculine variables in their speech.
- Testosterone may compromise healthy vocal functioning, including vocal range, intensity, and voice quality. Binders can also negatively affect health and potentially the voice.
- There is no one set of norms for masculine voice and communication that applies to all speakers. It depends on linguistic, social, cultural, time, and other factors in context.
- Currently, it is not possible to predict the magnitude of change in F0 as a result of pitch-lowering phonosurgery, and, in addition to voice therapy to maximize outcomes, corrections likely require revision surgery.
- Masculine voice training is recommended with or without pitch lowering from testosterone or phonosurgery, since there are many features of masculine communication, including resonance, intonation, articulation, loudness, speech rate, and non-verbal communication.

Diagnostic Considerations

Clinical work with the transmasculine client begins with a comprehensive assessment of the client's history, skills, and needs. In preparation, the clinician must come armed with ample knowledge of voice disorders, voice care, transgender health, and the common needs of the transgender community (Adler, Hirsch, & Mordaunt, 2012; Coleman et al., 2012; Dacakis, 2012; Davies & Goldberg, 2006; Pickering, Adler, Block, Helou, & Hirsch, 2014). Research and observations that pertain to the common needs of the transmasculine community were discussed in the section above. All of this information empowers the clinician, when conducting an assessment, to anticipate a specific range of possible needs of the transmasculine client. It can also shape the clinician's temperament when facing a client who may have been a victim of discrimination from outside or within the transgender community, or a client who has minimal understanding of the extent to which his needs can be met.

The client may be referred to the voice clinician through a variety of sources, including a transgender health specialist, a member of the transgender community, or himself. The timing of the referral can occur at any point in the person's journey toward a more masculine gender presentation. This is because a person's satisfaction with his voice and communication can vary depending on what gender expression choices he makes, what other gender expression services he seeks, what communication contexts he is involved in, and how his gender expression evolves. As mentioned in the above literature review section, these factors, as they relate to personal satisfaction with voice, can change within a transgender individual's life (Byrne, Dacakis, & Douglas, 2003; Dacakis, 2012) or across individuals. For example, a trans man, after having been on testosterone for years, may want to increase the masculine aspects of his voice as he starts a new vocally demanding job. In contrast, a masculine-identified genderqueer person, who is not on testosterone, may want to explore more masculine vocal expressiveness as he presents more often in public. Regardless of the circumstances that influence the client's needs, the voice clinician should be prepared to assess the person's potential for voice and communication change at the time. In this way, the clinician guides the client to make informed decisions for planning his path toward self-determination (Callen-Lorde Community Health Center, 2015; Coleman et al., 2012; Erickson-Schroth, 2014). Dacakis (2012) and Davies, Papp, and Antoni (2015) recommend a reassessment if there is a lag in time between assessment and therapy to account for any possible changes that may have occurred in the person's gender goals in the interim.

The following paragraphs outline the components of a transgender diagnostic evaluation as applied to the transmasculine client, which can assist the clinician in identifying individual needs for increasing the masculine aspects of voice and communication for the purpose of conversational speech. Because many of the same diagnostic issues apply to any transgender client, the reader is referred to Chapter 7 for additional discussion.

Laryngeal Imaging

Videostroboscopy continues to be the gold standard instrumental exam that is commonly available for visualizing the larynx and assessing vocal function of an individual. This exam, or other laryngeal imaging exams, such as the less available high-speed imaging system, is an essential component of the assessment of the transgender client if the client complains of dysphonia (Dacakis, 2012). As such, it can rule out vocal pathology that is most likely in the form of compensatory hyperfunction from testosterone administration or untrained behavioral manipulation of the voice. Thus, the examiner should pay close attention for supraglottic compression during sustained sounds and connected speech at different pitches.

If the client does not complain of dysphonia, a laryngeal imaging exam can still be used as a screening tool to rule out vocal pathology before therapy begins (Block, 2017). It can also provide an opportunity for teaching vocal anatomy and stressing the importance of vocal health. Changes in vocal fold mass before and with testosterone may be documented when possible. Access to laryngeal imaging often determines whether this approach is done and whether the laryngologist or speech-language pathologist (in consultation with the laryngologist) examines the client. The exam can be performed either before or after the rest of the diagnostic testing, provided that the purpose of each test is explained and rapport begins to develop as early as possible.

Case History

A key opportunity for building trust and establishing rapport with the transmasculine client occurs when taking case history. Asking the right questions in an informed and supportive way not only begins to develop a successful clinical relationship but also allows the clinician to elicit sensitive information that may be difficult for the client to disclose.

Contact Information

At the outset, the clinician should ask the client to identify his name, legal name (if different), and pronoun. The pronoun is likely 'he,' but it may be 'she' until masculine presentation emerges. Alternatively, a client may use a gender non-binary pronoun. The following are some of the more commonly used terms in the community at this time, relative to "he / his / him": "ze / zis / zim," "ve / vis / vim," or "they / their / them," respectively. The client's name and pronoun should be honored and used at all times except at particular times when permitted by the client, such as filing insurance claims when the policy is under the legal name (Simmons & White, 2014). The clinician should also verify that the phone, email, and mailing address are acceptable places to identify him/herself, in order to avoid disclosing voice services or unwittingly outing the client against his wishes.

Gender Expression History

The client's gender expression history, needs, and goals must first be identified before determining how voice and communication fit into that context. This information includes: (a) gender identity; (b) history of gender dysphoria; (c) history or upcoming plans of gender expression services that may have an impact on voice and communication, including psychotherapy, testosterone administration, chest compression clothing, chest reconstruction surgery, phonosurgery, legal services for name change, or other; and (d) history or upcoming contexts for the changing gender presentation, including where and to whom he has disclosed his identity, and how long, how

often, and in what contexts the person presents in a more masculine way.

When eliciting this information, the clinician should avoid assuming the answers to any questions, keeping in mind that there is no one way to transition or increase masculine aspects of gender expression (Antoni, 2015; Azul, 2015; Block, 2017; Coleman et al., 2012; Erickson-Schroth, 2014). Asking a trans man about his gender identity may seem unnecessary, but the client may have a specific cognitive interpretation of his masculinity—binary masculine, non-binary masculine, masculine genderqueer, or something else along the gender spectrum. This interpretation will be important for establishing how much of a voice change he needs. Similarly, the client may be able to specifically identify how much mental distress he has regarding a mismatch between gender identity and sex characteristics, and how that may have changed with psychotherapy or other transition services. The client may have more distress than he is willing or able to reveal in an initial interview, or he may have minimal or no mental distress at all. Knowing the extent of the client's dysphoria, the clinician can better predict whether psychosocial factors will affect his motivation in therapy.

Voice and Communication Complaints and Objectives

Once the gender expression history is disclosed, the clinician is ready to ask specific questions about the client's particular voice and communication needs for a more masculine gender presentation. This includes: (a) congruency of voice and communication with gender identity; (b) the impact of that (limited) congruency on social and professional activities; (c) previous attempts to communicate in a more masculine way;

(d) the role and timing of voice and communication in transition, such as coordination with hormone replacement therapy (HRT) or a coming out date; and (e) his overall goal(s) for working on voice and communication (Azul, 2015; Dacakis, 2012; Davies et al., 2015).

How clearly the client articulates this important information depends on the careful construction of the clinician's questions. Queries such as "How does voice fit in with gender expression?" "How do you feel about the sound of your voice?" or "What kind of masculine communicator do you envision yourself being?" can specify issues that the client may or may not have already considered fully. The client is likely primarily concerned about being gendered correctly by others, or in other words, be recognized as male. He may also have safety concerns related to voice or a great distaste for the sound of his voice, whether interacting with others or not (i.e., voice dysphoria). Issues such as these can inform goal setting and the role of vocal experimentation in therapy. Specific masculine voice complaints may include insufficient lowering of pitch with testosterone, sounding too young, difficulty speaking loudly, or difficulty being expressive.

Vocal health complaints may be the primary or even sole reason for seeking professional help. These may include dysphonia from testosterone, pitch-lowering phonosurgery, or attempts to manipulate the voice with or without testosterone, as discussed earlier in this chapter. Symptoms may include hoarseness, throat discomfort, vocal instability, reduced loudness level, voice fatigue, or vocal strain.

General vocal use questions are also covered, as with any voice patient, such as social and professional vocal demands, potential phonotraumatic behaviors (see Chapter 8 for further information), previous voice problems, and previous professional voice training (Andrews, 1999). These questions can uncover any dysphonia or vocal production knowledge that could influence therapy.

Social History

The client's social history can reveal factors that could affect progress toward his goals. For example, the client's living situation directly determines his opportunity to practice voice and speech exercises in comfort. He may cohabitate with someone who supports his journey, who doesn't support his journey, or who doesn't know about his gender identity. More generally, the client's overall level of personal support and integration in the transgender community can affect his level of stress and resilience throughout the therapy process. Before eliciting this information, the clinician should first explain the relevance of questions of this nature.

Medical History

A thorough medical history of the transmasculine client should be taken as with any voice patient, including, but not limited to, medical conditions, medications, and dietary risks for laryngopharyngeal reflux (Andrews, 1999). Particularly relevant information includes: (a) the possible administration of testosterone, including timeline and dosing; (b) history of depression or other mental distress related or not related to gender identity; (c) history of smoking; and (d) history of obstructive sleep apnea, daytime sleepiness, or snoring. In addition, height and weight (body mass index [BMI]) in relation to a gross observation of the size of the head and neck are relevant. For a discussion of this, see the sections on resonance and dysphonia below.

Perceptual Observations and Instrumental Measurements of Voice and Speech

During the case history, the clinician likely has already made some general observations of the client's voice and communication skills. The assessment then proceeds to more specific observations and measurements of the client's voice and speech in order to establish evidence for ruling out dysphonia and identifying gender markers as they relate to the client's particular masculine gender identity. In doing so, the clinician conducts diagnostic tasks for a typical clinical voice evaluation such that the client's current performance is compared with both the non-disordered patterns and gender markers of a cis man of a similar age and size (Dacakis, 2012). This information should suggest how well the client likely functions in daily life and how much potential he has for therapy, as it would with any client across the gender spectrum (Dacakis, 2012; Davies et al., 2015; Oates & Dacakis, 1997). The testing also provides a critical baseline for gauging progress in therapy (Andrews, 1999; King, Lindstedt, Jensen, & Law, 1999).

As in any clinical voice evaluation, the clinician takes audio samples of voice and speech during sustained sounds, reading, and spontaneous speech. If the client is comfortable, video samples may also be taken. In addition to doing tasks in the habitual voice, the client can be asked to read and speak spontaneously in "a more masculine way." This directive assists in determining potential hyperfunction, intuition about masculine communication, shyness when experimenting with voice, and potential for change. Because of this, it can serve as an early teaching moment for demonstrating to the client his pre-existing skills and exposing any initial self-impressions about working on his voice.

In this process, the clinician can focus their perceptual observations on speech and voice parameters, namely, pitch, intonation, resonance, vocal quality, loudness level, articulation, and speech rate. Observations may also target language parameters such as syntax, word choice, conversation style, and non-verbal communication. Azul et al. (2017), Davies et al. (2015), Freidenberg (2002), Oates and Dacakis (1997), and Pickering and Baker (2012) provide research reviews of how these parameters apply as gender markers for transgender individuals. In order to judge the client's performance on these parameters in an accurate and objective manner, the clinician must also have knowledge of culture-specific research about speech and voice norms of cisgender people, expected gender roles in communication, and various factors that are known to shape gender perception in communication, such as socioeconomic status, region, age, ethnicity, and power differences between the sexes. In addition to the above section of this chapter, literature reviews and seminal studies from speech science, sociolinguistics, and gender studies for the North American context include: Andrews (1999), Briton and Hall (1995), Cameron (2008), Coates (2004), Coleman (1976), Eckert (1989), Lakoff (2004), McConnell-Ginet (1988), Miller, Schutte, and Sulter, (1996), Mondorf (2002), Smith and Patterson (2005), and Titze (1989). These context-specific norms should not be used to make prescriptive judgments, but rather to compare with the client's view of his form of masculinity and thus inform prognosis for improving voice satisfaction. Particular sensitivity in this respect is required, since the literature shows (as discussed in the literature section above) that many transmasculine speakers are fundamentally uninterested in taking on linguistic expressions of normative masculinity. Nevertheless, even if the client does not eventually want to adopt a particular masculine feature, he will likely want to know how his production relates to applicable norms.

To further investigate the current level of client satisfaction and vocal health, the clinician, in addition to taking a case history, can also use vocal quality scales and client self-evaluation questionnaires to gather supplemental subjective judgments of the client's voice. Some commonly used items include the Consensus Auditory-Perceptual Evaluation of Voice (CAPE-V), the Voice Handicap Index-10, and the Voice-Related Quality of Life (V-RQOL) (American Speech-Language-Hearing Association, 2002; Hogikyan & Sethuraman, 1999; Rosen, Lee, Osborne, Zullo, & Murry, 2004). Though self-reporting survey studies on trans men have been conducted (see the literature review above), there currently is no clinical self-report measure that has been specifically designed for transmasculine individuals to appropriately investigate their vocal function and use. The clinician should avoid the impulse to use the Transsexual Voice Questionnaire (TVQ^{MtF}) by simply changing the gender markers in the items (Dacakis, Davies, Oates, Douglas, & Johnston, 2013). Dacakis argues in Chapter 7 that a new questionnaire needs to be developed from scratch and be psychometrically validated, with direct input from trans men, in order to capture transmasculine experiences that are unique from those of trans women. The reader is referred to Chapter 7 for further discussion.

In addition to perceptual judgments, acoustic measurements of speech and voice should be taken. These include: (a) mean fundamental frequency (F0); (b) mean conversational frequency range; (c) maximum phonation frequency range (of which the minimum pitch serves as the "pitch floor" mentioned in the literature review section above); and (d) mean intensity (Andrews, 1999; Baken & Orlikoff, 2000; Davies et al.,

2015). Other acoustic, aerodynamic, and electroglottographic measurements can be taken, when possible, to form a more comprehensive profile. Some may include mean cepstral peak prominence, cepstral/spectral index of dysphonia, a phonetogram, vowel formant measurements, perturbation, maximum phonation time, mean peak air pressure, mean expiratory airflow, closed quotient, or others (Andrews, 1999; Baken & Orlikoff, 2000; Davies et al., 2015; Mehta & Hillman, 2008; Peterson, Roy, Awan, Merrill, Banks, & Tanner, 2013; Sulter, Wit, Schutte, & Miller, 1994). In addition, forced expiratory volume and forced vital capacity measures, which are typically done by pulmonologists and allergists, could be done with and without a binder when possible.

Overall, the clinician can expect that perceptual observations and measurements may show, among other things, any of the following typical transmasculine patterns, as mentioned previously in this chapter: (a) pitch that is insufficiently low, with or without testosterone, (b) pitch variation that is either too monotone or too high when the client attempts to be expressive, (c) reduced maximum phonation frequency range, with or without testosterone, (d) resonance that is too "bright" or "small," resulting in sounding younger or more feminine regardless of possibly lower pitch, (e) difficulty speaking loudly in a lower pitch, (f) hoarseness, (g) vocal strain, or (h) harsh vocal onset. Later in this chapter, possible interventions for these problems will be discussed.

Diagnostic Therapy Tasks and Candidacy for Therapy

As the clinician advances to diagnostic therapy tasks, they synthesize the client's responsiveness with all of the information gathered so far to determine potential and readiness for therapy. In addition to previously asking the client to speak "in a more masculine way," the clinician can now help the client through modeling and audiovisual feedback to elicit pitch, resonance, or other target areas. Following the broad therapy objectives of improving and/or maintaining vocal health and client satisfaction, the clinician determines whether the client is a candidate for therapy. In general terms, he is eligible if he shows sufficient responsiveness to these tasks, has sufficient motivation, and has the opportunity to practice his new speaking skills, and use those skills, at least to a minimal extent, in daily life. The extent of these factors in relation to the client's current skills and physical qualities then shape prognosis with respect to the client's needs. As the clinician discusses next steps, they should send a clear message regarding realistic expectations, scheduling, and commitment while also reassuring him of the importance and relative changeability of his skills. This reassurance is typically necessary to begin empowering a client who is likely resigned to receiving relatively limited attention in the speech pathology field, the trans health community, and society at large (Adler et al., 2012; Azul, Nygren, Sodersten, & Neuschaefer-Rube, 2017; Block, 2017; Davies et al., 2015).

Therapeutic Considerations

When embarking on a therapy program to help the transmasculine client develop communication skills that are congruent with his gender identity, the clinician needs to carefully integrate the training of masculine skills with vocal health objectives and ample counseling. The following section explores how to proceed in this way in a Standard American English context, including some sample exercises.

Masculine Voice and Communication Skills

As the clinician approaches masculine training, they fully consider the client's desires, needs, and potential. In doing so, they should prioritize training targets on what makes the biggest difference first, since the client's quality-of-life needs are immediate. In this way, training can minimize, as soon as possible, any negative attention to the client's communication, either from himself or others, that may disrupt his daily activities. In addition, the clinician is faced with the difficult task of helping a client develop a unique skill set that nevertheless conforms, to a certain extent, to what is known or expected in social interactions. To do this, the clinician, first and foremost, should employ their knowledge of the locally relevant research while also navigating cultural stereotypes upon which the client may be relying and being judged against by others.

The following paragraphs are presented, in order, as the most essential and common voice and communication targets for increasing masculine aspects of conversational speech. They can serve as a short menu of possible technical skills from which to choose when working with the transmasculine client. This menu is by no means comprehensive, and does not include a full discussion of gender norms. For more background, see the literature review above and various citations in this clinical section of the chapter. Other chapters of this book, which primarily focus on transfeminine voice and communication, offer information about gender norms and communication of transgender individuals, which the reader may use to develop further ideas for working with the transmasculine client. For a discussion of singing for the transmasculine client, see Chapter 14.

Pitch

Even though pitch alone does not fully or sufficiently mark gender in voice, it is the most important factor for doing so (Freidenberg, 2002; Gelfer & Mordaunt, 2012; Gelfer & Schofield, 2000). While the transmasculine client is likely to be taking testosterone that results in sufficiently lower pitch, there are a number of cases where pitch can be a primary issue, namely, if: (a) the client has not chosen to, not yet chosen to, or cannot undergo testosterone administration; (b) the client is in the beginning stages of testosterone administration; or (c) pitch-lowering from testosterone is insufficient or behaviorally counteracted (Cosyns et al., 2014; Damrose, 2009; Papp, 2011; Talaat, Talaat, Kelada, Angelo, Elwany, & Thabert, 1987). In these cases, behavioral training of a lower average conversational pitch (F0) can be important (Davies et al., 2015; Nygren, 2014). For this purpose, the clinician must choose an appropriate target pitch. Currently, there are no studies that indicate an average conversational pitch at which transmasculine individuals can be recognized as male, so the clinician must rely on data about cisgender people and transgender women. Wolfe, Rutusnik, Smith, and Northrop (1990), Spencer (1988), and Gelfer and Schofield (2000) report that the lowest pitch at which their American-English-speaking transfeminine subjects were recognized as female was 155, 160, and 164 Hz, respectively. Wolfe et al. (1990) report their next lowest pitch at 145 Hz, which was perceived as male. Gorham-Rowan and Morris (2006) report as high as 174 Hz as a pitch at which their transfeminine subjects were judged as more masculine compared with subjects with a pitch of 180 Hz or higher. Based on these findings, target pitches of D3, D#3 or E3 (147–165 Hz) may be good choices for training a trans-

masculine client in North America, if the client's pitch is not already lower than that from testosterone. These pitches should significantly increase the client's ability to be perceived as masculine, or, at the very least, more masculine than feminine.

In addition, the target pitch must ensure that there is no hyperfunction, glottal fry, or decreased loudness level during connected speech (Stemple, Glaze, & Klaben, 2010). To ensure comfort for the transfeminine client, Gelfer and Mordaunt (2012) suggest choosing a conversational range of 12 semitones, calculated from an average target pitch, which falls within a total 24-semitone range for cisgender men. In this way, a conversational pitch range can be calculated for the transmasculine client. For example, if the target average pitch is D3 (147 Hz), the range would be A2–G#3 (110–208 Hz). This range can facilitate the avoidance of dysphonia, as it falls within the low end of a total cisfeminine conversational range of A2–G#4 (110–416 Hz), based on an average of 220 Hz. In addition, this range is likely to be perceived as masculine, given that it falls within a total cismasculine conversational range of B1–B3 (62–247 Hz), based on an average of 124 Hz. Figure 9–1 shows the overlap of these ranges.

Figure 9–1 also illustrates that there is some leeway at the high end of the cismasculine range for increasing the target average and/or conversational range. The reader is reminded that these ranges apply to a Standard American English context and are one possible set of examples.

To begin the training process, the clinician can elicit a sustained sound, such as "hmm" or "molm," by modeling a target pitch, playing the pitch with a guitar tuner, piano, smartphone app, or other device, or visually showing the pitch with pitch-tracking software (for example, Real-Time Pitch by KayPentax or VoicePrint from Estill Voice

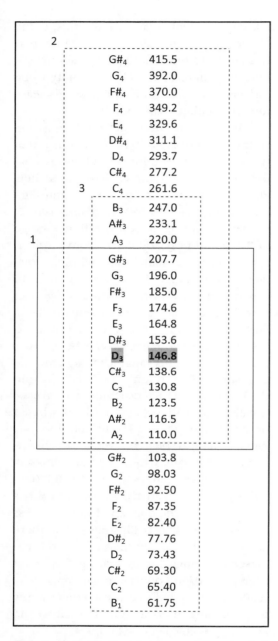

	G#$_4$	415.5
	G$_4$	392.0
	F#$_4$	370.0
	F$_4$	349.2
	E$_4$	329.6
	D#$_4$	311.1
	D$_4$	293.7
	C#$_4$	277.2
	C$_4$	261.6
	B$_3$	247.0
	A#$_3$	233.1
	A$_3$	220.0
	G#$_3$	207.7
	G$_3$	196.0
	F#$_3$	185.0
	F$_3$	174.6
	E$_3$	164.8
	D#$_3$	153.6
	D$_3$	**146.8**
	C#$_3$	138.6
	C$_3$	130.8
	B$_2$	123.5
	A#$_2$	116.5
	A$_2$	110.0
	G#$_2$	103.8
	G$_2$	98.03
	F#$_2$	92.50
	F$_2$	87.35
	E$_2$	82.40
	D#$_2$	77.76
	D$_2$	73.43
	C#$_2$	69.30
	C$_2$	65.40
	B$_1$	61.75

Figure 9–1. (1) Target transmasculine comfortable conversational range = A2–G#3 (110–208 Hz), 12 semitones, based on D3 (147 Hz) average. (2) Cisfeminine total conversational range = A2–G#4 (110–416 Hz), 24 semitones, based on A3 (220 Hz) average. (3) Cismasculine total conversational range = B1–B3 (62–247 Hz), 24 semitones, based on B2 (124 Hz) average.

International Inc.). For the client who is unresponsive to these tools, a countdown task can be useful, such that the client counts from three to one by intuitively making each number lower than the previous one. Once a lower pitch is achieved at the syllable level, the client can advance to phrases and sentences with a chant-to-speech exercise (Block, 2013) (see the section of sample exercises below). At the paragraph level, the client can attempt to maintain a lower pitch by thinking 'low' at the beginning of every phrase. For this, marking the phrases of a text with slashes can be helpful. As the client becomes more proficient in reading and spontaneous speech, he can benefit from audio and visual cues, such as hearing a target note that is played periodically as necessary or seeing pitch tracking software running on a computer in the background. Currently, there are no known smartphone apps that track pitch in connected speech in a reliable and user-friendly way.

A less direct approach to pitch may be more appropriate when the client is just starting to undergo testosterone administration and will reasonably be expected to experience some pitch lowering. In this case, the clinician can incorporate appropriately lower pitches into exercises that address other parameters, such as resonance.

Resonance

Resonance is typically the primary focus in transmasculine voice training, regardless of whether pitch work is required. This is due to a common transmasculine complaint of sounding "too feminine" or "too young," even when pitch is sufficiently lowered (Block, 2017). These percepts correspond to a classic transmasculine resonance, so to speak, that results from smaller laryngeal and upper airway cavities, particularly in the presence of lower pitch from large vocal fold mass as an effect of testosterone (Constansis, 2008; Cosyns, 2014; Damrose, 2009; Talaat et al., 1987) (see the literature review section above). This smaller supralaryngeal resonance chamber can, but not always, be influenced by reduced height relative to cis men. Increased weight (as measured with BMI), which can occur with testosterone, can also reduce the pharyngeal space. Luckily, as discussed in the literature section above, conscious and unconscious behavioral choices can shape the resonance system in a way that can balance or even override physiology. Thus, resonance work can help to address this transmasculine complaint of sounding "too feminine" or "too young," whether to compensate for a smaller resonance space and/or higher pitch range, or to further masculinize a voice that is already in an appropriately lower range.

Based on cisgender resonance patterns of Standard American English speakers (see the literature review section above), a useful approach to masculine resonance for an American client is to develop a "bigger," "darker," or richer tone by increasing open oral resonance. One way to achieve this is to increase articulatory excursion with a technique called "open mouth," in which the clinician instructs the client to open and move his mouth more, focusing on dropping the jaw. Another technique, called "open throat," can further increase open oral resonance by carrying the base-of-tongue (BOT) lower and farther back in the mouth, and raising the soft palate. This "open throat" technique is less intuitive for the client, so facilitation tasks may be necessary, such as: (a) a yawn-sigh ("ha!"); (b) imagining holding a ping-pong ball in the throat while producing a sound ("ah!"); (c) a Santa Claus–like "ho-ho-ho!" bellow; (d) producing opera-like "ha-ha-ha" sounds; or (e) making a sobbing sound (Klimek, 2014). In addition, the client can practice

three progressive stages of "open throat," from baseline (not open enough), to 'middle' posture (target), to yawn-stretch (too open). This exercise provides good negative practice for establishing a new, relaxed "open throat" posture during rest and speech. The "open mouth" and "open throat" techniques can be integrated with loudness level for a progressively "bigger" tone at the word, automatic speech, and phrase levels (Block, 2013) (see the section of sample exercises below). Exercises that utilize utterances and texts that contain low and back vowels, such as /a/ and /o/, are particularly useful before moving to more difficult high and front vowels, such as /i/ and /u/ /m/, and /n/ sounds can also be incorporated to avoid hyperfunction at the level of the larynx.

Chest resonance can also be targeted to achieve a 'heavier' or more masculine tone. The clinician should introduce this area with exercises for progressive relaxation and postural alignment of the head, neck, and shoulders to prevent tension in the upper body. Then, a series of exercises can be conducted to promote awareness of vibration and energy of the voice in the chest, such as producing sustained sounds with an open chest posture, with one hand on the back of a chair and one on the chest. The client can also learn to notice varying levels of a lowering laryngeal position in the neck during sustained sounds with different vowels. Once awareness and accuracy are established during sustained sounds, exercises can progress to words, phrases, and sentences.

Intonation

Intonation can also be an important target for achieving a more masculine voice. While the Pitch section above addressed how to establish a target average pitch and comfortable conversational pitch range, intonation training involves teaching various pitch contours and prosodic techniques within an established range, whether that range was naturally achieved with testosterone or artificially calculated for pitch training.

One important pitch contour in Standard American English, though not necessarily in other languages or dialects of English (see the literature review section above), is frequent downward pitch movement at the ends of utterances. This is to avoid what has been shown to be, in some contexts, a feminine intonation pattern that goes upward more often (Gelfer & Mordaunt, 2012; Gelfer & Schofield, 2000; Wolfe et al., 1990). The client can fortify this pattern with repetitive practice of single utterances, starting first with a list of common semantic pairs with identical syllabic and stress patterns, such as "black and white" and "on and off," and advancing to a list of declarative sentences such as "I'll see you tomorrow at 7:00 pm." More challenging are question-word questions. For example, wh- questions in English can end in a higher or a lower pitch, such as "Who is coming to the meeting?" or "What is your favorite food?"

Additional techniques apply when expressiveness is a particular concern. Specifically, the client may use inappropriately high pitch when being expressive. Alternatively, he may be speaking in a quieter and more monotone pattern, resulting in feeling insufficiently expressive or friendly. This pattern is a result of: (a) the client purposely dampening higher pitch movement in order to avoid sounding feminine; and/or (b) the client speaking at an uncomfortably low pitch range that limits loudness level and low pitch movement. To address this problem, the client can be taught different ways to be expressive while staying within an appropriate pitch range. The focus, then, would be on a maximum reference pitch—in other words, the top end of a comfortable conversational pitch range. This can be introduced to the client visually on a computer screen. The location of this pitch will depend on the location of the client's average pitch, lowered by testosterone, or where he is being trained to speak on average. For example, the client who is aiming for an average pitch of D3 (147 Hz) will try to stay within G#3 (208 Hz) for a comfortable 12-semitone range or even up to B3 (247 Hz), which is the high end of the total pitch range for cisgender men (see Figure 9–1). Showing a reference line at the maximum pitch, the clinician then trains the client on prosodic patterns below that maximum pitch. The patterns, namely, are productions of longer and louder syllables, which Standard American English speakers regularly use to stress words and ideas (Celce-Murcia, Brinton, & Goodwin, 1996). For example, the client practices an expressive utterance such as "That's unbelievable!" so that the third syllable of "unbelievable" is lengthened and/or louder rather than excessively high or higher than the maximum reference pitch. As the third syllable is lengthened or louder, the pitch can also quickly drop on that syllable for a more staccato-like or heavy effect. In this vein, the client can experiment with multiple ways of saying the same utterance in order to practice variations of expressiveness and emotions (see the sample exercises section below). Stretching a rubber band during a stressed syllable can be a useful facilitation task to notice vowel lengthening. At more advanced levels, the client can talk about topics that invite expressiveness or strong opinions, such as talking to a baby or a pet, or talking about a pet peeve.

Speech, Language, and Non-Verbal Communication

Non-voice linguistic parameters—speech rate, articulation, loudness level, syntax, semantics, pragmatics, body language—are typically secondary issues for the transmasculine client as for any transgender client, because they contain less salient gender markers compared with voice. This is likely due to there being more variation within and across individuals that is influenced by factors such as socioeconomic class, region, linguistic context, social context, culture, and/or age (Azul, 2015; Coates, 2004; Cameron, 2008) (see the discussion in the literature section above). Research in this area is, by design, very context specific, and stereotypes are often wrongly applied by non-researchers across a wider range of individuals and contexts. To avoid this, the clinician should carefully focus training on the client's specific interests and needs in a culturally appropriate context (Davies et al., 2015; see the literature review section earlier in this chapter) and avoid perpetuation of linguistic myths and sexism whenever possible. Below is a brief discussion of two of the most common areas for which the transmasculine client may need assistance, namely loudness level and workplace conversation style or discourse pragmatics.

Loudness level is a training target, regardless of testosterone administration, when the transmasculine client is speaking too quietly. This can affect the client's ability to be gendered correctly as masculine, since research shows that cisgender men speak more loudly than cisgender women (Baken & Orlikoff, 2000; Yanagihara, Koike, & von Leden, 1966), and since quiet talking can also hinder masculine resonance and expressiveness, as discussed above. Furthermore, quiet talking can affect the client's ability to be effective in contexts that require louder speech. Training can naturally be integrated into voice work that addresses efficient vocal production, particularly if the client is managing increased vocal fold mass from testosterone. The clinician may use standard voice therapy tasks with sustained sounds, such as a messa di voce vocalization or straw work (Titze, 2010), to control loudness level with proper breath control and breath support. When facilitating awareness of diaphragmatic breathing, such as putting one's hand on the abdomen to notice movement relative to the chest, the clinician should remain keenly aware of the presence of a binder or other compressive clothing that the client may be wearing. For additional discussion, see the literature review and dysphonia sections of this chapter. After sustained sounds, the client then can progress to words, phrases, and sentences. This can be done by repeating each item at varying loudness levels while avoiding overdriving or overthinking of inhalation. In addition, the clinician may combine loudness level with pitch work. Specifically, the clinician can visually display a maximum pitch to help the client be sufficiently loud within a target pitch range. Exercises that address resonance and intonation also can incorporate loudness level, as discussed in the above paragraphs. Lastly, the client can practice loudness level with particular phrases, sentences, and paragraphs that address safety and emotional health, such as yelling "Help!" or "No!" or reading the empowering poem "Posture" by Maureen Owen (Owen, 1996). This is particularly useful for the client who is speaking quietly because of shyness or clinical depression related to gender dysphoria.

Discourse pragmatics can be another area of masculine training in some cases. For example, the client may work in an environment that values a direct conversation style, and thus he may want and/or need to (further) develop such a style in that context. When approaching this issue, the clinician should not assume that a direct conversation style is a proven behavior in men in general, throughout one culture or across cultures, even though it is an active stereotype from which the client is judged by others. In fact, Deborah Cameron (2008) argues that men and women have been shown to both use various kinds of conversation styles—direct, cooperative, and others—depending on the situation. Thus, it is better for the clinician to focus very specifically on how to adapt as needed to the nature of the client's particular professional context. Training a more direct conversation style in Standard American English can typically be done in two ways, namely, varying word choice and using fewer words. One useful exercise is to instruct the client to formulate sentences for the workplace that convey the same meaning in a direct versus indirect way. For example, to disagree with a colleague, one could use a more direct, declarative statement, such as "I think there is a better way to do that" or use an indirect interrogative statement, such as "Are you sure you want to do it that way?" (Searle, 1970). Another example is interrupting one's boss, for which one could use fewer words, as in "Got a minute?" as opposed to using more words, as in "Could I talk to you for a minute?" The client can experiment in these ways, using specific workplace role-playing while making intuitive judgments regarding length, directness, and politeness of an utterance. The clinician should keep in mind that using fewer words in order to speak directly does not mean that the client must or should speak less about a topic, i.e., take shorter or fewer conversation turns. The client indeed may be given more time and attention to speak as a man with higher status in the workplace (Cameron, 2008; James & Drakich,

1993). The client should be encouraged to talk more without compromising the ability of others to do so as well.

In addition to training the client for speaking in a work environment, the clinician may need to address any of a myriad of other social contexts that prove to be challenging in the client's daily life. Careful self-observation and analysis can be useful in helping the client understand his own communication behavior in context, how his behavior relates to his other identities such as age, race, or region, and how his beliefs and behavior may change as his gender presentation changes. This awareness can, in turn, lead to communication skills that are not only more successful but also more culturally responsible. In an unpublished study entitled "Interview with Transmasculine Clients about Cultural Humility and Cultural Competence," Adler (2014) applied ASHA's mission of promoting cultural humility and cultural competence in speech-language pathologists to transmasculine clients themselves (ASHA, 2017). How can a transmasculine client understand and respectfully respond to the unique combination of cultural variables that he and his listeners bring to interactions (ASHA, 2017; Riquelme, 2013)? Through counseling and observations in daily situations, clients considered, among other things, how their thoughts and actions changed under a new set of masculine cultural demands and how they can communicate respectfully to others while being true to themselves. See the section of sample exercises below for further discussion of the study and an exercise based on it.

Dysphonia

In accordance with SOC7 of WPATH (Coleman et al., 2012), the clinician should address any pre-existing dysphonia before starting masculine training. Signs of dysphonia, such as hoarseness, vocal strain, vocal fatigue, reduced pitch range, or harsh vocal onset, can be expected from testosterone administration or from attempts to speak more masculine, as discussed earlier in this chapter. Possible weight gain from testosterone may also limit breath control. In addition, in compliance with post-surgical voice care (Coleman et al., 2012; Neumann & Welzel, 2004), the clinician should implement rehabilitative voice therapy immediately after pitch-lowering surgery to maximize and speed recovery. Standard rehabilitative voice therapy practices can be used to address dysphonia or post-surgical voice. Some include: (a) perceptual-motor learning principles (Titze & Verdolini-Abbot, 2012); (b) semi-occluded vocal tract techniques (Verdolini-Marston, Burke, Lessac, Glaze, & Calwell, 1995); (c) Vocal Function Exercises (Stemple, Lee, D'Amico, & Pickup, 1994); (d) stretch-and-flow phonation exercises (Watts, Diviney, Hamilton, Toles, Childs, & Mau, 2015); and (e) Estill figures for voice (Klimek, 2014). See the sample exercises section below and in Chapter 8 for some examples.

In addition to behavioral voice use and post-surgical voice, the wearing of binders or other compressive clothing may be associated with complaints of dysphonia. These include, as mentioned earlier in this chapter, reduced breath support and control, and musculoskeletal tension in the chest, neck, and shoulders. Instructions are readily available regarding proper fitting and use of binders, including avoiding wearing the binder an entire day (Reynolds & Goldstein, 2014). If the client is having complications, he may be willing to try a better-fitting binder or further limit wearing the binder in private. However, to prevent an increase in gender dysphoria, the clinician should not require that the client do so,

particularly when in public or in session, except in severe cases. Instead, the clinician should proceed with rehabilitation and masculine training with the binder in place. If the binder is confined to the chest, the clinician can guide the client to increase breath support by focusing on expansion and contraction of the abdomen below the binder while limiting it in the chest. However, if that is difficult for the client, or if the binder extends below the chest, then breath support will need to be addressed through negative practice, in other words, guiding the client to understand his limits of chest and abdominal expansion. From there, breath control exercises can be done within those limits. Some include rhythmic breathing, resistance breathing, maximum phonation time, utterances that increase in length, or stretch-and-flow phonation (Watts et al., 2015). The clinician can also provide compensatory strategies such as speaking with shorter breath groups, using proper posture, and getting up every 30 minutes when sitting for long periods. The client may be willing to do exercises at home when taking the binder off at the end of the day. In that case, he can be instructed to do any of the exercises mentioned above while focusing on further expansion of the chest cavity in order to further improve breathing and reduce tension. Additional intervention measures for tension include upper body stretches and self-massage, such as arm swings and palpation of the armpits, clavicle, and underside of the ribs (Reed, 2014).

Once dysphonia has been sufficiently addressed, or if dysphonia was never present, masculine voice training should progress in a manner that prevents dysphonia (Coleman et al., 2012; Davies et al., 2015). The clinician should integrate masculine training techniques with standard voice therapy practices to develop a healthy framework to develop a more masculine presentation. This can be done by including vocal warm-up exercises at the beginning of masculine voice practice routine and by being attentive to any sign of dysphonia as training is executed. In addition, the clinician can employ negative practice, in which the client performs a masculine technique that is hyperfunctional versus healthy. For example, the client can practice speaking too low, resulting in hoarseness or vocal strain, versus sufficiently low, without hoarseness or vocal strain. For further discussion of vocal health with the transgender client, see Chapter 8.

Therapy Progression and Counseling

Therapy with the transmasculine client typically progresses with frequent sessions, once per week, as with any voice client (Adler et al., 2012). As the clinician targets specific techniques, they use functional goals to set a framework for success in situations in which the client presents in a masculine way. As with any voice client, the clinician implements functional home practice exercises and real-life interactions during which the client tries to be mindful of his new techniques (Adams, 1971). It is important to frequently ask for updates from the client regarding presentation and transition activities in order to stay abreast of changing speaking contexts, effects on scheduling, or changes to his body that may influence communication, such as binding or mastectomy, which may cause upper body tension (Dacakis, 2012). Armed with information from the client, the clinician should continually consider various factors—mental, logistical, and societal—that may affect why and how the client's technical skills

are progressing in the way they are (Azul, 2015). Mental or psychological factors significantly influence therapy. This is mainly because gender identity shapes the goals and direction of therapy, which can shift within a therapy period. In addition, the client's emotional and functional needs may be heightened, since voice and identity have significant social consequences. Furthermore, the client's motivation in therapy may be diminished by depression and anxiety associated with gender dysphoria, transphobia in his community, internalized transphobia, or side effects from testosterone, such as weight gain and acne (Hembree et al., 2009). See Chapters 2 and 3, as well as Erickson-Schroth (2014) for a discussion of various psychosocial issues that impact transgender people.

If the client is not under the care of a mental health provider and he shows recurring signs of depression, anxiety, or other psychological issues, the clinician should refer him to one (Holland & Nelson, 2014), preferably a mental health provider who is a transgender specialist. However, the clinician, as with any voice client, should not shy away from discussing the client's feelings about his voice and communication skills. In fact, counseling is a critical part of successful therapy with the transmasculine client, as it directly addresses the link between voice and identity and ultimately to satisfaction with his voice. Counseling should begin in general terms by reviewing clinical expectations related to the effects of testosterone on the voice, the nature of behavioral training, and results from pitch-lowering surgery. Then, as the client develops technical skills, the clinician should facilitate an ongoing discussion of the client's mind–body connection to help him psychologically identify with those skills. This discussion will likely take on a more primary role as therapy progresses. Counseling issues that involve the mind–body connection, which can apply to any transgender client, have been discussed by Adler (2017), Block (2017), and Block, Langer, and Lipson (2016). Five primary themes will be introduced below, namely, identity development, inner versus outer voice, risk-taking, empowerment, and self-acceptance. For a more in-depth discussion of counseling issues, see Chapter 3.

Identity development lies at the heart of voice training for the transmasculine client. It is directly affected by how developed his gender identity already is as he embarks on voice work. Though the client will likely be clear about his masculine identity, voice work can help him to associate the kind of masculinity he feels and evokes through voice and communication, which can solidify as his skills develop. On the other hand, the client may be less clear about his identity when starting voice work, using it to check his feelings and decide whether to move forward with other transition activities that are irreversible. As the clinician guides the client in developing technical skills, they should regularly ask the client what he likes and doesn't like and why, with the goal of the client eventually 'owning' his best possible voice to the extent to be able to say "this is my voice" to himself and others. That takes a leap of faith with significant trust in the clinician. This trust must be built through continual respect of the client's interests in negotiation with what is possible.

When attempting to develop voice along with identity, the clinician facilitates experimentation and practice through a direct discussion of the inner voice versus the outer voice, in other words, his mental thoughts and authentic self versus his spoken thoughts and vocal expression. In doing so, the clinician helps the client tune into acoustic, proprioceptive, and interoceptive

aspects of the voice so that he can identify what changes he can relate to and feel positively about. The client may experience great difficulty in doing this, as he may be dissociated from his voice as a way to avoid dysphoria and/or he may feel dysphoria as he starts tuning in to aspects that may make him uncomfortable (Langer, 2016). He may also say that the skills seem fake, foreign, or otherwise strange, even when they objectively sound sufficiently masculine for his needs. This issue can be addressed by explaining the neurologic process of adopting new behavior. Does the voice feel strange because it is unnatural or because it is new? The client should be repeatedly reminded that his new skills may seem strange at first but they will gradually seem more natural and automatic as he experiences them over time and has success using them in daily life.

In addition to discussing inner and outer voice, the clinician should directly discuss risk-taking with the client if he is resistant to using his new skills out of fear of feeling silly or getting negative feedback from others. Because these fears may be as strong as the need to speak in a more masculine way, the client may need continual encouragement to carry over what he is learning. The clinician can do this by reminding him of his reasons for voice work, his likelihood of success, and his successful risk-taking in other ways in his life. The clinician can also ease the client into voice use outside session by first implementing conversations between the client and other people while in session, such as talking to on-site staff.

As the client uses his new skills more and more, counseling can be utilized to promote empowerment (Adler, 2017). As the client reflects on communication successes and failures, including moments of being gendered correctly or incorrectly, he can improve his understanding of how things go well or not well, what is and is not in his control, and how to modify his skills and emotions accordingly. Such reflections can lead to greater overall confidence, resilience, and optimism (Holland & Nelson, 2014), all of which could be diminished from gender dysphoria. In addition, the actual technical training itself, for "bigger" resonance, "heavier" intonation, increased loudness level, or a direct conversation style in certain work environments, can literally feel physically and emotionally powerful. Furthermore, empowerment can relate to the client actively considering how to responsibly use his new privilege as a man in society. The clinician can address this by discussing how to choose language that shows respect for both himself and others.

Empowerment and self-acceptance often go hand in hand, for as one changes, and hopefully increases, the other can as well. To directly address self-acceptance, the clinician should actively encourage the client to embrace his best possible self as a unique person within a masculine range (Adler, 2017; Block, 2017). One way this can be done is by simply demonstrating and celebrating diversity in masculinity and across the gender spectrum. The client can also be reminded that perfection is not necessary for happiness or success and that self-acceptance can lead to self-reliance and self-determination, which can, in turn, lead to more self-fulfillment in life. Additionally, the clinician should redirect any of the client's persistent comparisons of cisgender voices or feelings of inadequacy by focusing on improvement over time. Baseline and in-progress recordings can be a powerful tool in this case.

As the client becomes better at and more psychologically comfortable with his new skills, the therapy period can advance to its final stages. There is no proven optimal length of therapy for transgender men, which can vary widely depending on the client's individual needs and goals (Adler et al., 2012; Davies et al., 2015). As the client becomes more independent and 'lives his voice' in daily life, he should be able to rely on daily warm-up and mindful use of techniques to solidify his new skills and further the integration of those skills with his gender identity. After the initial therapy period is over, Davies et al. (2015) recommend follow-up maintenance or refresher sessions at three months, followed by periodic sessions every four to six months as needed. See Davies et al. (2015) and Chapter 16 for further discussion of general principles for habituation, carryover, maintenance, and discharge, which can apply to all transgender clients.

Sample Therapy Exercises

Exercise 1, Pitch

This exercise is adapted from the "Chant Your Pitch (voice feminization)" exercise by Christie Block in A. Behrman and J. Haskell's *Exercises for Voice Therapy*, 2nd edition (Block, 2013). It utilizes a common rehabilitative chant-to-speech exercise to establish and maintain a lower average pitch in single syllables, phrases, and sentences. The client is directed to chant a target pitch and then speak around that pitch at the onset of speech. This allows for an accurate target pitch as well as freedom of pitch movement within a natural range. Sufficient loudness level should also be maintained throughout all tasks. Masculine intonation contours, pitch range, or negative practice for glottal fry at low pitches may be introduced as well. One recommended target pitch is D3 (147 Hz), which can be modified depending on the client's needs (see the pitch section above for an explanation). The exercise integrates nasal sounds and syllables in order to prevent laryngeal tension with forward resonance. Pitch feedback tools can be particularly useful for this exercise, either for playing the target pitch or visually showing it with a reference line.

1. Say /m/ or /molm/ at D3 once for two or three seconds. Then count in a chant at D3: 1-2-3-4 breath 5-6-7-8 breath 9-10-11-12 breath 13-14-15-16 breath 17-18-19-20.
2. Say /m/ or /molm/ at D3 once for two or three seconds. Then count in a speaking voice around D3, thinking 'low' at the beginning of each set of four numbers: 1-2-3-4 breath 5-6-7-8 breath 9-10-11-12 breath 13-14-15-16 breath 17-18-19-20.
3. Chant a phrase or sentence at D3, then say the phrase or sentence around D3, thinking 'low.'
4. Chant a sentence at D3, then say the sentence around D3, thinking 'low.' Then make up another sentence to go with it, saying it around D3, thinking 'low.' As an alternative, the client could say /m/ or /molm/ once for two or three seconds instead of chanting the sentence first.

Exercise 2, Resonance

This exercise is adapted from the "Count big (voice masculinization)" exercise by Christie Block in A. Behrman and J. Haskell's *Exercises for Voice Therapy*, 2nd edition (Block, 2013). It is designed to establish and maintain a 'bigger,' 'darker,' or richer tone through increased open oral resonance and loudness level. The client is first directed to make more "open mouth" movements by dropping the jaw vertically, and then to create a more "open throat" feeling by raising the soft palate and moving the BOT farther down and back in the mouth. Once the client can accurately perform these postures in a single syllable, then he can progress to counting and phrases to practice a progressively 'bigger' sound with increased loudness level. Nasal sounds are integrated so that laryngeal tension is prevented as the size of the oral and pharyngeal cavities increase.

1. Say /ja/ repeatedly 5–10 times with an "open mouth," noticing your lips moving freely and your jaw moving down each time.
2. Make a yawn-sigh (/ha/!) with an "open throat," noticing your throat stretching. Finish the yawn-sigh by closing your lips while keeping that "open throat" posture. Hold that posture, with your lips closed, for 5 seconds, backing off slightly from a tight stretch to a more relaxed open feeling. Imagine holding a ping-pong ball in your throat if necessary. Do this three times.
3. Count to 5 ("1-2-3-4-5") twice with an "open mouth" for a bigger sound.
4. Count to 5 ("1-2-3-4-5") twice with an "open mouth" and an "open throat" together for an even bigger sound.
5. Count to 5 ("1-2-3-4-5!") twice with an "open mouth" and "open throat," getting increasingly louder and bigger from 1 to 5.
6. Say words and phrases (e.g., "now-now-now-now!" or "open in the door!") with an "open mouth" and "open throat," getting increasingly louder and bigger as you finish the utterance.

Exercise 3, Intonation

This exercise is adapted from the "Say it like you mean it" workshop by Christie Block presented at the Philadelphia Trans Health Conference (Block, 2014). It is designed to help the transmasculine client express emotion by producing a heavier and/or staccato-like stress pattern. The client is directed to expressively say words, phrases, and sentences by increasing the length or loudness level of stressed syllables/words without going too high in pitch. Visually displaying a maximum pitch with pitch-tracking software can be useful to help the client stay within masculine range. In addition, purposefully saying utterances in a feminine way can be useful, particularly when coupled with a reference line that illustrates how pitch is inappropriately high.

1. Say a word twice, making it more expressive the second time. Lengthen the stressed syllable, make it louder, and/or move the pitch quickly downward for a heavier or more staccato-like effect. Avoid going too high in pitch or punching the word with a harsh voice. For example, "Awesome! Awesome!!" or "Ridiculous! Ridiculous!!"

2. Repeat Step 1 with a phrase or sentence. For example, "Good job! Good job!!" or "I have so much work to do! I have so much work to do!!"

3. Repeat Step 1 with a phrase or sentence that you make up. For example, you won the lottery, you hurt your hand, or you ate too much.

Exercise 4, Cultural Humility and Cultural Competence

This exercise is designed to increase the transmasculine client's own cultural humility and cultural competence, as defined by Riquelme (2013) and ASHA (2017), while developing masculine voice and communication skills in context. It is adapted from an unpublished study at Minnesota State University entitled "Interview with Transmasculine Clients about Cultural Humility and Cultural Competence" (Adler, 2014). Some of the details of the study are outlined here as a preface to the exercise.

Thirty-five masculine-identified clients were each receiving individual and/or group sessions of transmasculine voice and communication therapy in a university clinic or LGBT community center as part of their transition to a more masculine presentation. In discussions with the clinician, the clients identified the identities, social groups, or "cultures" to which they felt they belonged and whether those changed before or since transition began. Some of the groups included female, male, lesbian, gay, college student, CPA, Catholic, and millennial. The clients then considered how their communication may or may not have changed or was expected to change in relation to group membership and communication context. In doing so, the clients performed observation tasks in particular situations that applied to them. Some included ordering lunch, getting help from a clerk at a shoe store, and discussing a topic with friends.

As a result of the observation tasks and discussions with the clinician, the clients increased their awareness and development of communication skills in context and in relation to their understanding of how they belong to a variety of cultures or social groups. At the end of the study, 85% of the clients noted that their outlook on communication had truly changed and they would continue to develop their thoughts on cultural competence as time passed. One client said, "I am more aware of the masculine culture now that I have emerged myself in these exercises; I think people expect me to stand a certain way, speak a certain way, and just be like society wants a man to be; but I have learned that it is 'me' who I am speaking about and I will develop competence that fits into my own cultural picture: male, doctor, city dweller, middle class, senior, and . . . well, just me."

The following exercise is a recurring homework assignment that was adapted from the approach and methodology of this study.

The client first chooses one or two contexts from his daily life to write under the "Activity" column, and during those situations, he observes and practices (or eventually practices) masculine voice and communication skills specific to those situations. After the activity is conducted, the client writes comments in the "Observations" column regarding his own or others' communication behavior and how it may relate to gender, other relevant identities, or other aspects of the social situation. The client may look out for *any* form of communicative behavior or focus specifically on one or more parameters, such as word choice, word frequency, communication style, non-verbal communication, pitch, intonation, etc. In the "Next week" column, the client decides what to target for the next session. By making these decisions, the client shapes the task in terms of what is relevant and important to him. The clinician may need to guide the client in making choices, particularly in terms of interpreting and understanding what is known about gendered behavior, gender norms, and gender expectations. The following are questions that could be posed before and/or after any occurrence of the assignment:

- What cultures or social groups do you feel you belong to?
- How have those cultures changed before and since you started to present more masculine?
- How have your communication skills changed or not changed before and since you started to present more masculine?

- How does your communication style change across situations?
- What factors and identities influence the way you talk in a particular situation? Is gender always relevant or the most important factor?
- Does your communication style show respect for the culture(s) of your listeners?

Using questions like these, the clinician can guide the client in becoming more aware of masculine behavior and how that changes or shifts in importance depending on the context. In doing so, he can understand the nuances and complex interactions of different identities in order to avoid stereotypes and develop his own form of functional masculine communication. In this process, he also develops cultural humility and cultural competence that promotes understanding and openness as a man in society. Table 9–5 illustrates a number of examples of contexts and observations, some of which were adapted from Adler (2014).

Case Studies

Each of the following case studies is a composite profile of a variety of clients from the authors' clinical and research practices. They represent some of the most common and diverse aspects of transmasculine experiences and illustrate many of the areas of testing and therapy that are discussed earlier in this chapter. These cases are discussed in a Standard American English context with KayPentax systems (Laryngeal Strobe Model 9400, Computer Speech Lab Model 4500) as the chosen measurement tools. See the diagnostic and therapeutic sections above for more specific descriptions of tasks that are referenced in the discussion.

Table 9–5. Examples of Cultural Humility and Cultural Competence Observations

Activity	Observations	Next week
Talking to a young child	Age and body size and gender were important; I spoke more sweetly and gently with my words which is more feminine but ok because it's a child; tried hard to not touch the child	Maybe try lower pitch if my words are more feminine; stay aware that some people think a man shouldn't touch a child
Ordering at a restaurant	Minimum amount of description; not too much enthusiasm; watch my voice tone . . . it could change my meaning	A more stoic voice tone is needed
Visiting a friend in the hospital	Listened to her; when she was tired, I tried to talk more to cheer her up; spoke quietly; same as I would before transition	Not sure if I need to change this; would men and women both act the same in this situation?
Speaking to a new person	Need to project voice; be aware of how I am standing and how close I am to this person; are my hand gestures appropriate; do my choice of words match my body language?	Need to be more aware of how I am standing and how many gestures I am using; seems like I use too many gestures and not enough words?
Calling the phone company	Direct and authoritative; it's the phone company so not really because I'm a man; I was annoyed with my bill so I could've been more friendly; the person had a foreign accent but it wasn't a problem	Try to be friendly without being too high with my pitch or my words; don't assume a person isn't competent if they have an accent
Talking at a meeting	I'm surprised I talked more than usual; it felt good but did my female colleague not talk because I talked too much?	I don't want to be that guy who talks too much in meetings; how do I find a balance?

■ Speaking to someone at a support group that I have not spoken to before

■ Asking a stranger for directions

■ Participating in lunchtime discussions

■ Joining a book club and speaking out about the book

■ Going to the motor vehicle bureau to change my name

Case Study 1

Case History and Testing

PK is a 38-year-old trans man who sought professional help to increase the masculine features of his voice and communication skills. He had been presenting with a more masculine gender expression full-time for 14 months, including clothing, hair, legal name change, pronoun change, and body changes from testosterone, including pitch lowering and significant weight gain. Despite having a lower pitch, his voice still seemed feminine to him. He felt he sounded like a "little boy" and "too girly" when joking around with friends. He had mild voice dysphoria and believed that his voice was a primary reason for being misgendered by others, which occurred approximately 40% of the time. In addition, he had difficulty being heard in loud environments. He also wanted to be more assertive at his job as a financial broker, where he felt less confident as a transgender person despite being a competent professional. His vocal load was moderate. He had been seeing a psychotherapist for gender dysphoria, depression, and anxiety once per week and he had a mastectomy one year prior to the voice exam. He had been on testosterone for 9 months and experienced three or four temporary periods of hoarseness and vocal strain, each of which lasted three to five days. Each period occurred when his dose of testosterone was administered, the most recent one occurring approximately three weeks prior to the exam. He had environmental allergies to dust, mold, and pollen. He had no history of difficulty breathing, dysphagia, or upper body tension. His medications were testosterone (0.3 mL injection per week) and a corticosteroid nasal spray as needed.

Perceptual observations revealed normal vocal quality except for mild strain when loudness level was increased. PK's resonance was viewed to be mild to moderately feminine, with a notably "small" and "bright" tone. This appeared to be a result of behavioral resonance placement as well as a smaller physical supralaryngeal space relative to a cis man. Influencing this smaller space was PK's height and weight, which he reported to be 5 feet 4 inches and 160 pounds (due partially to significant weight gain). Intonation patterns were mildly feminine, which was indicated by the pitch frequently moving upward at the ends of expressive utterance. Speech rate, articulation, language use, and non-verbal communication were not saliently feminine in conversation. PK was responsive to a variety of cues and feedback modalities during diagnostic training tasks.

Acoustic measurement and analysis of PK's sustained phonation and connected speech were performed. Fundamental frequency (F0) was within masculine range at 130 Hz. Mean conversational frequency range was also within masculine range at 13 semitones (ST) (92–195 Hz). Maximum phonation frequency range was decreased within masculine range: 35 ST (81–622 Hz). Other measurements were within normal limits (WNL), including cepstral measures during sustained phonation and connected speech, mean intensity during connected speech, and maximum phonation time. Videostroboscopy showed mild supraglottic compression with all pitches during sustained phonation and connected speech, which appeared to be behavioral rather than compensatory to vocal pathology.

Therapy

PK was seen for 10 skill-building sessions over 13 weeks, followed by 4 maintenance sessions over 11 months. PK's signs of dysphonia—mild strain during increased loudness level, occasional periods of hoarseness with testosterone administration, reduced maximum phonation frequency range, and mild supraglottic compression—were addressed directly in the entire first session and indirectly in masculine training after that. This was done through vocal hygiene directives, stretches for the face and upper body, postural alignment, vocal warm-up vocalizations and glides, rehabilitative breath control tasks, and semi-occluded vocal tract exercises. B2 (124 Hz) was used as a reference pitch for vocal warm-up, but pitch was not a masculine training target. Rather, resonance was the primary target in masculine training via open oral resonance exercises for a 'bigger' and 'darker' tone. This included a yawn-stretch exercise that was implemented repeatedly in order to develop a new, consistent resting and speech posture that involved a lower BOT. Intonation was also addressed by increasing the amount of downward intonation at the ends of utterances and by increasing expressiveness within a masculine pitch range through vowel lengthening, increased loudness, and staccato-like downward pitch movement. Useful tools for practicing expressiveness at the conversation level were baby pictures and fun topics that PK would typically discuss with friends. Loudness level was integrated into vocal warm-up, resonance, and intonation exercises in order to increase vocal control and flexibility for loud environments and to increase the salience of masculine patterns.

Once resonance, intonation, and loudness level were significantly improved, PK practiced being assertive at work by producing more direct utterances with different word choices and fewer words based on situations in his specific professional environment. This included, for example, roleplaying in which he asked for help, gave

feedback, or proposed an idea. As PK progressed to a maintenance level in all target areas, reading and conversation tasks were used to troubleshoot situations that arose in PK's social and professional life. Throughout therapy, PK was also given daily homework and mindfulness strategies to employ in daily life, which PK was able to do regularly. Particularly useful cues for mindfulness were "open up," "down," and "direct" for resonance, intonation, and pragmatics, respectively. Audio recordings were also made periodically to increase vocal awareness and demonstrate progress. A significant amount of counseling was necessary to supplement technical skill-building. Topics of discussions that arose included: (a) misgendered moments, (b) being direct and being likable are not mutually exclusive, (c) accepting that his best voice, though not perfect, is much improved, and (d) his communicative success is much more likely than communicative failure.

Outcome

PK significantly improved on all targets within 13 weeks and maintained that improvement over 11 more months. His F0 decreased slightly to 128 Hz at 13 weeks and 126 Hz at 14 months. Maximum phonation frequency range increased to 36 ST due to an increase in the upper end to 710 Hz at 13 weeks and 709 Hz at 14 months. PK was able to increase loudness level more efficiently and successfully overall and in noise without vocal strain. The temporary hoarseness did not recur while he continued to take testosterone. Most significantly, his resonance was 'bigger' and his intonation was 'heavier' and more staccato-like within a masculine range. PK felt he sounded more like his age, which he felt gained him more respect. PK had difficulty staying mindful of intonation when talking to one particular friend, but when he was mindful, he was able to sound sufficiently masculine. At work, he felt better able to speak directly about 75% of the time. He was misgendered only once, on the phone, in the final 5 months of therapy. Overall, PK was pleased with his improvement and felt more confident as a communicator. When he faced challenges, particularly at work, he felt able to successfully adjust his technique.

Case Study 2

Case History and Testing

TJ is a 21-year-old masculine-identified genderqueer person who wanted to sound more masculine while talking. TJ had been presenting with androgynous and slightly masculine gender expression full-time for eight months, including clothing, binding, packing, hair, name change, and pronoun change ("ze"). Ze had attempted to speak in a more masculine way by taking up smoking and by speaking "lower and monotone," which was more difficult to do when spending time with zis friends. Ze was a university student in his third year, majoring in psychology with a plan to become a social worker. Zis vocal load was moderate. Ze came out eight months prior to the voice exam as a "genderqueer transguy" to his teachers, classmates, friends, and close family members. Ze was not concerned about zis language use, because ze felt it was sufficiently masculine. TJ had no history of gender dysphoria. While ze felt zis voice didn't cause zim distress, ze considered zis voice an "annoyance" that bothered zim more than being misgendered by others. Ze had no intentions of seeking psychotherapy, HRT, or surgery. Ze was taking no medications and had no history of dysphonia or dysphagia. Ze did have occasional

shortness of breath and chest and shoulder tension from binding. Ze had been smoking one pack of cigarettes per week for nine months.

Perceptual observations showed mild signs of dysphonia, including intermittent glottal fry, reduced intonational variety, and reduced loudness level from attempts to speak more masculine. In addition, there was reduced breath support and control, and chest and neck tension from wearing a binder. TJ's voice and speech patterns appeared to be gender neutral overall. Pitch and resonance were mildly feminine, being relatively high and "small" or "bright" in tone, respectively. The resonance appeared to be influenced primarily by behavioral placement and less so by the physical size of TJ's head and neck or his height or weight, which were reported by TJ to be 5 feet 7 inches and 135 pounds. Intonation was mildly masculine, moving downward at the ends of most sentences. Speech rate, articulation, language use, and non-verbal communication were not particularly feminine or masculine in conversation. TJ was responsive to a variety of cues and feedback modalities during diagnostic training tasks.

TJ's sustained phonation and connected speech were measured and analyzed acoustically. Fundamental frequency (F0) was 180 Hz, which was above masculine range and below feminine range for TJ's age. Mean conversational frequency range was reduced within masculine range: 9 ST (141–243 Hz). Maximum phonation frequency range was WNL and overlapped feminine and masculine ranges: 36 ST (113–906 Hz). Maximum phonation time was decreased at 13 secs at 179 Hz. Mean intensity during connected speech was at the low end of normal at 67 dB. Cepstral measures during sustained phonation and connected speech were WNL. Videostroboscopy showed mild supraglottic compression with all pitches during sustained phonation and connected speech, which appeared to be behavioral. Also, there were signs of reduced hydration, which was likely related to smoking.

Therapy

TJ participated in 8 skill-building sessions over 8 weeks, and 2 maintenance sessions over 6 months. Therapy began by addressing TJ's tension, breathing limitations, and glottal fry via chest and neck stretches, diaphragmatic, rhythmic, and resistance breathing exercises, postural alignment, vocal warm-up vocalizations and glides, and semi-occluded vocal tract exercises. These tasks were performed at the beginning of each session. TJ wore zis binder at all times, and therapy techniques were adjusted around it as needed. After initial rehabilitative exercises, each session proceeded with exercises that targeted masculine pitch, resonance, and intonation. Using a KORG guitar tuner and Real-time Pitch computer software, D3 (147 Hz) was employed as the new average pitch (F0) during a chant-to-speech exercise, which progressed from words to phrases to sentences to two sentences to one or two spontaneous sentences. As TJ advanced beyond two-sentence spontaneous utterances, ze practiced aiming "low," around D3, at the beginning of every phrase when reading or speaking in monologue or conversation. Resonance was addressed with open oral resonance and chest resonance exercises. A hand gesture was used to facilitate an "open throat" posture during sustained sounds and reading. Downward glides with common utterances such as "oh no," "yep," and "yeah" were used periodically to check pitch, resonance, and glottal fry simultaneously. TJ also worked on how to be more expressive within masculine range without compromising vocal quality, loudness

level, or pitch range. Ze expressed a variety of emotions when reading single sentences, bringing out the meaning through different combinations of vowel lengthening, increased intonational variety within masculine range, increased loudness, and staccato-like downward pitch movement. Negative practice was used to help TJ be aware of the amount of expressiveness ze needed to achieve a healthy and efficient voice. TJ liked to read comic books, which were a particularly useful tool for advancing beyond single sentences. School assignments, i.e., readings and a presentation, were also utilized for practice. TJ was given daily homework for all targeted areas and ze was encouraged to do the stretching, breathing, vocal warm-up as well as self-massage tasks without the binder at home when possible. Ze was able to practice three or four times per week, and ze did self-massage without the binder every evening. Ze attempted to stay mindful of low pitch, "darker" resonance, and more expressiveness by thinking "low" and "big." A moderate amount of counseling was provided throughout therapy, particularly regarding the following topics: (a) smoking cessation, (b) the importance of addressing dysphonia, (c) identifying the level of masculine patterns ze desired, and (d) the importance of regular practice and mindfulness. Audio recordings were useful tools for counseling, vocal awareness, and documentation of progress.

Outcome

TJ's overall speech and voice presentation was more masculine within eight weeks and was maintained over six more months. Zis F0 decreased by three semitones to 152 Hz at eight weeks and 153 Hz at eight months, closer to masculine range. Mean conversational frequency range increased to 12 ST at eight weeks (118–236 Hz) and eight months (121–248 Hz) within masculine range. Maximum phonation time was WNL at 17 seconds at 162 Hz at eight weeks and 16 seconds at 159 Hz at eight months. Mean intensity during connected speech was increased to WNL by 3 dB to 70 dB at eight weeks and maintained at 71 dB at eight months. TJ reported having less chest and neck tension and no more difficulty breathing. Glottal fry was consistently absent since the third session. TJ's resonance was 'bigger' and ze employed a wider range of expressions within a lower pitch range. Ze came to realize that expressiveness was a problem and ze felt better able to "talk like I mean it" without dampening down his emotions. While ze took vocal health more seriously than ze had before therapy began, his vocal health was still at risk, since he did not attempt to smoke less and did home exercises only sporadically. Nevertheless, ze was able to be mindful of zis voice techniques when talking, which was zis best method of maintaining gains in session. Overall, TJ was more satisfied with zis voice and ze felt able to adjust it as needed in daily life.

Case Study 3

Case History and Testing

LC is a 46-year-old trans man who complained of persistent vocal effort, persistent throat tightness, and intermittent hoarseness for approximately 10 years. He could not recall any illness, injury, phonotraumatic event, or increased vocal load at initial onset. These symptoms worsened in recurrent periods of 4–5 days over 6 months when he started taking testosterone 3 years prior to the voice exam. He could not recall if the changes in symptoms coincided with each

testosterone administration or change in dosage. His testosterone dosage was 0.5 mL injection every 10–14 days for the past 2.5 years. He was seeing a laryngologist and an allergist for laryngopharyngeal reflux and environmental allergies, respectively, which were controlled with a reflux diet, an H2 blocker as needed at dinner or bedtime, and a corticosteroid nasal spray as needed. He had finished immunotherapy treatment 4 years prior to the exam. He complained of tension in his neck and shoulders, and he occasionally got a massage to address it. He had no history of shortness of breath, daytime sleepiness, dysphagia, heartburn, throat burn, or globus sensation, though he did start snoring occasionally since taking testosterone. He worked as a digital marketing specialist and rated his vocal load and stress level, professionally and socially, as moderate. He was rarely in loud environments. At the time of the exam, he rated his vocal health overall at 75%. His laryngologist had recommended voice therapy one year prior to the exam, but he had not had the time to follow up.

He had minimal complaints regarding gender presentation. He had been presenting in a more masculine way full-time for 3.5 years with changes in clothing and hair, legal name change, pronoun change, and body changes from testosterone. He felt that his voice lowered sufficiently with testosterone, and he communicated in a sufficiently masculine way in terms of how he felt and how others treated him. He was misgendered approximately 25% of the time when talking on the phone. He was never misgendered when speaking face-to-face. His priority was to decrease his dysphonia, but he was also interested in improving his ability to be recognized as male on the phone. He had had a mastectomy 2.5 year prior to the exam and did not complain of stiffness or tension in the chest. He had been under the care of a mental health specialist 3 years prior to the exam for 1.5 years for gender dysphoria and anxiety, both of which had resolved.

Perceptual observations showed intermittent mild hoarseness and trace to mild persistent vocal strain. Articulatory excursion was mildly limited. Breath control was mildly reduced. Pitch and intonation were sufficiently masculine. Resonance was mildly feminine (i.e., "bright" in tone) due to high tongue carriage from lingual tension rather than healthy forward placement. Without efficient placement, the vocal strain and visible musculoskeletal tension of the neck occurred. Gross observation of the size of LC's head and neck, and relatedly, his height and weight, which he reported to be 5 feet 10 inches and 210 pounds, suggested that LC's physical supralaryngeal space was not a significant factor in shaping the mildly feminine resonance. Loudness level, speech rate, articulation, language use, and non-verbal communication were not saliently feminine during conversation. LC had moderate to severe musculoskeletal tension in the neck and shoulders. LC was responsive to a variety of cues and feedback modalities during diagnostic training tasks.

Acoustic measurement and analysis were taken of LC's sustained phonation and connected speech. Fundamental frequency (F0) was 122 Hz and within masculine range. Mean conversational frequency range and maximum phonation frequency range were decreased and within masculine range: 11 ST (94–175 Hz), and 32 ST (90–580 Hz), respectively. Additional measurements—cepstral measures during sustained phonation and connected speech, mean intensity during connected speech, and maximum phonation time—were WNL. Videostroboscopy confirmed that laryngopharyngeal reflux was controlled. Mild to moderate supraglottic compression was observed with all pitches during sustained phonation and connected speech, which appeared to be behavioral in etiology. The structure of the upper airway did not indicate testing for sleep apnea.

Therapy

LC was seen for five sessions over 12 weeks, the first three of which occurred weekly, followed by two maintenance sessions 3 and 6 weeks later. Therapy focused almost entirely on dysphonia by implementing the following: vocal hygiene directives, stretches for the tongue, face, neck, and shoulders, laryngeal massage, postural alignment, vocal warm-up vocalizations and glides, diaphragmatic and rhythmic breathing tasks, straw phonation, and semi-occluded vocal tract exercises. Resonance was targeted by using nasal consonants in combination with back and/or low vowels, such as "molm," "mom," "nine," "moan," or "mine," in order to shift the energy away from the neck, avoiding hyperfunction, while increasing open oral resonance. LC was instructed to first notice vibration in the mask of the face and later add in increased mouth movement. Once he could achieve sufficient awareness and accuracy with words, he formed spontaneous sentences with the words. Open oral resonance was further increased from there with the "Get Big" exercise to increase articulatory movement and lower the BOT. LC read words, phrases, and sentences with varying levels of forward resonance placement, jaw dropping, and lower BOT to achieve the appropriate balance of fronted and oral resonance for healthy, efficient, and masculine resonance and vocal quality. LC was cued to maintain the energy of his voice fixed at the level of his eyebrows while he simultaneously increased the "bigness" of his voice by opening up his mouth and throat. In this way, LC could avoid any mental focus at level of the neck, where he was apt to activate tension. Instead he was mindful of aiming his vocal energy forward, looking straight ahead at his listener, while using a broader range of movement of the tongue and jaw. Sobbing was also used to facilitate release of laryngeal tension while increasing masculine resonance. In addition to resonance, strategies for phone use were discussed. LC was instructed to focus on "nailing the first sentence" with low pitch and "big" resonance. Saying and spelling his name was also a recommended strategy for facilitating correct gender reference on the phone. Along with daily home practice of rehabilitative and masculine resonance exercises, LC was instructed to make phone calls regularly, first as phone messages to the clinician then to random businesses. These were recorded and/or reviewed together. LC used the cues "eyes and mouth" and "loose" to stay mindful of resonance and relaxation during daily conversational interactions. Audio recordings were taken three times to increase vocal awareness and demonstrate progress. Occasional counseling was necessary to address the following topics: (a) efficient vocal production, (b) variations of feminine and masculine resonance, and (c) the interaction of vocal health with gender markers in voice and speech.

Outcome

LC's dysphonia was resolved, and his resonance was more masculine within three sessions and maintained over 12 weeks. His vocal quality and breath control were WNL. F0 remained essentially unchanged within masculine range at 123 Hz. Mean conversational frequency range remained at 11 ST at 95–175 Hz but maximum phonation frequency range increased to WNL within masculine range at 36 ST (85–674 Hz). LC had

less musculoskeletal tension in the neck and shoulders, he no longer felt throat discomfort, and he did not get misgendered on the phone since therapy began. He understood how vocal health and masculine voice could affect each other. He was particularly surprised that the absence of vocal strain not only felt better but sounded more masculine too. He felt he was able to adjust his voice for smooth vocal quality as well as increase how 'big' he sounded for an added masculine effect.

Conclusion

The voice and communication needs of the transmasculine speaker have often been overlooked, oversimplified, or misrepresented by the research and clinical communities. This chapter has set out to shed light on what is known so far in the research and offer an approach to what actually is a unique and complex set of clinical issues. Despite many transmasculine individuals benefiting from successful pitch-lowering that often results from testosterone administration, a significant number of speakers do not fall into this category or experience dysphonia. Simply put, there is a need for voice care.

The transmasculine client, like any client on the gender spectrum, deserves an attentive clinician who is both clinically and culturally competent at addressing his specific needs. While interested in understanding normative masculine behavior in context, he is more likely to be focused on using that information to develop his own interpretation of it. In doing so, he may require guidance in pitch, resonance, or other communication skills, though the approach is not always the exact opposite as that for the transfeminine client. In addition, he may need counseling about a number of issues, such as acceptance or conceptualization of his vocal identity, which may be similar to or different from some other transgender clients, or entirely unique to himself. It is a rewarding challenge.

As transgender research and clinical practice grows, transmasculine issues will gain more traction, which, in turn, will promote more awareness and more extensive and improved clinical service. For now, this chapter has aimed to serve as a catalyst, one clinician at a time.

References

Adams, J. A. (1971). A closed-loop therapy of motor learning. *Journal of Motor Behavior, 3*(2), 111–149.

Adler, R. K. (2014). *Interview with transmasculine clients about cultural humility and cultural competence*. Unpublished manuscript.

Adler, R. K. (2017). The SLP as counselor for the transgender client. *SIG 10 Perspectives in Higher Education, 20*(2), 92–101.

Adler, R. K., Constansis, A. N., & Van Borsel, J. (2012). Female-to-male transgender/transsexual considerations. In R. Adler, S. Hirsch, & M. Mordaunt (Eds.), *Voice and communication therapy for the transgender/transsexual client: A comprehensive clinical guide* (2nd ed.) (pp. 153–185). San Diego, CA: Plural Publishing.

Adler, R. K., Hirsch, S., & Mordaunt, M. (2012). *Voice and communication therapy for the transgender / transsexual client: A comprehensive clinical guide* (2nd ed.). San Diego, CA: Plural Publishing.

American Speech-Language Hearing Association (2002). Consensus auditory-perceptual evaluation of voice (CAPE-V). Special Interest Group 3, Voice and Voice Disorders. http://www.asha .org.

American-Speech-Language-Hearing Association (2017, December 7). *Cultural competence*. Retrieved from http://www.asha.org/PRPSpecific Topic.aspx?folderid=8589935230&section=Key _Issues

Andrews, M. L. (1999). *Manual of voice treatment: Pediatrics through geriatrics*. San Diego, CA: Singular Publishing.

Antoni, C. (2015). Service delivery and the challenges of providing service to people who are transgender. *Perspectives of the ASHA Special Interest Groups, 25* (SIG3), 59–65.

Antoszewski, B., Zadzinska, E., & Foczpanski, J. (2009). The metric features of teeth in female-to-male transsexuals. *Archives of Sexual Behavior, 38*(3), 351–358.

Azul, D. (2015). On the varied and complex factors affecting gender diverse people's vocal situations: Implications for clinical practice. *Perspectives on Voice and Voice Disorders, 25,* 75–86.

Azul, D., Nygren, U., Sodersten, M., & Neuschaefer-Rube, C. (2017). Transmasculine people's voice function: A review of the currently available evidence. *Journal of Voice, 31*(2), 261.e9–261. e23.

Baken, R., & Orlikoff, R. (2000). *Clinical measurement of speech and voice* (2nd ed). Clifton Park, NY: Thomson Delmar Learning.

Baker, J. (1999). A report on alterations to the speaking and singing voices of four women following hormonal therapy with virilizing agents. *Journal of Voice, 13*(4), 496–507.

Barbieri, R. L., Evans, S., & Kistner, R. W. (1982). Danazol in the treatment of endometriosis: Analysis of 100 cases with a 4-year follow-up. *Fertility and Sterility, 37*(6), 737–746.

Benjamin, B. J. (1981). Frequency variability in the aged voice. *Journal of Gerontology, 36,* 722–726.

Block, C. (June, 2011). *A vocal health diagnostic protocol for transgender individuals*. Presentation at the World Professional Association for Transgender Health Biennial International Symposium, Atlanta, GA.

Block, C. (2013). *Chant your pitch (voice feminization), and count big (voice masculinization)*. In A. Behrman & J. Haskell (Eds.), Exercises for voice therapy (2nd ed, p. 177–180). San Diego, CA: Plural Publishing.

Block, C. (2014, June). *Say it like you mean it*. Workshop presented at the Philadelphia Trans Health Conference, Philadelphia, PA.

Block, C. (2017). Making a case for transmasculine voice and communication training. *Perspectives of the ASHA Special Interest Groups, 2* (SIG3), 33–41.

Block, C., Langer, S. J. & Lipson, J. (June 2016). *Voice and identity: Perspectives and intervention approaches across three disciplines.* Presentation at the World Professional Association for Transgender Health Biennial International Symposium, Amsterdam, the Netherlands.

Boothroyd, C. V., & Lepre, F. (1990). Permanent voice change resulting from Danazol therapy. *Australian and New Zealand Journal of Obstetrics and Gynaecology, 30*(3), 275–276.

Bouman, W. P., Suess Schwend, A., Motmans, J., Smiley, A., Safer, J., & Deutsch, M. (2017). Language and trans health. *International Journal of Transgenderism, 18*(1), 1–6.

Briton, N. J., & Hall, J. A. (1995). Gender-based expectancies and observer judgments of smiling. *Journal of Nonverbal Behavior, 19*(1), 49–65.

Bultynck, C., Pas, C., Defreyne, J., Cosyns, M., den Heijer, M., & T'Sjoen, G. (2017). Self-perception of voice in transgender persons during cross-sex hormone therapy. *Laryngoscope, 127*(12), 2796–2804.

Byrne, L. A., Dacakis, G. & Douglas, J. M. (2003). Self-perceptions of pragmatic communication abilities in male-to-female transsexuals. *Advances in Speech-Language Pathology, 5*(1), 15–25.

Callen-Lorde Community Health Center (2015). *Protocols for the provision of hormone therapy.* https://issuu.com/callenlorde/docs/tg_protocols_2014_v.5?e=8526609/10794494

Cameron, D. (2008). *The myth of Mars and Venus: Do men and women really speak different languages?* New York, NY: Oxford University Press.

Celce-Murcia, M., Brinton, D. M., & Goodwin, J. (1996). *Teaching pronunciation: A reference for teachers of English to speakers of other languages.* New York, NY: Cambridge University Press.

Chowdhury, K., Saha, S., Pal, S., & Chatterjee, I. (2014). Effects of type 3 thyroplasty on voice quality outcomes in puberphonia. *Philippine Journal of Otolaryngology—Head and Neck Surgery, 29*(1), 6–10.

Coates, J. (2004). *Women, men and language: A sociolinguistic account of gender differences in language* (3rd ed.). New York, NY: Routledge.

Coleman, E., Bockting, W., Botzer, M., Cohen-Kettenis, P., DeCuypere, G., Feldman, J. . . . Zucker, K. (2012). Standards of care for the health of transsexual, transgender, and gender nonconforming people, version 7. *International Journal of Transgenderism, 13*, 165–232.

Coleman, R. (1976). A comparison of the contributions of two voice quality characteristics to the perception of maleness and femaleness in the voice. *Journal of Speech and Hearing Research, 19*(1), 168–180.

Constansis, A. (2008). The changing female-to-male (FtM) voice. *Radical Musicology, 3.* Retrieved from http://www.radical-musicology.org.uk/2008/Constansis.htm

Cosyns, M., Van Borsel, J., Wierckx, K., Dedecker, D., Van de Peer, F., Daelman, T. . . . & T'Sjoen, G. (2014). Voice in female-to-male transsexual persons after long-term androgen therapy. *Laryngoscope, 124*(6), 1409–1414.

Dacakis, G. (2012). Assessment and goal setting: Revisited. In R. Adler, S. Hirsch, & M. Mordaunt (Eds.), *Voice and communication therapy for the transgender / transsexual client: A comprehensive clinical guide* (2nd ed.) (pp. 111–138). San Diego, CA: Plural Publishing.

Dacakis, G., Davies, S., Oates, J., Douglas, J., & Johnston, J. (2013). Development and preliminary evaluation of the transsexual voice questionnaire for male-to-female transsexuals. *Journal of Voice 27*(3), 312–320.

Damrose, E. J. (2009). Quantifying the impact of androgen therapy on the female larynx. *Auris, Nasus, Larynx, 36*(1), 110–112.

Davies, S., & Goldberg, J. M. (2006). Clinical aspects of transgender speech feminization and masculinization. *International Journal of Transgenderism, 9*(3–4), 167–196.

Davies, S., Papp, V. G., & Antoni, C. (2015). Voice and communication change for gender nonconforming individuals: Giving voice to the person inside. *International Journal of Transgenderism, 16*(3), 117–159.

Deuster, D., Matulat, P., Knief, A., Zitzmann, M., Rosslau, K., Szukaj, M., & Schmidt, C.-M. (2016). Voice deepening under testosterone treatment in female-to-male gender dysphoric individuals. *European Archives of Otorhinolaryngology, 273*(4), 959–965.

Deuster, D., Vincenzo, K. D., Szukaj, M., Zehnhoff-Dinnesen, A. A., & Dobel, C. (2016). Change of speech fundamental frequency explains the satisfaction with voice in response to testosterone therapy in female-to-male gender dysphoric individuals. *European Archives of Otorhinolaryngology, 273*(8), 2127–2131.

Dorreen, K. (2017). *Fundamental frequency distributions of bilingual speakers in forensic speaker comparison.* (Unpublished master's thesis). University of Canterbury.

Eckert, P. (1989). The whole woman: Sex and gender differences in variation. *Language Variation and Change, 1*(3), 245–267.

Erickson-Schroth, L. (2014). *Trans bodies trans selves.* New York, NY: Oxford University Press.

Fairbanks, G. (1960). *Voice and articulation drillbook.* (2nd ed.) New York: Harper & Row.

Fitch, W. T., & Giedd, J. (1999). Morphology and development of the human vocal tract: A study using magnetic resonance imaging. *Journal of the Acoustical Society of America, 106*(3), 1511–1522.

Fogel, R. B., Malhotra, A., Pillar, G., Pittman, S. D., Dunaif, A., & White, D. P. (2001). Increased prevalence of obstructive sleep apnea syndrome in obese women with polycystic ovary syndrome. *Journal of Clinical Endocrinology and Metabolism, 86*(3), 1175–1180.

Freidenberg, C. B. (2002). Working with male-to-female transgendered clients: Clinical considerations. *Contemporary Issues in Communication Science and Disorders, 29*, 43–58.

Gelfer, M., & Schofield, K. (2000). Comparison of acoustic and perceptual measures of voice in male-to-female transsexuals perceived as female versus those perceived as male. *Journal of Voice, 14*(1), 22–33.

Gelfer, M. P., & Mikos, V. A. (2005). The relative contributions of speaking fundamental frequency and formant frequencies to gender identification based on isolated vowels. *Journal of Voice, 19*, 544–554.

Gelfer, M., & Mordaunt, M. (2012). Pitch and intonation. In R. Adler, S. Hirsch, & M. Mordaunt (Eds.), *Voice and communication therapy for the transgender / transsexual client: A comprehensive clinical guide* (2nd ed., pp. 187–223). San Diego, CA: Plural Publishing.

González, J. (2004). Formant frequencies and body size of speaker: A weak relationship in adult humans. *Journal of Phonetics, 32*(2), 277–287.

Gorham-Rowan, M., & Morris, R. (2006). Aerodynamic analysis of male-to-female transgender voice. *Journal of Voice, 20*(2), 251–261.

Hancock, A. B., Childs, K. D., & Irwig, M. S. Trans male voice in the first year of testosterone therapy: Make no assumptions. *Journal of Speech, Language and Hearing Research, 60*(9), 2472–2482.

Hembree, W., Cohen-Kettenis, P., Delemarre-Van de Wall, H. A., Gooren, L. J., Meyer III, W. J., Spack, N. P., . . . & Montori, V. M. (2009). Endocrine treatment of transsexual persons: An Endocrine Society clinical practice guideline. *Journal of Clinical Endocrinology and Metabolism, 94*, 3132–3154.

Henton, C. G. (1989). Fact and fiction in the description of female and male pitch. *Language and Communication, 9*, 299–311.

Herbst, L. (1964). *Untersuchungen zur Indifferenzlage der Sprechstimme. Studien zur Problematik des physiologischen Hauptsprechtonbereichs* (Unpublished doctoral dissertation). Universität Halle-Wittenberg.

Hoffman, M. R., Devine, E. E., Remacle, M., Ford, C. N., Wadium, E., & Jiang, J. J. (2014). Combined type IIIB with bilateral type I thyroplasty for pitch lowering with maintenance of vocal fold tension. *European Archives of Otorhinolaryngology, 271*(6), 1621–1629.

Hogikyan, N. D. & Sethuraman, G. (1999). Validation of an instrument to measure voice-related qualify of life (V-RQOL). *Journal of Voice, 13*(4), 557–569.

Holland, A., & Nelson, R. (2014). *Counseling in communication disorders: A wellness perspective.* San Diego, CA: Plural Publishing.

Howard, D. M., & Angus, J. A. S. (2017). *Acoustics and psychoacoustics.* (Fifth ed.) New York, NY: Routledge.

Hudson, A. I., & Holbrook, A. (1981). A study of the reading fundamental vocal frequency of young black adults. *Journal of Speech and Hearing Research, 24*, 197–201.

Hudson, A. I., & Holbrook, A. (1982). Fundamental frequency characteristics of young black adults: Spontaneous speaking and oral reading. *Journal of Speech and Hearing Research, 25* (1), 25–28.

Irwig, M. S., Childs, K. D., & Hancock, A. B. (2017). Effects of testosterone on the transgender male voice. *Andrology, 5*(1), 107–112.

Isshiki, N. (2000). Progress in laryngeal framework surgery. *Acta Oto-Laryngologica, 120*, 120–127.

Isshiki, N., Taira, T., & Tanabe, M. (1983). Surgical alteration of the vocal pitch. *Journal of Otolaryngology, 12*(5), 335–340.

James, D., & Drakich, J. (1993). Understanding gender differences in amount of talk. In D. Tannen (Ed.), *Gender and conversational interaction* (pp. 281–312). New York, NY: Oxford University Press.

Jessen, M. (2007). Speaker classification in forensic phonetics and acoustics. In C. Müller (Ed.),

Speaker Classification (1) (Vol. 4343, pp. 180–204). Springer.

Johnson, K. (2006). Resonance in an exemplar-based lexicon:The emergence of social identity and phonology. *Journal of Phonetics, 34*(4), 485–499.

Johnson, K. (2007). Speaker normalization in speech perception. In D. Pisoni & R. Remez (Eds.), *The Handbook of Speech Perception* (pp. 363–89).Wiley-Blackwell.

Killick, R., Wang, D., Hoyos, C. M., Yee, B. J., Grunstein, R. R., & Liu, P. Y. (2013). The effects of testosterone on ventilatory responses in men with obstructive sleep apnea: A randomised, placebo-controlled trial.*Journal of Sleep Research, 22*(3), 331–336.

King, A., Ashby, J., & Nelson, C. (2001). Effects of testosterone replacement on a male professional singer. *Journal of Voice, 15*, 553–557.

King, J. B., Lindstedt, D. E., Jensen, M., & Law, M. (1999).Transgendered voice: Considerations in case history management. *Logopedics, Poniatrics, Vocology, 24*(1), 14–18.

Klatt, D.H., & Klatt, L.C. (1990). Analysis, synthesis, and perception of voice quality variations among female and male talkers.*Journal of the Acoustical Society of America, 87*, 820–857.

Klimek, M. M. (2014). *Estill voice training: Figures for voice control.*Two-day workshop presented at New York University, New York, NY.

Koçak, I., Doğan, M., Tadihan, E., Cakir, Z. A., Bengisu, S., & Akpinar, M. E. (2008). Window anterior commissure relaxation laryngoplasty in the management of high-pitched voice disorders. *Archives of Otolaryngology, 134*(12), 1263–1269.

Lakoff, R.T., & Bucholtz, M. (2004). *Language and woman's place: Text and commentaries.* New York, NY: Oxford University Press.

Langer, S. J. (2016). Trans bodies and the failure of mirrors. *Studies in Gender and Sexuality 17*(4), 306–316.

Lee, S., Potamianos,A., & Narayanan, S. (1999).Acoustics of children's speech:Developmental changes of temporal and spectral parameters. *Journal of the Acoustical Society of America, 105*(3), 1455–1468.

Li, G. D., Mu, L., & Yang, S. (1999).Acoustic evaluation of Isshiki Type III thyroplasty for treatment of mutational voice disorders. *Journal of Laryngology and Otology, 113*(1), 31–34.

Loth, S. R., & Henneberg, M. (2000). Gonial eversion: Facial architecture, not sex.*Homo, 51*, 81–89.

Mackenzie, S., & Wilkinson, C. (2017). Morphological and morphometric changes in the faces of female-to-male (FtM) transsexual people. *International Journal of Transgenderism, 18* (2), 172–181.

McConnell-Ginet, S. (1988). Language and gender. In F. Newmeyer (Ed.), *The Cambridge Survey 4: The socio-cultural context* (pp. 75–99). Cambridge, UK: Cambridge University Press.

Meier, S. C., Fitzgerald, K. M., Pardo, S.T., & Babcock, J. (2011).The effects of hormonal gender affirmation treatment on mental health in female-to-male transsexuals.*Journal of Gay and Lesbian Mental Health, 15*, 281–299.

Mercaitis, P.A., Peaper, R. E., & Schwartz, P.A. (1985). Effect of danazol on vocal pitch: A case study. *Obstetrics and Gynecology, 65*(1), 131–135.

Mehta, D. D., & Hillman, R. E. (2008). Voice assessment: Updates on perceptual, acoustic, aerodynamic, and endoscopic imaging methods. *Current Opinion in Otolaryngology and Head and Neck Surgery, 16*(3), 211–215.

Miller, D., Schutte, H., & Sulter. A. (1996). Standardized laryngeal videostroboscopic rating: Differences between untrained and trained male and female subjects, and effects of varying sound intensity, fundamental frequency, and age. *Journal of Voice, 10*(2), 109–213.

Mondorf, B. (2002). Gender difference in English syntax. *Journal of English Linguistics, 30*(2), 158–180.

Moore, B. C., & Glasberg, B. R. (1983). Suggested formulae for calculating auditory filter bandwidths and excitation patterns. *Journal of the Acoustical Society of America, 74*, 750–753.

Nakamura, K., Tsukahara, K., Watanabe, Y., Komazawa, D., & Suzuki, M. (2013).Type 3 thyroplasty for patients with mutational dysphonia. *Journal of Voice, 27*(5), 650–654.

Neumann, K., & Welzel, C. (2004).The importance of voice in male-to-female transsexualism. *Journal of Voice, 18*(1), 153–167.

Newman, D., & Forbes, K. (1993). The effects of danazol on vocal parameters—is an objective prospective study needed? *Medical Journal of Australia, 19*(8), 575.

Nygren, U. (2014).*Effects of increased levels of androgens on voice and vocal folds in women with congenital adrenal hyperplasia and female-to-male transsexual persons.* Stockholm, Sweden: Karolinska Institutet PhD dissertation.

Nygren, U., Nordenskjöld, A., Arver, S., & Södersten, M. (2016). Effects on voice fundamental frequency and satisfaction with voice in trans men during testosterone treatment—a longitudinal study. *Journal of Voice, 30*(6), 766.e23–766.e34.

Oates, J., & Dacakis, G. (1997). Voice change in transsexuals. *Venereology, 10*(3), 178–187.

Owen, M. (1996). Posture. In J. Blum, B. Holman, & M. Pellington (Eds.), *The united states of poetry* (p. 159). New York, NY: Harry N. Abrams Inc.

Papp, V. (2011). *Speaker gender: Physiology, performance and perception.* Houston, TX: Rice University PhD dissertation.

Papp, V. G. (2011). *The female-to-male transsexual voice: Physiology vs. performance in production* (Unpublished doctoral dissertation). Rice University, Houston, TX.

Pattie, M. A., Murdoch, B. E., Theodoros, D., & Forbes, K. (1998). Voice changes in women treated for endometriosis and related conditions: The need for comprehensive vocal assessment. *Journal of Voice, 12*(3), 366–371.

Pegoraro-Krook, M. I., & Castro, V. C. (1994). Normative speaking fundamental frequency (SFF) characteristics of Brazilian male subjects. *Brazilian Journal of Medical and Biological Research, 27*(7), 1659–1661.

Peitzmeier, S., Gardner, I., Weinand, J., Corbet, A., & Acevedo, K. (2017). Health impact of chest binding among transgender adults: A community-engaged, cross-sectional study. *Culture, Health and Sexuality, 19*(1), 64–75.

Peterson, E., Roy, N., Awan, S., Merrill, R., Banks, R., & Tanner, K. (2013). Toward validation of the cepstral spectral index of dysphonia (CSID) as an objective treatment outcomes measure. *Journal of Voice, 27*(4), 401–410.

Pickering, J., Adler, R., Block, C., Helou, L., & Hirsch, S. (November 2014). *Promoting effective services for transgender speakers in the United States: Applying WPATH's Standards of Care.* Presentation at the American Speech-Language-Hearing Association Annual Convention, Orlando, FL.

Pickering, J., & Baker, L. (2012). A historical perspective and review of the literature. In R. Adler, S. Hirsch, & M. Mordaunt (Eds.), *Voice and communication therapy for the transgender / transsexual client: A comprehensive clinical guide* (2nd ed., pp. 1–34). San Diego, CA: Plural Publishing.

Proctor, D. F. (1980). *Breathing, speech, and song.* Vienna, Austria: Springer-Verlag.

Reed, F. (2014). *Self-massage for those who bind.* Workshop presented at the Philadelphia Trans Health Conference, Philadelphia, PA.

Remacle, M., Matar, N., Verduyckt, I., & Lawson, G. (2010). Relaxation thyroplasty for mutational falsetto treatment. *Annals of Otology, Rhinology, and Laryngology, 119* (2), 105–109.

Reynolds, H. M., & Goldstein, Z. G. (2014). Social transition. In L. Erickson-Schroth (Ed.), *Trans bodies trans selves* (pp. 124–154). New York, NY: Oxford University Press.

Riquelme, L. (2013). Signature's: Evolving expressions of culture. *ASHA Leader, 18* (SIG N), pp. 52–55.

Rose, P. (1991). How effective are long term mean and standard deviation as normalisation parameters for tonal fundamental frequency? *Speech Communication, 10*, 229–247.

Rosen, C., Lee, A., Osborne, J., Zullo, T., & Murry, T. (2004). Development and validation of the Voice Handicap Index-10. *Laryngoscope, 114*, 1549–1556.

Searle, J. R. (1970). *Speech acts: An essay in the philosophy of language.* Cambridge, UK: Cambridge University Press.

Shahar, E., Redline, S., Young, T., Boland, L. L., Baldwin, C. M., Nieto, F. J., . . . Robbins, J. A. (2003). Hormone replacement therapy and sleep-disordered breathing. *American Journal of Respiratory and Critical Care Medicine, 167*(9), 1186–1192.

Simmons, H., & White, F. (2014). Our many selves. In L. Erickson-Schroth (Ed.). *Trans bodies trans selves* (pp. 3–23). New York, NY: Oxford University Press.

Simpson, A. P. (2009). Phonetic differences between male and female speech. *Language and linguistics compass, 3*(2), 621–640.

Slavit, D. H., Maragos, N. E., & Lipton, R. J. (1990). Physiologic assessment of Isshiki Type III thyroplasty. *Laryngoscope, 100* (8), 844–848.

Smith, D. R., & Patterson, R. D. (2005). The interaction of glottal-pulse rate and vocal tract length in judgements of speaker size, sex, and age. *Journal of the Acoustical Society of America, 118*(5), 3177–3186.

Söderpalm, E., Larsson, A., & Almquist, S.-Å. (2004). Evaluation of a consecutive group of transsexual individuals referred for vocal intervention in the west of Sweden. *Logopedics, Phoniatrics, Vocology, 29*(1), 18–30.

Spencer, L. E. (1988). Speech characteristics of male-to-female transsexuals: A perceptual and acoustic study. *Folia Phoniatrica, 40*(1), 31–42.

Stemple, J., Glaze, L., & Klaben, B. (2010). *Clinical voice pathology* (4th ed.). San Diego, CA: Plural Publishing.

Stemple, J., Lee, L., D'Amico, B., & Pickup, B. (1994). Efficacy of vocal function exercises as a method of improving voice production. *Journal of Voice, 8*(3), 271–278.

Stoicheff, M. L. (1981). Speaking fundamental frequency characteristics of nonsmoking female adults. *Journal of Speech, Language, and Hearing Research, 24* (3), 437–441.

Sulter, A. M., Wit, H. P., Schutte, H. K., & Miller, D. G. (1994). A structured approach to vocal range profile (phonetogram) analysis. *Journal of Speech and Hearing Research, 37*(5), 1076–1085.

Szakay, A. (2006). Rhythm and pitch as markers of ethnicity in New Zealand English. In P. Warren & C. Watson (Eds.), *Proceedings of the 11th Australian International Conference on Speech Science and Technology* (pp. 421–426).

Talaat, M., Talaat, A. Kelada, I., Angelo, A., Elwany, S., & Thabert, H. (1987). Histological and histochemical study of effects of anabolic steroids on the female larynx. *Annals of Otology, Rhinology, and Laryngology, 96*(4), 468–471.

Titze, I. R. (1989). Physiologic and acoustic differences between male and female voices. *Journal of the Acoustical Society of America, 85*(4), 1699–1707.

Titze, I. R. (2000). *Principles of voice production.* (2nd ed.) Iowa City, IA: National Center for Voice and Speech.

Titze, I. R. (2006). Voice training and voice therapy with a semi-occluded vocal tract: Rational and scientific underpinnings. *Journal of Speech, Language, and Hearing Research, 49*, 448–459.

Titze, I. R., & Verdolini-Abbot, K. (2012). *Vocology: The science and practice of voice habilitation.* Salt Lake City, UT: National Center for Voice and Speech.

Van Borsel, J., de Cuypere, G., Rubens, R., & Destaerke, B. (2000). Voice problems in female-to-male transsexuals. *International Journal of Language and Communication Disorders, 35*(3), 427–442.

van Dommelen, W., & Moxness, B. (1995). Acoustic parameters in speaker height and weight identification: sex-specific behaviour. *Language and Speech, 38*(3), 267–287.

Verdolini-Marston, K., Burke, M. K., Lessac, A., Glaze, L., & Calwell, E. (1995). Preliminary study of two methods of treatment for laryngeal nodules. *Journal of Voice, 9*(1), 74–85.

Vorperian, H. K., Kent, R. D., Lindstrom, M. J., Kalina, C. M., Gentry, L. R., & Yandell, B. S. (2005). Development of vocal tract length during early childhood: A magnetic resonance imaging study.

Journal of the Acoustical Society of America, 117(1), 338–350.

Vorperian, H. K., Wang, S., Chung, M. K., Schimek, E. M., Durtschi, R. B., Kent, R. D., . . . Gentry, L. R. (2009). Anatomic development of the oral and pharyngeal of portions of the vocal tract: An imaging study. *Journal of the Acoustical Society of America, 125*(3), 1666–1678.

Wardle, P. G., Whitehead, M. I., & Mills, R. P. (1983). Non-reversible and wide ranging voice changes after treatment with danazol. *British Medical Journal, 287*(1), 946–946.

Watts, C., Diviney, S., Hamilton, A., Toles, L., Childs, L., & Mau, T. (2015). The effect of stretch-and-flow voice therapy on measures of vocal function and handicap. *Journal of Voice, 29*(2), 191–199.

Wolfe, V., Rutusnik, D., Smith, F., & Northrop, G. (1990). Intonation and fundamental frequency in male-to-female transsexuals. *Journal of Speech and Hearing Disorders 55(1)*, 43–50.

Yanagihara, N., Koike, Y., & von Leden, H. (1966). Phonation and respiration: Functional study in normal subjects. *Fonia Phoniatr, 18*(5), 323–340.

Zimman, L. (2012). *Voices in transition: Testosterone, transmasculinity, and the gendered voice among female-to-male transgender people* (Unpublished doctoral dissertation). University of Colorado.

Recommended Readings

Awan, S. N. (1993). Superimposition of speaking voice characteristics and phonetograms in untrained and trained vocal groups. *Journal of Voice, 7*(1), 30–37.

Britto, A. I., & Doyle, P. C. (1990). A comparison of habitual and derived optimal voice fundamental frequency values in normal young adult speakers. *Journal of Speech and Hearing Disorders, 55*(3), 476–484.

Brown, W. R., Morris, R. J., Hicks, D. M., & Howell, E. (1993). Phonational profiles of female professional singers and nonsingers. *Journal of Voice, 7*, 219–226.

Brown, W. R., Morris, R. J., Hollien, H., & Howell, E. (1991). Speaking fundamental frequency characteristics as a function of age and professional singing. *Journal of Voice, 5*, 310–315.

Chen, S. H. (2007). Sex differences in frequency and intensity in reading and voice range profiles for

Taiwanese adult speakers. *Folia Phoniatrica et Logopaedica, 59,* 1–9.

Cowan, M. (1936). Pitch and intensity characteristics of stage speech. *Archives of Speech* (Supp. 1).

de Pinto, O., & Hollien, H. (1982). Speaking fundamental frequency characteristics of Australian women: then and now. *Journal of Phonetics, 10*(4), 367–375.

Fitch, J. L. (1990). Consistency of fundamental frequency and perturbation in repeated phonations of sustained vowels, reading, and connected speech. *Journal of Speech and Hearing Disorders, 55*(2), 360–363.

Fitch, J. L., & Holbrook, A. (1970). Modal vocal fundamental frequency of young adults. *Archives of Otolaryngology, 92,* 379–382.

French, P., Saxena, M., Harrison, P., & Künzel, H. J. (1998). Normative F0 data for Panjabi and Urdu: preliminary report on male speakers over telephone lines. In *International Association for Forensic Phonetics and Acoustics Annual Meeting 1998.* Voorburg, Netherlands.

Garofolo, J. S., Lamel, L. F., Fisher, W. M., Fiscus, J. G., Pallett, D. S., Dahlgren, N. L., & Victor, Z. (1993). *TIMIT Acoustic-phonetic continuous speech corpus.* (Published: Linguistic Data Consortium, Philadelphia, PA)

Gilmore, S. I., Guidera, A. M., Hutchins, S. L., & van Steenbrugge, W. (1992). Intra-subject variability and the effect of speech task on vocal fundamental frequency of young adult Australian males and females. *Australian Journal of Human Communication Disorders, 20,* 65–73.

Hanley, T., & Snidecor, J. C. (1967). Some acoustic similarities among languages. *Phonetica, 17,* 97–107.

Hollien, H., & Paul, P. A. (1969). A second evaluation of the speaking fundamental frequency characteristics of post-adolescent girls. *Language and Speech, 12,* 119–124.

Hollien, H., & Shipp, T. (1972). Speaking fundamental frequency and chronological age in males. *Journal of Speech and Hearing Research, 15*(1), 155–159.

Hollien, H., Hollien, P. A., & de Jong, G. (1997). Effects of three parameters on speaking fundamental frequency. *Journal of the Acoustical Society of America, 102*(5 Pt. 1), 2984–2992.

Hollien, H., Tolhurst, G. C., & McGlone, R. E. (1982). *Speaking fundamental frequency as a function of vocal intensity* (Tech. rep.). IASCP Report 027-82 submitted to the Dreyfuss Foundation, University of Florida, Gainesville.

Hudson, T., de Jong, G., McDougall, K., Harrison, P., & Nolan, F. (2007). F0 statistics for 100 young male speakers of Standard Southern British English. In J. Trouvain & W. Barry (Eds.), *Proceedings of the 16th International Congress of Phonetic Sciences, 6–10 August 2007, Saarbrücken* (pp. 1809–1812). Saarbrücken, Germany.

Izadi, F., Mohseni, R., Daneshi, A., & Sandughdar, N. (2012). Determination of fundamental frequency and voice intensity in Iranian men and women aged between 18 and 45 years. *Journal of Voice, 26*(3), 336–340.

Jessen, M. (2009). Forensic phonetics and the influence of speaking style on global measures of fundamental frequency. In G. Grewendorf & M. Rathert (Eds.), *Formal linguistics and law* (pp. 115–140). Mouton de Gruyter.

Lass, N. J., & Brown, W. R. (1978). Correlational study of speakers' heights, weights, body surface areas, and speaking fundamental frequencies. *Journal of the Acoustical Society of America, 63*(4), 1218–1220.

Lindh, J. (2006). Preliminary descriptive F0-statistics for young male speakers (Technical report). *Lund University Working papers, 52,* 89–92.

Linke, C. E. (1953). *A study of pitch characteristics of female voices and their relationship to vocal effectiveness* (PhD dissertation). The University of Iowa, Iowa City, IA.

Linke, C. E. (1973). A study of pitch characteristics of female voices and their relationship to vocal effectiveness. *Folia Phoniatrica et Logopaedica, 25*(3), 173–185.

Michel, J. F., Hollien, H., & Moore, P. (1966). Speaking fundamental frequency characteristics of 15, 16 and 17 year-old girls. *Language and Speech, 9,* 46–51.

Moon, K. R., Chung, S. M., Park, H. S., & Kim, H. S. (2012). Materials of acoustic analysis: sustained vowel versus sentence. *Journal of Voice, 26*(5), 563–565.

Morris, R. J., Brown, W. R., Hicks, D. M., & Howell, E. (1995). Phonational profiles of male trained singers and nonsingers. *Journal of Voice, 9* (142–148).

Murray, E., & Tiffin, J. (1934). An analysis of some basic aspects of effective speech. *Archives of Speech, 1*(1), 61–83.

Nolan, F., McDougall, K., de Jong, G., & Hudson, T. (2006). A forensic phonetic study of "dynamic" sources of variability in speech: The DyViS project. In P. Warren & C. Watson (Eds.), *Proceedings of the 11th SST Conference* (pp. 13–18). Auckland, NZ.

Oates, J. (2012). Evidenced-based practice in voice therapy for transgender/transsexual clients. In R. Adler, S. Hirsch, & M. Mordaunt (Eds.), *Voice and communication therapy for the transgender / transsexual client: A comprehensive clinical guide* (2nd ed., pp. 45–68). San Diego, CA: Plural Publishing.

Pemberton, C., McCormack, P., & Russell, A. (1998). Have women's voices lowered across time? A cross-sectional study of Australian women's voices. *Journal of Voice, 12*(2), 208–213.

Schiwitz, A. C. (2011). *The effect of task type on speaking fundamental frequency in women* (MSc thesis). Auburn University, Alabama.

Snidecor, J. C. (1951). The pitch and duration characteristics of superior female speakers during oral reading. *Journal of Speech and Hearing Disorders, 16,* 44–52.

Weaver, A. T. (1924). Experimental studies in vocal expression. *Journal of Applied Psychology, 8*(2), 159–186.

Yamazawa, H., & Hollien, H. (1992). Speaking fundamental frequency patterns of Japanese women. *Phonetica, 49*(2), 128–140.

10

Pitch and Intonation

Marylou Pausewang Gelfer, Jack Pickering,
and Michelle Mordaunt

Introduction

As our conceptualization of gender, gender identity, and gender expression evolve, so too does our intervention for voice and communication for people who are transgender. Historically, speech-language pathologists (SLPs) have worked primarily with trans women, clients transitioning from male to female. However, the spectrum of gender diverse individuals seeking voice and communication services has broadened. Moving forward, we will likely see more transgender men, individuals who prefer a gender ambiguous vocal presentation, and those who may seek both feminine and masculine communication presentation depending on the context (Azul, Nygren, Sodersten, & Neuschaefer-Rube, 2017; Davies, Papp, & Antoni, 2015).

In all cases, these clients will need to be assessed carefully to determine their communication needs and wants. It will also be important for speech-language pathologists and other professionals to develop cultural competence in lesbian, gay, bisexual, and transgender (LGBT) populations, to understand the contexts, environments, and challenges that affect our clients' communication (Hancock, 2015; Kelly & Robinson,

2011). Finally, an overarching goal of all of our intervention with this population must be to maintain and enhance vocal health and well-being. Careful assessment, cultural competence, and vocal hygiene have always been important in our provision of speech-language services, but we will need to attend more closely to our clients' unique individual perspectives in planning effective treatment (Hancock, 2015). For clients whose communication does not require the consistent perception of a female speaker, a variety of treatment targets may be appropriate. However, trans women are likely to remain a large percentage of the gender diverse clients on our caseload, and these individuals need a comprehensive approach to voice modification or voice feminization.

Most commonly, the transfeminine[1] client comes to the clinic with the foremost concern being pitch or speaking fundamental frequency (SFF). Understandably, for many trans women, the perception and means of

---

[1]Voice modification is necessary for both transfeminine and transmasculine clients; however, therapy for the transfeminine population will be more prominently addressed in this chapter. The methods discussed in this chapter might be applied to the transmasculine population with some modification. Voice and communication therapy for transmasculine clients is discussed in depth in Chapter 9.

attaining a more feminine voice is to use a "higher pitch." However, a woman's voice is not simply a higher-pitched version of man's voice. Recent studies have indicated that a higher SFF is not in itself sufficient to create the perception of a female voice (Gelfer & Bennett, 2013; Gelfer & Schofield, 2000; Hillenbrand & Clark, 2009). Furthermore, a higher-pitched voice does not correlate strongly with ultimate client satisfaction with voice therapy (Hancock, Krissinger, & Owen, 2011; McNeil, Wilson, Clark, & Deakin, 2008). Hence, the goal of voice therapy may be different than what the transfeminine client initially expects. It is the clinician's responsibility to work with the client to develop realistic goals that address the client's presenting concerns, while maintaining flexibility to also include individual differences and the client's evolving sense of gender presentation through voice.

While pitch is not the only element of voice change for transfeminine clients, studies have indicated that it is necessary to raise the SFF to at least a "gender-acceptable pitch" to assist with voice feminization (Davies et al., 2015; Hancock & Garabedian, 2013; Holmberg, Oates, Dacakis, & Grant, 2010). The details on gender-acceptable pitch will be discussed at length later in this chapter. However, during the voice feminization process, as pitch is increased, intonation and pitch variation must also be addressed. This is in part due to the fact that women's voices tend to be approximately one octave higher than men's voices, and in order to achieve a "higher" pitch, the intonation range must be shifted upward as well. As clients begin to target increased pitch, intonation patterns may initially become monotone or excessive. The client may sacrifice intonation and natural prosody, considered standard across all genders, in order to achieve the desired pitch and pitch range. The clinician will have to help the client maintain, or in some cases

regain, the intonation patterns typically used in American English that will allow her to have the most natural-sounding speech. Finally, when targeting pitch for voice feminization, it is imperative to recognize that a forward focus resonance, light quality, and other aspects of communication feminization will impact the client's ability to successfully alter pitch.

In this chapter, the focus will be on approaches to establishing a more feminine sounding pitch and appropriate pitch range for transfeminine individuals, while retaining natural intonation patterns within a variety of contexts. It is important to remember, as in any goal setting, that the examples given are guidelines and should be individualized as needed. Just as there are numerous voice modification approaches, there are a number of ways to establish pitch, prosody, and a feminine voice. The following outlined approaches have proven successful for the authors. Clinicians should feel free to extrapolate and further develop techniques that are effective within their own scope of practice. Any clinician, voice or otherwise, should understand that skills are not taught to 100% mastery, and that the client's feminine voice will evolve with practice. Given this assumption, when achieving a new pitch and pitch range, produced with natural prosody, clients may end up sounding feminine with a pitch, pitch range, or intonation pattern not targeted or identified in this chapter.

Pitch

Speaking Fundamental Frequency

Speaking fundamental frequency (SFF) generally refers to the mean or average of the frequencies produced in a connected speech sample by a speaker (Colton, Casper, & Leonard, 2011). Because SFF can vary with intensity, phonemic content, and the intent of the message (Colton et al., 2011), an individual can use a range of average SFFs in different communication situations. The *habitual* SFF is the most commonly used average frequency that the individual produces in connected speech. This SFF can be a partly learned behavior, and partly based on the client's anatomical structures. For example, mothers and daughters can tend to sound similar, and people within the same age group may have similar habitual speaking fundamental frequencies.

The habitual SFF used by individuals may or may not be at their *physiologically normal pitch*, or the pitch that is produced by an individual if his or her phonatory physiology is normalized (Colton et al., 2011). In general, it is most beneficial for people to speak at or near their physiologically normal SFF, so that the habitual and physiologically normal SFFs are similar. In the general population, adopting a speaking pitch that deviates from the physiologically normal SFF can be a potential risk factor for the individual in developing problems with his or her voice (Stemple, Glaze, & Klaben, 2010), if proper voice modification techniques are not implemented. Thus, changing pitch in the gender diverse population must be undertaken with care, as in most cases clinicians will *not* be attempting to target a speaking fundamental frequency that the client would produce in a normal, relaxed phonatory position. Traditional voice therapy techniques may be similar, but the concept of attaining the most physiologically appropriate speaking fundamental frequency may not be possible (although determining this frequency will help define and establish the transfeminine client's eventual feminine target pitch).

Obviously, when altering pitch for this population, both a feminine-sounding voice and a healthy laryngeal mechanism are important goals.

Determining Speaking Fundamental Frequency

To determine habitual speaking fundamental frequency for a transfeminine client, the KayPentax Visi-Pitch, Multi-Speech, SonaSpeech™, or Computerized Speech Lab (CSL™) can be used, as well as any other acoustic analysis system to which the clinician has access. Acoustic measures of fundamental frequency for the following tasks should be documented:

1. Sustained phonation on the vowels /i/, /a/, and /u/
2. Reading a standardized passage, such as the Rainbow Passage (Fairbanks, 1960)
3. Spontaneous speech sample of 40 to 60 seconds

The unit of measure for SFF is hertz (Hz), or cycles per second. This measure is an acoustically determined approximation of the number of vocal fold openings and closings per second. However, Hz values do not necessarily correspond well to perceptions of pitch. Most normal-hearing listeners perceive pitch only as accurately as the unit of the musical half-step, or *semitone*. If the clinician is working with a tone-producing app, piano, or pitch pipe or with a client who has a musical background, it may facilitate communication with the client if Hz values are converted into semitones, each representing a half-step on the musical scale. Table 10–1 presents a conversion standard for Hz into semitones or musical notes. Gallena (2007) presents this conversion directly on a piano keyboard.

Table 10–1. Conversion Table Indicating Semitone and Hertz Values

Semitone Value	Hertz Value	Semitone Value	Hertz Value
A_1	55.0	F_3	174.6
$A^{\#}_1$	58.26	$F^{\#}_3$	185.0
B_1	61.75	G_3	196.0
C_2	65.40	$G^{\#}_3$	207.7
$C^{\#}_2$	69.30	A_3	220.0
D_2	73.43	$A^{\#}$	233.1
$D^{\#}_2$	77.76	B_3	247.0
E_2	82.40	C_4	261.6
F_2	87.35	$C^{\#}_4$	277.2
$F^{\#}_2$	92.50	D_4	293.7
G_2	98.03	$D^{\#}_4$	311.1
$G^{\#}_2$	103.8	E_4	329.6
A_2	110.0	F_4	349.2
$A^{\#}_2$	116.5	$F^{\#}_4$	370.0
B_2	123.5	G_4	392.0
C_3	130.8	$G^{\#}_4$	415.5
$C^{\#}_3$	138.6	A_4	440.0
D_3	146.8	$A^{\#}_4$	466.2
$D^{\#}_3$	153.6	B_4	493.9
E_3	164.8		

Source: Adapted from M. L. Andrews (1999), *Manual of Voice Treatment: Pediatrics Through Geriatrics* (2nd ed.). San Diego, CA: Singular.

Determining Physiologically Appropriate Speaking Fundamental Frequencies

Determining the client's physiologically appropriate SFFs will give the clinician valuable information as to where to begin working on altering the client's habitual SFF. To determine these measures, have the client do one or more of the following techniques, after ensuring that the client is in a relaxed state and is sitting or standing in an erect posture for good breath support. An acoustic analysis system should be used to document acoustic measures of the frequencies produced.

1. Throat clear into sustained phonation (usually the ultimate "no-no" for voice!)
2. "Uh-uh" as in a response to a question
3. Hum spontaneously with no-pitch model

In the techniques described above, the frequency or range of frequencies produced by the client are usually physiologically appropriate.

1. Count from 1 to 5, starting at a comfortable pitch and going up the scale in even steps (as if on a tone scale). If the client can get to "5" and still feel comfortable and produce a phonation of good

quality, then "1" or "2" are usually at physiologically appropriate frequencies.

Gender-Acceptable Pitch

Many trans women may have difficulty achieving an SFF that is at or near the mean for ciswomen of their chronological age, but this does not preclude them from achieving a perceptually feminine voice. Normative data on women's connected speech reveal that a variety of SFFs are typical. Research literature reports mean SFFs that include 224 Hz for females ages 20 to 29 years (Stoicheff, 1981) during reading, and 221 Hz in extemporaneous speech (Ovesky, 2004). For older female speakers, a mean SFF of 187 Hz has been reported during reading in the 40 to 50-year age range (Saxman & Burk, 1967), and 189 Hz in extemporaneous speech (Ovesky, 2004). Fortunately for older transfeminine clients, SFF for females tends to decrease with age (Boone, McFarlane, Von Berg, & Zraick, 2014). Although women in their 20s may be expected to speak at frequencies in excess of 200 Hz, women in their 30s, 40s, and 50s are reported to be below 200 Hz (Colton et al., 2011), which may be more attainable for the transfeminine client. In fact, when the range of SFFs is examined in some of the normative studies, some female subjects have SFFs as low as 143 Hz (for a female in the 60- to 69-year-old group [Stoicheff, 1981]), or 147 Hz (for a female in the 40- to 50-year group [Ovesky, 2004]). Thus, achieving the "mean" SFF for the client's age group should not necessarily be the goal.

The target pitch for transfeminine clients should fall within a gender-acceptable Hz range. This is the pitch at which the speaker's gender is correctly identified as female some or most of the time, based on voice alone. Studies have provided various recommendations for a gender-acceptable pitch. Gelfer and Schofield (2000) found that the three transfeminine participants in their study who were consistently perceived as female had a mean SFF of 187 Hz; however, one subject in this group had an individual SFF of 164 Hz. Previous studies (Spencer 1988; Wolfe, Ratusnik, Smith, & Northrup, 1990) have suggested a gender-acceptable pitch is attainable for this population at speaking fundamental frequencies as low as 155 to 160 Hz, based on observations that subjects within this frequency range were frequently or consistently perceived as female based on voice alone. Extensive reviews of the available literature by Davies et al. (2015), Oates and Dacakis (2015), and King, Brown, and McCrea (2011) suggest that the SFF target for the transfeminine individual must move above the cismale range (100–140 Hz) and approach the cisfemale range (180–220 Hz). At this time, it is evident that there is some discrepancy for gender-acceptable pitch, but a range may be defined as an SFF between 150 and 185 Hz.

Working toward a gender-acceptable pitch may initially and continually be a concern for the client, as this pitch may fall short of the client's expected female pitch as a target goal. As the client becomes more comfortable with developing a "natural" voice as opposed to merely a "higher" voice, she usually begins to understand the wisdom in setting this more realistic goal of gender-acceptable pitch. For example, the "natural" pitch should allow ample room for upward inflections of pitch during connected speech. The mean speaking fundamental frequency is only one aspect of the voice/communication feminization process.

Vocal Tension and Quality

The involvement of various laryngeal muscles in fundamental frequency elevation is complex (Behrman, 2013). We typically think of an increase in SFF as requiring increased contraction of the cricothyroid muscle, which stretches the vocal folds, causing both length and tension to be increased passively (that is, without added tension in the vocal fold muscles, the thyroarytenoids, themselves; Behrman, 2013). However, contraction of the thyroarytenoid muscles can also assist in raising pitch, especially at moderate to high intensities (Behrman, 2013). It is possible that this additional tension can add an element of vocal hyperfunction to the process of pitch elevation. When deviating significantly from an individual's physiological pitch, it is crucial to confirm that the client is not tensing the vocal muscles excessively during the process. Clients should be made aware of the dangers of excessive laryngeal muscle tension and have ways of reducing it, if present. Using the following tasks to measure and/or monitor vocal tension while altering habitual SFF will help to provide the client with a healthy approach to working on this aspect of voice feminization:

1. Visual cues (Boone et al., 2014)
2. Laryngeal palpation and/or massage (Aronson, 1990)
3. Progressive relaxation (Boone et al., 2014)
4. Yawn-sigh (Boone et al., 2014)
5. Confidential voice (Boone et al., 2014).

The clinician may not always be able to begin working directly on feminine voice and communication, and may be called upon to deal with correcting the client's maladaptive vocal behaviors in therapy (see Chapter 8 for additional information on vocal health). Some transfeminine clients may have adopted unfavorable voice qualities such as excessive tense breathiness that must be addressed. Tense breathiness is produced with excessive tension in the lateral cricoarytenoid muscles which compress the anterior part of the vocal folds together, with a posterior gap that allows turbulent air to be forced through, giving the voice a strained and breathy sound. Other common voice qualities found within this population include harshness, hoarseness, strain, glottal fry, and hard glottal attacks, which may also need attention. Traditional techniques to reduce the impact of poor voice quality include:

1. /h/ onsets (an extension of yawn-sigh; Boone et al., 2014)
2. Vocal Function Exercises (Stemple, Glaze, & Klaben, 2010)
3. Resonance approaches, e.g., Lessac-Madsen's Resonant Voice Therapy Approach (see Chapter 11)
4. Straw phonation and other semi-occluded vocal tract techniques (Kapsner-Smith, Hunter, Kirkham, Cox, & Titze, 2015)

Experience has shown that increasing pitch and modifying pitch variation in tandem with a resonant voice therapy approach will provide the client with many of the tools necessary for settling into a comfortable, natural, easy pitch range, without introducing excessive vocal tension or unfavorable voice qualities. Approaches that support and modify resonance are described in Chapter 11.

Client Perception

It is crucial to train clients to accurately monitor all aspects of their progress. The clinician needs to pay attention to possible inconsistency in the client's self-perception of pitch, tension, fatigue, and other auditory and tactile sensations.

As the transfeminine client works to alter her habitual SFF, it is important for the client to be able to self-monitor her habitual SFF. Awareness of habitual SFF must begin as soon as this area is targeted. The following processes may be used to increase and maintain client awareness of habitual SFF and vocal tension.

1. Provide visual feedback for pitch using an acoustic analysis system or one of a growing number of apps developed for tablets and smart phones.
2. Increase awareness of overall body tension.
3. Record and play back video samples using smartphone and tablet technology to increase awareness of voice quality.
4. Match speaking pitch to electronic guitar tuners, electronic keyboards, or even an old-fashioned pitch pipe, if the client has good pitch-matching skills.

Pitch Therapy

Establishing Target Speaking Fundamental Frequency

Establishing a client's target speaking fundamental frequency is a dynamic process. After considering the client's physiological and habitual speaking fundamental frequencies as well as vocal tension, voice quality, and client perception, the next step is to establish an initial or "starting frequency" during the first few sessions of therapy. This starting frequency will be an easy production of an "m-humm" or sustained "ah" at a frequency that is above the client's physiological SFF. Although this point will vary across clients, a frequency of 150 to 160 Hz is not unreasonable (corresponding to the

notes D3 to E3 on a piano keyboard; see Table 10–1 for conversions from Hz to semitones or notes). As therapy progresses, the target SFF will most likely change upward until it rests at what will be the client's final SFF goal. Progression toward the final goal will be influenced by other voice parameters addressed in voice feminization therapy, and more significantly by the client's ability to participate and modify her voice. Varying degrees of feedback and support will be necessary, with increased feedback needed in the early stages of therapy. A typical progression toward the final goal may include:

1. "m-humm"
2. "m-vowel" (e.g., /mi/, /mu/)
3. To enhance tactile feedback, use straw phonation, which will establish good lip vibration and facilitate forward resonance.
4. Syllable production, beginning with syllables initiated by /m/
5. Word production, again focusing on /m/- and also /n/-initiated syllables
6. Phrase production, initially with lots of /m/- and /n/-onset words, but gradually normalizing phonemic context
7. Sentence production of increasing length
8. 10-second monologue
9. 30-second monologue
10. 2- to 5-minute conversation

Progression toward the target SFF is not necessarily perfectly linear or methodical for each client. The particular relationship with the above approach may shift to accommodate each client's individual needs, but the overall approach will remain similar. The ultimate objective is for the client to use a comfortable, perceptually feminine voice that matches her personality and lifestyle, in a variety of situations and with a variety of communication partners. Monitoring clients' feelings about their voice and their satisfaction will be important, so the application of counseling skills will be a necessary aspect of your therapy (see Chapter 3). Although the client's voice may occasionally be mistaken for male when no visual cues are present (such as over the telephone), the voice plus the client's physical appearance should ultimately be recognized consistently as feminine.

Establishing a Range for Speaking Fundamental Frequency

It is unrealistic to expect the client to target a specific SFF at all times. Each client has a range for her average SFF within which her voice resonates with a comfortable tone. Once a client's individual SFF has been established within the gender-acceptable or feminine speaking range (e.g., 175 Hz, or F3), a plus/minus one-semitone area is established around the given SFF. This range will allow flexibility when targeting the established SFF. For instance, targeting 175 Hz exactly and consistently is not realistic. Time of day, allergies, general physical health, emotional state, fatigue, and stress are all factors that may influence the SFF on any given day or time of day. These influences will make a specific SFF target difficult to maintain. One or more semitones may be necessary above or below the established SFF to create a range for the average SFF. This range will be determined in part by the client's vocal potential. As illustrated in Figure 10–1, for a 175 Hz (F3) SFF (gender-acceptable), the average range using a target of one semitone above and below would be 165 Hz (E3) to 185 Hz (F#3).

A "real-life" test for voice feminization is essential prior to final discharge from any therapy program. Progress toward the final target SFF will take time and effort on the part of the client, although it has been our experience that younger clients tend to have an easier time with voice feminization. The

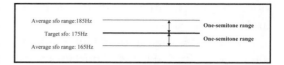

Figure 10–1. Range for average speaking fundamental frequency.

process of altering pitch will have tremendous impact on the client's self-esteem and overall progress in voice therapy. Although SFF may be addressed separately at first, habitual pitch, intonation and pitch range, and resonance will eventually be addressed together as the client moves into phrases, sentences, and extemporaneous speech.

Conversational Pitch Range

Comfortable Conversational Pitch Range

After establishing the average SFF and a range of average SFFs for a client, the *comfortable* conversational range needs to be determined. The comfortable conversational pitch range is the range that will be easily available to the client during normal, everyday speech. This differs from the conversational pitch range described in previous studies, called here the *total* conversational pitch range, which refers to the complete pitch range a client may use during connected speech, including the frequencies that may be produced only as artifacts. For example, the total conversational pitch range (or speaking fundamental frequency range) as measured in previous studies may have included very low frequencies, momentarily produced during voicing offsets and vocal fry (Cumbers, 2013). The comfortable conversational pitch range is also different from the maximum (total) phonational frequency range, which refers to every frequency an individual can phonate with maximum effort, from the lowest tone in modal register to the highest tone in falsetto register (Boone et al., 2014). Maximum phonational frequency range will not be discussed in this chapter because it goes well beyond the frequencies used in speech and does not strongly inform clinical decision making for transfeminine clients.

Male and female *total* conversational pitch ranges have been found to include 16 to 27 semitones (Iwen, 2010; Linke, 1973; Mysak, 1959; Ovesky, 2004; Snidecor, 1951). However, the work of Gelfer and Schofield (2000) indicates that for transfeminine clients, conversational variability of approximately 12 semitones is typically used; thus, this will be considered the *comfortable* conversational range for this population.

For their female-perceived subjects with a mean SFF of 187 Hz (F#3), Gelfer and Schofield (2000) found a comfortable conversational range from 138 Hz (C3) to 301 Hz (approximately D4). This may serve as a convenient target range if an SFF of 187 Hz is set; however, it may be desirable for the clinician to calculate his or her own range for a different SFF. Based on an average SFF of 220 Hz for a cis-woman and a calculation of 12 semitones around this SFF, the potential comfortable conversational pitch range for this woman would be 165 Hz to 311 Hz, or E3 to D#4, a total range of 146 Hz. This calculation is made with 6 semitones above and below the target SFF of 220 Hz. It is important to keep in mind, however, that 6 semitones equally above and below may not necessarily be the final target or realistic for the client. Based on the client's vocal potential, any variation of the division of the semitone range is possible (e.g., 8 above and 4 below). The comfortable conversational pitch range for a speaker with an SFF of 220 Hz is illustrated in Table 10–2. In contrast, a target SFF of 180 Hz (F-F#3), as shown in Table 10–3, which is considered a gender-acceptable pitch, would result in a 12-semitone range of 131 Hz (C3) to 247 Hz (B3). The total pitch range would be 116 Hz for a gender-acceptable pitch of 180 Hz.

It is important to note that although the client with an SFF of 220 Hz *appears* to have a larger range (146 Hz) than the client with the SFF of 180 Hz (116 Hz), in fact both have the *same* range perceptually. That is, both have a range of 12 semitones, or one octave. For this reason, it is important to always convert a speaker's pitch range measures into semitones, which provide perceptually stable units regardless of top or bottom limits of the client's conversational range. Why? The ear is nonlinear in

Table 10–2. 12-Semitone Female Conversational Pitch Range for an SFF of 220 Hz (A3)

Hertz Value	Semitone Value
311 Hz Highest	D#4 Highest
220 Hz Average	A3 Average
165 Hz Lowest	E3 Lowest

Table 10–3. 12-Semitone Gender Ambiguous Conversational Pitch Range for an SFF of 180 Hz (F-F#3)

Hertz Value	Semitone Value
247 Hz Highest	B3 Highest
180 Hz Average	F-F#3 Average
131 Hz Lowest	C3 Lowest

its perception of pitch. It is more sensitive to frequency changes in lower frequencies compared with higher frequencies. For example, we are easily able to hear the difference between voices of 100 Hz and 200 Hz; however, if the 100 Hz difference was between 1000 Hz and 1100 Hz, we would not perceive the difference as clearly (Behrman, 2013). Given this nonlinearity in sensitivity, the 146 Hz around an SFF of 220 Hz sounds the same to the human listener as the 116 Hz surrounding an SFF of 180 Hz. In fact, Hz doubles for each perceived octave. If we relied on Hz to measure range, it would appear that speakers with high-frequency voices have larger ranges than speakers with low-frequency voices, although both ranges would be identical perceptually.

Using 12 semitones as the standard comfortable conversational range, and given client variability, and allowing for some flexibility and individual variation, it is reasonable to assume a 10- to 14-semitone target comfortable conversational range. As illustrated in Figure 10–2, using a 12-semitone conversational range around a target SFF of 180 Hz would result in an upper limit target of 247 Hz and a lower limit target of 131 Hz. As previously stated, this equal and balanced semitone relationship (i.e., 6 semitones above and below) is not necessarily realistic or the same for each client, but will be used for demonstration purposes.

The frequency levels for 10, 12, and 14 semitone comfortable conversational ranges at the targeted gender-acceptable SFF have now been established. From this point on, the client will be able to target a reasonable conversational range that is appropriate for female speakers and allows adequate variability to express a variety of emotional states: a realistic goal. However, using the new conversational range in a perceptually natural manner is deceptively difficult and requires commitment and many hours of practice.

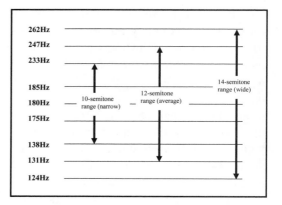

Figure 10–2. 10- to 14-semitone comfortable conversational range with a gender-acceptable pitch of 180 Hz.

Stress, Intonation, and Pitch

Stress and intonation are part of what we call the *suprasegmental* aspects of speech—that is, their execution covers more than a single phoneme. Suprasegmentals are applied to the syllable, word, phrase, or sentence levels (Raphael, Borden, & Harris, 2011).

Stress occurs at the syllable and word levels. Stress in English is conveyed by using a higher pitch, louder intensity, and longer duration on the stressed syllable or word. Words like RECord and reCORD can actually have different meanings, depending on which syllable is stressed (Raphael et al., 2011). Stress is particularly important for transfeminine clients, as it gives them an opportunity to use a momentary pitch elevation or upward inflection that can help signal a female speaker.

Intonation patterns, on the other hand, are pitch changes that are typically imposed at the phrase and sentence level. They are less predictable than stress, but are important in conveying the meaning of the speaker's message. They are also important in conveying the attitudes and feelings of the speaker. Sentences such as "The book is yours" can be understood by a listener as either a statement or a question, depending on the speaker's intonation pattern (falling vs. rising). Similarly, a sentence such as "That was a great game" can be understood as either an enthusiastic observation or a sarcastic comment that reveals that the speaker's feelings are the exact opposite of the surface meaning of the sentence (Raphael et al., 2011).

The intonation patterns of the English language, as distinct from intonation patterns that characterize other languages, can cross the voice boundaries that define genders and can be, at least in some cases, considered gender neutral. When altering pitch and pitch range, these linguistically appropriate stress and intonation patterns do not necessarily change, as men and women tend to use generally similar patterns during conversation. However, some clients may find it difficult to maintain their original and natural speech rhythms once pitch and pitch range have been altered. It is important for clients to understand that whereas a higher SFF is desirable, attaining a higher pitch by changing intonation and stress patterns is not recommended. Eventually, clients may wish to alter their speech patterns and style of their own accord, but it is not a requirement to either attain a higher pitch or achieve a more feminine voice. This is important, as some clients may closely identify with their intonation as a defining aspect of who they are as individuals.

Intonation and the Message

Although stress, intonation, and pitch are clearly part of the same final voice therapy goal, stress and intonation need separate consideration. These suprasegmental features impact the entire pattern of an utterance, and are necessary to add meaning

to clarify or reinforce a sentence. English, like all languages, has a melody that distinguishes it from other tongues; however, in English, unlike some other languages, changes in that melody may alter meaning slightly. Change the meaning of the following sentences by stressing the words in bold. Be sure to use simultaneous changes in pitch, loudness, and duration.

> *I want that hat.*
> *I **want** that hat.*
> *I want **that** hat.*
> *I want that **hat**.*

Use of stress and intonation can influence how a message is conveyed or received, and has been the cause of many "misunderstandings." It can also serve to add emphasis and impact to a conversation. Each language or dialect can be defined by basic stress and intonation patterns. There are also certain elements of these features that differentiate women from men. However, for the most part, the standard English stress and intonation patterns apply equally to both genders.

In English, we utilize primary levels of emphasis and secondary levels of emphasis, applied to words in a sentence that are important to the sentence's overall meaning. Nouns tend to be the primary conveyors of meaning. Verbs are usually secondary means of emphasis, followed by adjectives and adverbs. The use of varied emphases in a sentence can alter the meaning of the intended message. Figure 10–3 uses one sentence to illustrate how use of intonation or stress can change the message of the sentence.

Male versus Female Intonation

The English language, as just described, uses standard intonation patterns that cross gender boundaries. However, subtle differences in intonation patterns might cue the

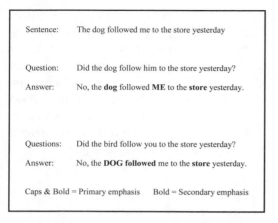

Sentence:	The dog followed me to the store yesterday
Question:	Did the dog follow him to the store yesterday?
Answer:	No, the **dog** followed **ME** to the **store** yesterday.
Questions:	Did the bird follow you to the store yesterday?
Answer:	No, the **DOG followed** me to the **store** yesterday.

Caps & Bold = Primary emphasis   Bold = Secondary emphasis

Figure 10–3. Impact of varied intonation/stress on a sentence.

perception of speaker gender, although exact differences between genders have been difficult to pin down. Several studies have compared the intonation patterns of transfeminine speakers perceived as female versus those perceived as male (Gelfer & Schofield, 2000; Hancock, Colton & Douglas, 2014; Wolfe et al. 1990). A recent study by Hancock et al. (2014) found that "speakers with a larger percentage of utterances with *upward intonation* and larger *ST (semitone) range* are perceived as female" (p. 206). This finding is consistent with research by Wolfe et al. (1990), who noted that the transfeminine participants perceived as females tended to have more upward inflections in pitch than participants who were perceived as males.

Gelfer and Schofield (2000) did a similar study and found that in their female-perceived group of transfeminine participants, there were a greater number of upward shifts in pitch. Hancock et al. (2014) also noted that transfeminine speakers who did not pass as female in their study appeared to use fewer upward and more downward intonations than either cisfemale speakers or transfeminine speakers perceived as female.

This was interpreted by Hancock et al. (2014) as suggesting that females and female-perceived speakers use more upward intonation, but that males and male-perceived speakers are not necessarily monotone. A problem with all of these studies is that the small numbers of participants makes it difficult to generalize the results to the entire population of trans women. Hancock et al. (2014) suggested that perhaps there is some percentage of upward intonations that is "enough" for a speaker to be perceived as female, vs. how many downward intonations are "too much"; in fact, they hypothesized that there may be a threshold effect that has yet to be explored.

Clearly, there is much to be learned about the subtleties of intonation characteristics of males versus females and male-perceived versus female-perceived gender diverse individuals. However, the results to date do suggest that the production of more inflections (especially upward) in females has some basis in the literature. The concept that increased use of intonation is a more perceptually female trait can be linked to how women use language. For example, greater use of intonation can provide a more effective delivery of a message, as its use conveys emotion and emphasis without implying aggression or forcefulness. Furthermore, whereas greater intonation use can be more dramatic, greater intonation is socially less acceptable for men in Western cultures.

Standard American Intonation Pattern

Using appropriate intonation patterns in conjunction with appropriate pitch range (approximately 12 semitones) allows for a natural voice with expression and flexibility.

Additionally, using an appropriate 10 to 14 semitone pitch range with a standard (or perhaps emphasized) intonation pattern will increase the perception of a feminine voice, facilitating successful voice feminization.

It is important to think about pitch range and intonation as the music of the language. When considering individuals for whom English is spoken as a second language, or who speak a different dialect of English, it is likely that differences in pitch range and intonation patterns will be noted. Beyond rate of speech and sounds being phonemically produced differently in these individuals, the "melody" of the language is different. This "melody" can be defined by pitch changes, as well as stress and intonation patterns.

Walk-Jump-Step-Fall

Using the Walk-Jump-Step-Fall (WJSF) intonation approach demonstrated by Edwards and Strattman (1996), intonation can systematically be applied to adjust a client's voice to be more perceptually feminine. The WJSF intonation pattern is the root of all intonation in the American English language and variations of this pattern are used throughout speech. It is important to remember that this pattern is just the *basis* of intonation and must be varied to create successful intonation use. The WJSF can be used in varied order to create natural and realistic intonation. Refer to Figure 10–4 to view the original WJSF pattern.

Walk. In our interpretation of the Edwards and Strattman (1996) model, the WALK of the WJSF pattern would utilize the client's target SFF prior to the word that is to be emphasized. The word emphasized will vary from sentence to sentence, thus varying the length of the extent of the WALK

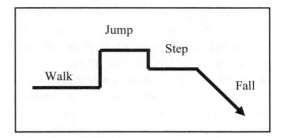

Figure 10–4. Standard American intonation pattern—WJSF.

phase or the use of the target SFF. The client and clinician should note that each new sentence gives the client a chance to "reset" her SFF to the appropriate target level.

Jump. After the WALK, it is necessary to JUMP on the prominent syllable of the word to be emphasized. In order to JUMP, pitch must be increased, thereby adding emphasis to the sentence. This pitch should be within the comfortable conversational pitch range previously described.

Step. After the JUMP, it is necessary to STEP down in pitch, but down to the pitch level of the initial WALK (the target SFF). This STEP tends to be the element most commonly avoided during voice feminization, as it requires more precise and small pitch change increments.

Fall. Finally, for declarative sentences, it is typical for the pitch to FALL below the pitch level of the initial WALK. The FALL, or the decrease of pitch at the end of the sentence, can provide listeners with acoustic cues that help them segment the flow of speech into sentences or mark grammatical structure (Lieberman, Katz, Jongman, Zimmerman, & Miller, 1985). Many clients will try to avoid the FALL in order to avoid approximating the more masculine-sounding pitch levels or registers. However, in order to produce appropriate intonation in English, it is necessary to drop SFF somewhat at the end of declarative sentences. It is important for clients to understand and recognize a feminine lower limit to target, within their comfortable conversational pitch range, as opposed to where their voice may no longer be considered acceptably feminine with regard to pitch.

Applying Natural Intonation Patterns to Comfortable Conversational Range

In addition to varying the WJSF pattern itself, the pattern may vary as it is applied to the comfortable conversational pitch range. Even when using a 10 to 14 semitone comfortable conversational range, if intonation use is reduced or "nonstandard," the amount of "expression" in the

voice and the intended meaning is limited. If the pitch is monotone and high (e.g., a Minnie Mouse voice) and does not use a 10 to 14 semitone speaking pitch range, the overall voice can be perceived as high, "flat," and "unnatural." In contrast, if there is too great a pitch range, one that consistently exceeds 14 semitones, the voice will sound "artificial" and "excessive." In order to reduce unnatural intonation patterns, the WJSF is used across various conversational pitch ranges to provide meaning and emphasis.

High Pitch Target

When it is necessary to strongly emphasize a point using an increased pitch, the JUMP will extend to the highest frequency value of the conversational pitch range. Figure 10–5 illustrates the use of emphasis with a high pitch target. This pattern may be used when saying a sentence such as "I **want** to go!"

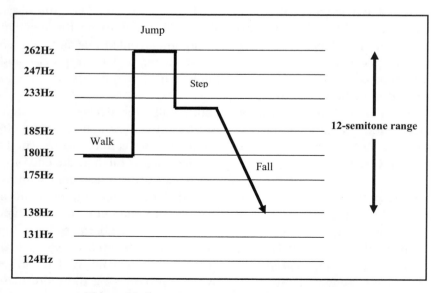

Figure 10–5. Using high pitch for emphasis with WJSF.

Low Pitch Target

Likewise, at times it is necessary to drop pitch down to provide emphasis. Figure 10–6 shows the WJSF pattern with a low pitch emphasis. Apply the sentence "I **won't** go there" to this pattern.

Increased Pitch Range Use

When extreme emphasis is needed to convey meaning, the WJSF pattern can be applied to the 14 semitone conversational range. This is illustrated in Figure 10–7 and a sentence such as "I **love** your hat!"

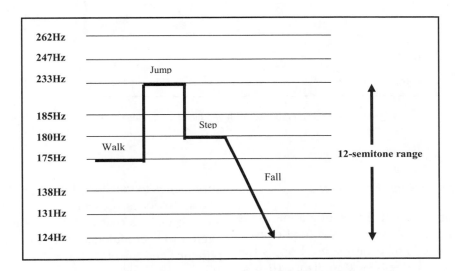

Figure 10–6. Using low pitch for emphasis with WJSF.

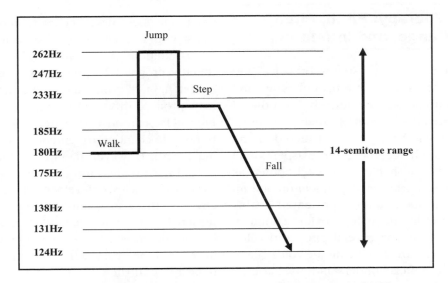

Figure 10–7. Using extreme pitch variation for emphasis with WJSF.

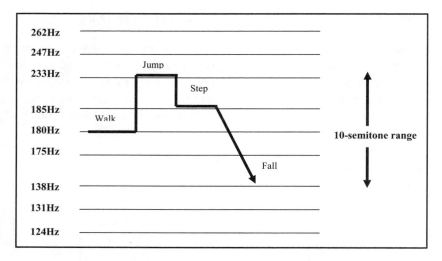

Figure 10–8. Using reduced pitch variation for emphasis with WJSF.

Decreased Pitch Range Use

Finally, at times when less intonation use is optimal, the lower end of the total conversational pitch range can be used. Apply the sentence "My **dog** is sick" to Figure 10-8 to illustrate decreased pitch range.

Therapy: Pitch, Pitch Range, and Intonation

Although all three aspects of voice and speech feminization, pitch, pitch range, and stress/intonation are initially introduced and targeted separately in therapy, eventually they will have to be considered in unison. At discharge, these three aspects will be indistinguishable from each other, as they are so intricately dependent on one another. The methodology presented in this chapter is intended to provide a foundation and basis for general pitch and voice alteration for the transfeminine voice client. Once the clinician understands the basics, it is possible to implement novel and unique

approaches to voice feminization. The therapy approaches presented in this chapter are suggestions that may be modified and altered to accommodate the clinician's experience and the client's need.

General Therapy Considerations

Once objectives have been set, therapy for transfeminine clients progresses as it would for a traditional voice or speech/language therapy program. The hierarchy of therapy for pitch, pitch range, and stress/intonation may proceed from humming and changing pitch or intonation patterns to words/phrases, to chanting, to sentences of increasing length. However, therapy in one area should not progress too far when other areas remain at a lower level within the hierarchy, as all these areas must be considered in unison. Furthermore, the ultimate goal must be considered as the objectives progress. For instance, if the final pitch goal is anticipated to be approximately 175 Hz, it will not serve the client to linger at 150 Hz at the sentence level. It would be better to revert to a lower level, either the phrase or word level, increasing the pitch level gradually toward the final goal of 175 Hz. At this level within the hierarchy, while a higher pitch is being targeted, stress/intonation, pitch range, and all other elements of voice and communication therapy may also be addressed.

Speaking Fundamental Frequency Target Therapy

When targeting SFF, a safe and appropriate starting place may be 10 to 15 Hz above the client's physiological speaking fundamental frequency. For example, if the client's physiological pitch is measured at 130 Hz, therapy may start with sustained /a/ production at 140 to 145 Hz (Figure 10-9). If this frequency proves to be relatively easy and stress/strain free, the client may quickly, within a session or two, progress to 155 Hz. It is customary, but not always necessary, to raise pitch in increments of 10 Hz. The

10 Hz value is used because in the typical target frequencies for voice feminization therapy, 10 Hz is approximately one semitone, which is usually perceptually salient for the client. The most important considerations with SFF therapy is that the productions be easy and relaxed and that the client is able to produce the SFF in multiple environments and at varying loudness levels. Although the quiet loudness levels might be easy for the client, the moderate, loud, and very loud levels may prove more challenging, as these require laryngeal tension and increased subglottal pressure that can bring strain, harshness, and hoarseness to the voice quality.

Conversational Pitch Range Therapy Process

When conducting SFF therapy, it may seem logical to target the goal SFF and have the client produce speech at this specific target SFF. However, it is often unrealistic to

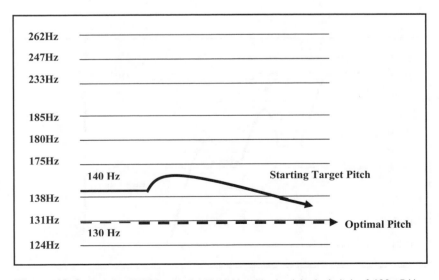

Figure 10–9. Starting SFF target of 140 ±5 Hz with physiological pitch of 130 ±5 Hz.

expect the client to speak at a specific SFF target, even when provided a range of 5 to 10 Hz (see Figure 10–2). Why then be so concerned about determining a target SFF? First, determining the SFF target is essential in establishing a target 10 to 14 semitone comfortable conversational pitch range (see Figure 10–2) for therapy. Second, once the conversational pitch range has been established, therapy can proceed by having the client work within the 10 to 14 semitone range, *while maintaining the average SFF*. It is necessary that the range and the SFF are established in conjunction with each other. If conversational range is used by itself without maintaining the determined SFF, the client can easily access the target 10 to 14 semitone range by speaking at a consistently low or high pitch, and then producing one syllable or word at the opposite pitch extreme to create a false conversational range that looks good on the equipment but sounds very unnatural. For example, if the client has a target of 175 ±10 Hz and a conversational range of 130 to 250 Hz, the client might speak at 150 Hz (not the target SFF), but then inappropriately "jump" to a high 250 Hz frequency so as to create a false comfortable conversational range as seen on the acoustic analysis system. Many clients will attempt to manipulate their acoustic measures in this manner. In order to eliminate this strategy, the client must not only produce the 10 to 14 semitone range, but must ultimately average the target SFF that was used to establish the conversational range in the first place (Figure 10–10).

When starting conversational pitch range therapy, the client may begin with upward and downward glissandos (pitch glides), sirens, and accents, and progress to using musical scale steps (do-re-mi, etc.) up and down to explore pitch range. Using an app to identify starting frequencies and mapping change with a Visi-Pitch, for example, can be helpful in establishing the extent and limitations of the conversational pitch range. It is important for the client to be able to reach the comfortable range available (12 semitones) but know when she is exceeding this range.

Once the range is established with glissandos and scales, the client can self-monitor

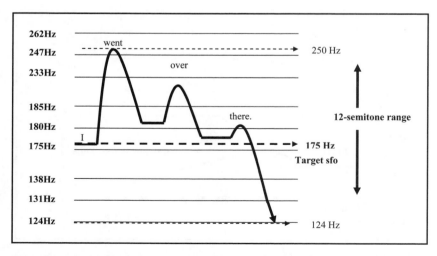

Figure 10–10. Conversational pitch range therapy target of 124 to 250 Hz, which is the range for SFF target of 175 ±10 Hz (e.g., "I went over there").

progress by counting up and down four to five half-notes, or semitones. As the client becomes more accustomed to the SFF, the conversational range will be the natural progression up and down from the SFF starting point. For instance, if the client's SFF is 160 Hz, he or she may be able to count five half-steps or musical notes up, and six down, to create an approximate conversational pitch range that can be used and self-monitored without the visual feedback of an acoustic analysis system (e.g., the Visi-Pitch or Multi-Speech). Acoustic analysis programs with visual feedback serve as an excellent resource and reference during therapy, but quickly challenging the client to rely on *self*-monitoring and pitch judgment once good awareness is established is crucial. The client will only have herself for feedback during discharge and maintenance (see Chapter 16). If clients become too dependent on the acoustic analysis system or fixated on the pitch and pitch range "numbers" (Hz), their success and ultimate independence with voice therapy may be compromised.

When the client is able to successfully and safely produce 10 to 14 semitones around the target SFF, the hierarchy can resume, continuing with automatic speech, phrases, sentences, and so on. As before, the clinician should be sure to pace SFF shifts realistically. Try to advance the client to her maximum SFF and conversational range potential before having the client move up too far on the hierarchy. As therapy progresses, resources like voice and diction texts/workbooks (e.g., Glenn, Glenn, & Forman's *Your Voice and Articulation*, 1998) and websites (e.g., www.whysanity.net/monos/ and www.10-minute-plays.com/scenes/scenes_two_women.html) that contain monologues and dialogues can facilitate conversational practice opportunities. Ultimately, functional, day-to-day conversation can be used in voice training and during outside practice.

Pitch and Conversational Pitch Range Case Study

The client is a trans woman who has been in transition for eight years. Client reports that pitch and the naturalness of her intonation are her biggest concerns regarding her voice. Probes of minimum and maximum pitch indicated that the client was able to produce a minimum pitch of 74 Hz and a maximum high pitch of 266 Hz when performing glissandos on the vowel /a/. This total pitch range is equivalent to 22 semitones, which is within normal limits for total pitch. Probes of client's ability to use the targeted SFF of 175 ±5 Hz with a sustained /a/ yielded 49% accuracy across two sessions following calibration with visual feedback. She was able to identify when she was at the target SFF with 70% accuracy. When provided with an auditory example of her targeted SFF on an electronic keyboard, she was able to match it with /a/ with 100% accuracy and identify when she had matched it with 83% accuracy. Several random samples of client's pitch were taken during conversational speech and yielded an average of 120 Hz. Her habitual speaking fundamental frequency did not fall within the targeted gender-acceptable 12-semitone pitch range of 130 to 250 Hz.

Pitch Objective. Client will use an average fundamental frequency of 175 ±10 Hz during a 1-minute conversation with 80% accuracy.

Progress: This goal was discontinued after the first few sessions, as it encouraged the client to use unnatural intonation patterns and extreme pitch changes in an attempt to bring up the average fundamental frequency measure. Client experienced more success when focusing on speaking within a specified pitch range rather than on maintaining a specific fundamental frequency.

Conversational Pitch Range Objective. Client will use a 12-semitone range (130 to 250 Hz)[2] in a 1-minute conversation with 80% accuracy.

Progress: Objective in progress. Client was able to use a 12-semitone range of 130 to 250 Hz in 10-second monologues with 82% accuracy and identify when she had used it with 88% accuracy.

Discussion. Targeting SFF directly did not work for this client, but when it was targeted by providing the client with a comfortable conversational range within which to speak, she was able to have more success at attaining her target SFF *as well as* her conversational range. However, this approach may not work for all clients. Contrary to the client in this situation, some clients may benefit from direct therapy targeting the SFF, with the addition of the comfortable conversational pitch range as a secondary feature. Finally, it was also noted that the client in this example was able to better match pitch with auditory versus visual feedback. These variations and modifications demonstrate the need to understand the voice and pitch therapy techniques, and then the need to apply them individually to each unique circumstance and client, versus instituting a select "program" or "protocol."

Intonation Therapy

Re-establishing Natural Intonation

During the pitch and pitch range alteration process of voice therapy, the transfeminine client may lose, or, in a sense, sacrifice, her natural intonation patterns. As discussed, intonation patterns should exist within the

client's comfortable conversational range, which has been established as approximately 12 semitones for both genders. If a client is using a conversational range that is too high, i.e., a range that is displaced upward, the intonation will be flat or monotone, as the client cannot use higher pitch for emphasis. In some cases, an elevated comfortable conversational pitch range will actually result in diminishing the available semitones for upward inflection. For example, if a client with an SFF target of 175 ±10 Hz and a conversational pitch range target of 130 to 250 Hz starts attempting an elevated range that is approximately 143 to 293 Hz, she may have difficulty achieving the desired upward inflections, and may consequently avoid "dropping" pitch in order to compensate. This could result in a reduced conversational pitch range, say 220 to 262 Hz, which is only three semitones but is higher than normal and artificial. Figure 10–11 demonstrates a reduced but elevated conversational pitch range.

In contrast, a client who has a conversation pitch that is below the eventual target conversation pitch may use upward intonation as a means to attempt to achieve the desired target pitch. In this case, the client will tend to use awkward, artificial, and inappropriate rises in intonation. These may occur anywhere within the utterance, but tend to be more prominent at the end of sentences. This constant upward wave-like pattern may indeed create the desired numbers calculated on the acoustic analysis system for the target SFF, and even raise the SFF. However, the speech pattern sounds unnatural. With this particular intonation pattern, the average SFF is raised, but the semitone range is reduced.

This pattern is endearingly referred to as *Dracula speech*, due to the pattern sounding similar to that used in old movies where the vampire says, "I **want** to **suck** your **blood**." The upward intonation on "want,"

---

[2]The conversational pitch range noted above was determined based on a 175 Hz pitch target.

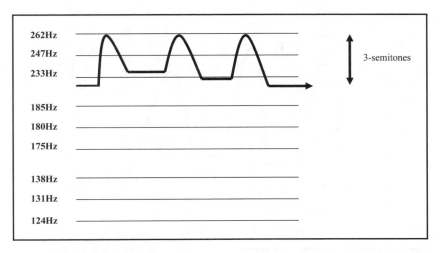

Figure 10–11. Flat intonation pattern due to the conversation target being too high and having reduced semitone and total conversational pitch range.

"suck," and "blood" sounds unnatural, but will be successful in raising the overall SFF of the sentence. Figures 10–12A and 10–12B show the unnatural intonation pattern that is created when the client tries to adjust the average SFF by inserting inappropriate intonation "jumps." Figure 10–12C shows how the pitch range and average SFF can be within normal limits when the intonation pattern is natural and follows the WJSF method.

Intonation Therapy Process

When re-establishing intonation at a different pitch, the first step is to begin with humming within the target conversational pitch range. The straw technique or other semi-occluded vocal tract activities might also be productive (Kapsner-Smith et al., 2015). An acoustic analysis system will give the client both visual and auditory feedback necessary to make modifications to either pitch or intonation patterns. Furthermore, humming allows the client to maintain gentle, forward phonation and will also allow the client to start imitating a conver-

sation pattern that is natural (e.g., humming spoken conversation or dialogues). The client will begin to realize the effort necessary and the possibility of using her voice within the target range.

As the client progresses from humming all the way to conversation, it is important to keep both conversational range and "natural" intonation as targets simultaneously. Some clients can become so concerned with or fixated on intonation patterns that they are no longer able to work within the targeted conversational pitch range. When this occurs, it is time to implement a more subjective method for evaluating intonation, eliminating objective measurements provided by the acoustic analysis system. This can be done by using the rating scale similar to the one below, where the target is "3" during a conversation within the target conversational pitch.

1 = Monotone/inappropriate
2 = Somewhat monotone
3 = Natural/appropriate
4 = Somewhat excessive
5 = Excessive/inappropriate

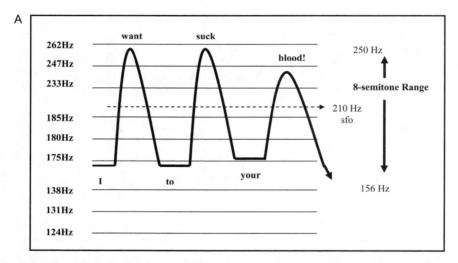

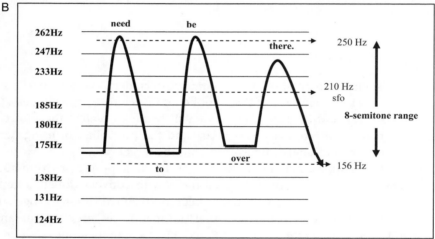

Figure 10–12. **(A)** "Dracula Speech" pitch pattern used to artificially increase overall SFF (e.g., as the vampire from the old movies would say, "I want to suck your blood!"). Although the average SFF is raised (210 Hz), the comfortable conversational range is reduced (8 semitones), and the intonation pattern is not natural. **(B)** "Dracula Speech" pitch pattern used to artificially increase overall SFF during sentence production (e.g., "I need to be over there"). The comfortable conversational range is approximately 8 semitones (reduced), but the average SFF is artificially elevated to approximately 210 Hz. **(C)** Natural pitch pattern used with 12-semitone comfortable conversational range and an approximate SFF of 182 Hz during sentence production (e.g., "I need to be over there").

It should be noted that there are times that a "2" or "4" rating, or even a "1" or "5" rating, may be appropriate. For instance, giving bad news to a friend may require a more monotone voice, whereas rejoicing over a new job may require more excessive intona-tion. This is why it is necessary to consider intonation in terms of "naturalness" as well as "appropriateness," and modify the scale accordingly.

As the client moves toward discharge, he or she must be able to rate his or her own

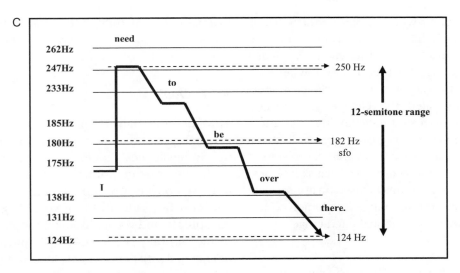

Figure 10–12. (*continued*)

intonation in terms of naturalness and appropriateness. This can be accomplished by increasing the client's awareness of intonation use, and making sure that the client's rating of intonation matches the clinician's rating of intonation for the client.

"Natural" Intonation Case Study. Client is a 37-year-old trans woman in transition for 2 years, and currently presenting as a woman 100% of the time. Client is being seen for ongoing voice and communication feminization training. Acoustic measures revealed an average SFF of 174 Hz. Probe measures revealed that the client had maintained appropriate SFF across treatments, but that comfortable conversational pitch range and intonation were not being maintained. Therefore, sessions focused on regaining awareness of target conversational pitch range and re-establishing appropriate intonation patterns. A realistic conversation outside the clinic with a novel communication partner was used to probe the client's skills using perceptual rating scales for client satisfaction and client's overall rating of feminine voice presentation.

Objective: Client will rate herself as "4"[3] or above on a feminine voice scale during conversation with a novel partner while maintaining the following characteristics, with a rating of "3" in agreement with the clinician's rating: resonance, intonation, nonverbal communication, lexical choices, pitch range, and intensity.

Progress: Client self-ratings and clinician's ratings were in 86% agreement (10 out of 12 opportunities), with ratings of "3" on all characteristics and the client's overall self-rating of feminine voice at "4" in both situations.

Discussion. Treatment sessions focused on establishing speech behaviors in the target conversational range and using the client's SFF across the domains of resonance, intonation, nonverbal communication, lexical choices, pitch range, and appropriate intensity, and combining these skills during

---

[3]Five-point femininity scale, where 5 is most feminine presentation, 4 is target feminine presentation, 3 is acceptable feminine presentation, 2 is less acceptable feminine presentation, and 1 is not an acceptable feminine presentation.

conversations with various partners (familiar and unfamiliar) in various environments. This approach is used as clients approach discharge (see Chapter 16). Following each activity, the client and the clinician independently rated the client's performance, and then discussed their findings. Occasionally, when client progress probes indicated a regression in a specific area, an entire session was spent on remediation of that skill (for example, some sessions focused on appropriate resonance or pitch range in addition to SFF and target conversational pitch range).

Other Therapy Considerations

As indicated in the example above, when considering pitch, pitch range, and intonation patterns, there are many other areas of voice and communication feminization that must be taken into account.

Loudness

Loudness level can impact the ability to alter pitch, and pitch can impact the ability to use varied loudness. It is difficult to shout to a friend across the street if the pitch being used is too high within the total pitch range. Keeping the conversational pitch within a realistic and appropriate range will allow the client greater flexibility in altering loudness, both for increased as well as decreased loudness. It is important that the client be able to have varied loudness levels within the targeted conversation pitch range. This is further discussed in Chapter 11.

Resonance

It is the impression of the authors that appropriate forward focus resonance will assist in achieving the targeted conversational pitch range and will also assist in

maintaining a natural intonation pattern. The role of resonance is further discussed in Chapter 11.

Vocal Quality

Throughout therapy for pitch alteration, vocal quality is of paramount concern. Under no circumstances should the vocal health of the client be compromised to achieve a targeted conversational pitch range. The client must be made aware of vocal hygiene (Chapter 8) and vocal physiology so that he or she may fully understand the implication of changed pitch and what is involved with voice and intonation alteration. However, the clinician should not rely solely on client reports for dependable information regarding vocal quality or health. Some clients, in their desire to achieve a "higher pitch," will not disclose vocal discomfort or pain. The clinician should be thorough in his or her observation and assessment of vocal health and voice production throughout the voice feminization process. For example, if the client begins to sound strained during production of higher pitches, the clinician should make a note immediately, and follow up with the client if the strain persists. Other behaviors that indicate challenges to vocal health, such as frequent throat-clearing or an expressed need for frequent sips of water during speech, should likewise not be ignored. If necessary, the conversational pitch range can be rebalanced in order to maintain a healthy vocal mechanism.

Summary

In addressing the pitch and intonation aspects of voice feminization therapy, it cannot be stressed enough that there must be an agreement between the clinician and the client as to the ultimate objective for

SFF alteration. There may also exist differing opinions of what constitutes a "natural" feminine intonation pattern. The client's desired goals may diverge considerably from the clinician's idea of the eventual target SFF, conversational pitch range, and intonation pattern use. This incongruence can cause a problem, as the client may have limited satisfaction with the end results of the voice therapy process that the clinician considers successful. It is imperative to frequently discuss the reasons for targeting the specific gender-acceptable SFF that was chosen, and why a higher target frequency may not necessarily benefit the client. It is important for the transfeminine client to realize that the contributions of pitch, pitch range, and intonation must be combined with the other target areas of voice and communication in order to successfully attain a feminine voice.

References

10-Minute Plays.com (2006). Acting scenes for two women. Retrieved September 30, 2017, from: http://www.10-minute-plays.com/scenes/scenes_two_women.html.

Andrews, M. L. (1999). *Manual of voice treatment: Pediatrics through geriatrics* (2nd ed.). San Diego, CA: Singular.

Aronson, A. (1990) *Clinical voice disorders: An interdisciplinary approach* (3rd ed.). New York, NY: Thieme Inc.

Azul, D., Nygren, U., Sodersten, M., & Neuschaefer-Rube, C. (2017). Transmasculine people's voice function: A review of the currently available evidence. *Journal of Voice, 31*(2), 261.e9-261.e23.

Behrman, A. (2013) *Speech and voice science* (2nd ed.). San Diego, CA: Plural.

Boone, D. R., McFarlane, S. C., Von Berg, S. L., & Zraick, R. (2014). *The voice and voice therapy* (9th ed.). Boston, MA: Pearson Education.

Colin's Movie Monologue Page. (2009). Retrieved September 30, 2017 from: http://www.whysanity.net/monos/.

Colton, R., Casper, J., & Leonard, R. (2011). *Understanding voice problems: A physiological perspective for diagnosis and treatment* (4th ed.). Baltimore, MD: Lippincott, Williams & Wilkins.

Cumbers, B. (2013). *Perceptual correlates of acoustic measures of vocal variability.* Master's thesis, University of Wisconsin–Milwaukee, Milwaukee, WI.

Davies, S., Papp, V., & Antoni, C. (2015). Voice and communication change for gender nonconforming individuals: Giving voice to the person inside. *International Journal of Transgenderism, 16*, 117-159.

Edwards, E. T., & Strattman, K. H. (1996). *Accent modification manual: Materials and activities.* San Diego, CA: Singular.

Fairbanks, G. (1960). *Voice and articulation drillbook* (2nd ed.). New York, NY: Harper and Brothers.

Gallena, S. K. (2007). *Voice and laryngeal disorders: A problem-based clinical guide with voice samples.* Maryland Heights, MI: Elsevier Mosby.

Gelfer, M. P. & Bennett, Q. (2013). Speaking fundamental frequency and vowel formant frequencies: Effects on perception of gender. *Journal of Voice, 27*, 556-566.

Gelfer, M. P., & Schofield, K. J. (2000). Comparison of acoustic and perceptual measures of voice in male-to-female transsexuals perceived as female versus those perceived as male. *Journal of Voice, 14*, 22-33.

Glenn, E., Glenn, P., & Forman, S. (1998). *Your voice and articulation* (4th ed.). Boston: Allyn and Bacon.

Hancock, A. (2015). The role of cultural competence in serving transgender populations. *Perspectives on Voice and Voice Disorders, 25*(2), 37-42.

Hancock, A., Colton, L, & Douglas, F. (2014). Intonation and gender perception: Applications for transgender speakers. *Journal of Voice, 28*, 203-209.

Hancock, A., & Garabedian, L. (2013). Transgender voice and communication treatment: A retrospective chart review of 25 cases. *International Journal of Communication Disorders, 48*, 54-65.

Hancock, A., Krissinger, J., & Owen, K. (2011). Voice perceptions and quality of life of transgender people. *Journal of Voice, 25*, 553-558.

Hillenbrand, J., & Clark, M. (2009). The role of f0 and formant frequencies in distinguishing the voices of men and women. *Attention, Perception and Psychophysics, 71*, 1150-1166.

Holmberg, E., Oates, J., Dacakis, G., & Grant, C. (2010). Phonetograms, aerodynamic measurements, self-evaluations, and auditory perceptual ratings of male-to-female transsexual voice, *Journal of Voice, 24,* 511–522.

Iwen, M. (2010). *Normative data on speaking fundamental frequency in young and middle age men.* Master's thesis, University of Wisconsin–Milwaukee, Milwaukee, WI.

Kapsner-Smith, M. R., Hunter, E. J., Kirkham, K., Cox, K., & Titze, I. R. (2015). A randomized controlled trial of two semi-occluded vocal tract voice therapy protocols. *Journal of Speech Language Hearing Research, 58*(3), 535–49.

Kelly, J., & Robinson G. C. (2011). Disclosure of membership in the lesbian, gay, bisexual, and transgender community by individuals with communication impairments: A preliminary Web-based survey. *American Journal of Speech-Language Pathology, 20*(2), 86–94.

King, R., Brown, G. & McCrea, C. (2011). Voice parameters that result in identification or misidentification of biological gender in male-to-female transgender veterans. *International Journal of Transgenderism, 13,* 117–130.

Lieberman, P., Katz, W., Jongman, A., Zimmerman, R., & Miller, M. (1985). Measures of the sentence intonation of read and spontaneous speech in American English. *Journal of the Acoustical Society of America, 77*(2), 649–657.

Linke, C. (1973). A study of pitch characteristics of female voices and their relationship to vocal effectiveness. *Folia Phoniatrica, 25,* 173–185.

McNeil, E., Wilson, J., Clark, S., & Deakin, J. (2008). Perception of voice in the transgender client. *Journal of Voice, 22,* 727–733.

Mysak, E. (1959). Pitch and duration characteristics of older males. *Journal of Speech and Hearing Research, 2,* 46–54.

Oates, J., & Dacakis, G. (2015). Transgender voice and communication: Research evidence underpinning voice intervention for male-to-female transsexual women. *SIG 3 Perspectives on Voice and Voice Disorders, 25*(2), 48–58.

Ovesky, R. (2004). *Speaking fundamental frequency characteristics in young and middle-age adults during spontaneous speech and reading.* Master's thesis, University of Wisconsin–Milwaukee, Milwaukee, WI.

Raphael, L., Borden, G., & Harris, K. (2011). *Speech science primer: Physiology, acoustics and perception of speech.* Philadelphia: Wolters Kluwer/Lippincott, Williams & Wilkins

Saxman, J., & Burke, K. (1967). Speaking fundamental frequency characteristics of middle-age females. *Folia Phoniatrica, 19,* 167–172.

Snidecor, J. (1951). The pitch and duration characteristics of superior female speakers during oral reading. *Journal of Speech and Hearing Disorders, 16,* 44–52.

Spencer, L. (1988). Speech characteristics of male-to-female transsexuals: A perceptual and acoustic study. *Folia Phoniatrica, 40,* 31–42.

Stemple, J., Glaze, L., & Gerdeman, B. (2000) *Clinical voice pathology: Theory and management* (3rd ed.). San Diego, CA: Singular Thompson Learning.

Stemple, J., Glaze, L., & Klaben, B. (2010). *Clinical voice pathology* (4th ed.). San Diego, CA: Plural.

Stoicheff, M. (1981). Speaking fundamental frequency characteristics of nonsmoking female adults. *Journal of Speech and Hearing Research, 24,* 437–441.

Wolfe, V. L., Ratusnik, D. L., Smith, F. H., & Northrop, G. E. (1990). Intonation and fundamental frequency in male-to-female transsexuals. *Journal of Speech and Hearing Disorders, 55,* 43–50.

11

The Art and Science of Resonance, Articulation, and Volume

Sandy Hirsch, Marylou Pausewang Gelfer, and Joan Boonin

Resonance and Articulation: Supralaryngeal Phenomena

In Chapter 10, the pitch and intonation characteristics of voice that are discussed are both *laryngeal* phenomena; that is, they are the result of activity in the intrinsic (and in some cases, extrinsic) muscles of the larynx. But let us consider for a moment the "big picture" in terms of the speech production systems. According to Raphael, Borden, and Harris (2011), speech production can be conceived of as including a power supply (the respiratory system), an oscillator that generates a periodic tone (the vocal folds), a noise generator that generates an aperiodic signal (the articulators), and a resonator that modifies the output of both the periodic and aperiodic sources (the supralaryngeal vocal tract). It is clear that we have thus far addressed only the output of the oscillator. This is logical, because there are well-known differences between the laryngeal characteristics of male and female speakers (Behrman, 2013; Zemlin, 1998) and the resulting vocal signal. In order to

assist gender diverse speakers in achieving the voice of the target gender, altering the output of the oscillator, or vocal fold vibratory characteristics, is absolutely crucial.

However, male and female speakers also have well-documented differences in the *resonator* component of the speech production system, or the supralaryngeal vocal tract (Behrman, 2013; Rendall, Vokey, & Nemath, 2007). The longer and larger male vocal tract, from the laryngopharynx to the lips, amplifies the lower frequencies present in the complex acoustic output emanating from vocal fold vibration. The smaller and narrower female vocal tract amplifies higher frequencies within the complex acoustic output of vocal fold vibration. In fact, differences in size between male and female supralaryngeal vocal tracts also result in somewhat different acoustic characteristics for aperiodic output as well, resulting in differences between genders for even voiceless speech sounds (Schwartz, 1968). The challenge to the speech-language pathologist working with the gender diverse population is to assist these clients in modifying the characteristics of the "resonator" to enable the client to achieve the speech attributes of the target gender to the greatest extent possible. The combination of clinical and artistic methods will be illustrated as one successful method for training gender diverse clients in reaching a tone that comfortably matches their gender identity. As has already been discussed in Chapter 10, a balanced relationship between habitual frequency and intonation is critical. Resonance may be considered the third portion of the vocal triumvirate[1] that contributes to a male/female *sound* differentiation, and subjectively may actually be the most telling.

In this chapter, we will begin with a review of resonance as a component of the overall quality of a voice, and one which can presumably contribute to perception of speaker maleness or femaleness. We will then continue with a review of articulation, or the formation of speech sounds, to consider what changes in articulatory movements might be facilitative for achieving the attributes of a male or female speaker. We will conclude with an examination of vocal intensity, or volume, and its role in gender identification.

Resonance and Clinical Tradition

Resonance can be defined as "selective amplification and filtering of the complex laryngeal tone by the cavities of the vocal tract after that tone has been produced by vibration of the vocal folds" (Boone, McFarlane, Von Berg, & Zraick, 2014, p. 290). This selective amplification and damping make each voice unique and distinctive (Stemple, Glaze, & Klaben, 2010). However, clinical application of this concept has not generally addressed the issue of how resonance defines a speaker.

Traditionally speech-language clinicians have discussed resonance within a framework of voice and speech *disorders*, specifically nasality disorders, that may have a variety of etiologies ranging from anatomical to neurological (Boone et al., 2014; Stemple et al., 2010). The clinician typically uses the term "resonance disorders" when describing the speech and voice of an individual who has difficulty controlling the coupling and de-coupling of the nasal cavities from the vocal tract. In such cases the clinician must measure the hypernasality or hyponasality present in the voice, using such instrumentation as a Nasometer®.

Over the past 20 years or so, "resonant voice" and "tone focus" are terms that also have been used in the treatment of hyperfunctional voice disorders (Chen, Hsiao, Hsiao, Chung, & Chiang, 2007; Roy, Weinrich, Gray, Tanner, Stemple, & Sapienza, 2003; Verdolini, Druker, Palmer, & Samawi, 1998), and have been used within the singing tradition for many years (Lessac, 1967; Miller, 1993, 1996; Verdolini-Madsen, Burke, Lessac, Blaze, & Caldwell, 1995; Verdolini et al., 1998). In these contexts, *"Resonant voice has been defined as a vocal quality that projects well, is easy to produce, and involves a sensation of vibration in the area of the face around the nose and mouth, called the <u>mask</u>"* (Ferrand, 2012, p. 184). It is within the latter framework that the application of resonant voice therapy approaches to gender diverse voice and communication training will be discussed in this chapter.

---

[1]While this specific triad of vocal parameters has not been shown scientifically to contain the make-or-break markers of vocal femininity, experience suggests that it is these three qualities that make a listener say, "She *sounds* feminine." . . . or "he *sounds* masculine."

The Challenge of Training Resonance across the Gender Continuum

As has been mentioned in Chapter 6 of this text, the vast majority of research studies on communication function and therapy for transgender (TG) and gender diverse individuals has been conducted with trans women (Azul, Nygren, Sodersten, & Neuschaefer-Rube, 2017; Davies, Papp, & Antoni, 2015). This is certainly true in the resonance area, where there have been several reports of the role of resonance modification in voice therapy and training for the transfeminine individual (e.g., Carew, Dacakis, & Oates, 2007; Hancock & Garabedian, 2012). However, publications focused on transgender voice modification are increasingly targeting the importance of resonance training for transmasculine clients (e.g., Block, 2017; see also Chapter 9). Therefore, while this chapter may emphasize resonance in terms of voice feminization, transmasculine applications are considered to be of equal importance, as suggested by Block (2017).

The objective of resonance training with the transfeminine client is to bring the focus of the tone of the voice up into the facial mask and head, so as to diminish the perception of a "chestier" sound associated with the male voice. Many transfeminine clients are able to maintain an adjusted fundamental frequency within a feminine range and successfully learn feminine intonation patterns, rate, volume, semantics, and feminine nonverbal communication styles. However, learning and maintaining a feminine resonance or tone is perhaps the most difficult portion of voice and communication modification. It requires teaching what Miller (1996) calls "hearing the voice" (p. 46), as well as feeling the sensations

that it produces. It requires teaching the difference in subtle adjustments, and listening for "color" nuances in the vocal quality. Unlike the measurement of resonance *disorders*, resonant quality, i.e., tone, cannot be reliably measured instrumentally; it has to be judged subjectively (Case, 1996). This fact is initially not always comfortable for many well-trained, scientifically minded clinicians.

Experienced clinicians have found that trans women who successfully develop a natural feminine voice must start with an average speaking fundamental frequency (SFF) in the "gender fluid" range of 155–185 Hz. Previous studies (Gelfer & Schofield, 2000; Spencer 1988; Wolfe, Ratusnik, Smith & Northrup, 1990) have found that transfeminine subjects within this frequency range have the potential to be perceived by listeners as female, based on voice alone. However, in the clinical judgment of the authors, it is may also be important for clients to establish consistently feminine intonation patterns, and maintain a forward focus resonance with a "headier" sound without dark undertones if they are to be confidently perceived as female. By contrast, clients who have successfully shifted their habitual frequency to an average SFF for young females of 220 Hz (not necessarily recommended, since it narrows the potential margin for intonation; see Chapter 10), but have not fully grasped the intonational and resonance aspects of voice training, are less likely to be recognized as female. These clients tend to perceive themselves as sounding "like a man with a high voice." A brief replaying of a sample of "before" and "after" recordings is evidence for them to understand the importance of studying and modifying resonance. Indeed, many clients have already learned this from internet blogs and forums about voice modification.

Clients have reported that this is one of the most challenging goals in therapy, but agree that once they master the skill, it provides a strong foundation to which they can return repeatedly whenever the new voice begins to unravel, especially in challenging contexts of high cognitive or emotional load. Eventually being able to speak confidently is achieved across all contexts, but this is often long after the course of therapy is complete. Clients have consistently reported that having an understanding of the inherent acoustic challenges, and learning the possible solutions in voice modification, has given them the confidence to continue learning independently after discharge from therapy.

The abstract concept of "resonance" can be made somewhat more concrete if we remember that "resonance" relates directly to the acoustic characteristics of speech, which are impacted by the changing shape of the vocal tract (articulation). For example, vowels, which are relatively long-duration speech sounds, have well-known acoustic characteristics called formant frequencies. These formant frequencies signal the identity of the vowel as well as (presumably) some speaker-specific information, and will be discussed in greater detail later in the chapter.

Formant Frequencies versus Speaking Fundamental Frequency

At this point, it may be useful to affirm the independence of vowel formant frequencies and SFF (described previously in Chapter 10). Speaking fundamental frequency is an acoustic measure that reflects the number of vocal fold vibrations per second, as measured in hertz (Hz). In connected speech, the

average speaker may use a 1.5- to 2-octave range of frequencies around their central tendency (SFF), but the average SFF value is useful as a general indication of how high or low a voice might be perceived to be. In general, men have average SFFs of approximately 110–130 Hz, while women have average SFFs of 180–230 Hz (Ferrand, 2012). Regardless of SFF, however, both genders generate a *laryngeal spectrum* when the vocal folds vibrate. This laryngeal spectrum encompasses a large number of frequencies generated by the complex vibratory pattern of the vocal fold cover, and includes harmonics (whole-number multiples) of the SFF, usually measured up to 8000 Hz (Raphael et al., 2011).

The Role of Vowel Formants

Formant frequencies result from the amplification and damping of patterns of harmonics in various frequency regions within the laryngeal spectrum. More specifically, vowel formants are regions of energy concentration in the acoustic signal, occurring primarily between 300 and 3000 Hz. These regions of energy concentration at various points in the acoustic spectrum are determined by the size and shape of vocal tract cavities that amplify or dampen the frequencies that pass through them.

Physiologically speaking, the articulatory positions assumed by the vocal tract determine which frequencies will be resonated. The first formant is thought to be affected by the size of the pharyngeal cavity, from the glottis to the point of maximum constriction of the tongue. When the posterior tongue is retracted, the back cavity is smaller and the first formant frequency (F1) is higher. When the posterior tongue is advanced, the larger back cavity results in a lower F1 (Raphael et al., 2011). The second formant (F2) is believed to be due to the size of the oral cavity, from the point of maximum constriction of the tongue to the lips. Adding length to the oral cavity through lip-rounding will decrease the frequency of F2; retracting the lips and therefore shortening the length of the oral cavity will increase the frequency of F2. The third formant (F3) varies in response to front versus back constriction. Although numerous additional formants can be identified for each vowel, the first three are the most important to vowel recognition (Raphael et al., 2011), and are the most clearly related to articulatory gestures.

In fact, each vowel has a characteristic pattern of formants that allow us to instantly recognize it ("ee" vs. "oo," for example). This pattern is recognizable even if displaced upward (as it would be for a child's vocal tract with its smaller dimensions) or downward (as it would be for a large male vocal tract with its larger dimensions). In musical terms, this is analogous to a major chord versus a minor chord being recognized, no matter where it is played on the piano keyboard (high notes or low notes). A major chord would still be recognized as a major chord (let us say, the vowel "ah"), and not a minor chord (let us say, the vowel "aw"), whether it is played at the high end of the piano or the low end. The *pattern* of formants within the frequency spectrum is currently believed to be one of the defining attributes for recognition of the vowel sounds (Raphael et al., 2011).

Since vowel formant patterns are so crucial to our understanding of speech, changing them too much would result in the listener hearing a different vowel other than the one intended by the speaker (for example, "uh" instead of "oo"). But *slight* changes in formant frequencies may affect only the perceived *quality* of the voice, a

phenomenon known as "formant tuning," utilized by singers (Behrman, 2013). If the entire pattern is moved up or down somewhat in frequency, then gender perception may also be affected. Presumably, listeners might be able to detect the lower formant frequencies typically heard in male speech (due to a larger vocal tract), as opposed to the somewhat higher formant frequencies typically heard in female speech (due to a smaller vocal tract). Thus, the challenge for the gender diverse client is to learn to make small changes in formant structure that do not interfere with speech intelligibility but result in formant frequencies that are more similar to those of the target gender. These small changes will be discussed in detail later in the chapter.

Do changes in formant frequencies actually result in altered perception of speaker gender? This has not been an easy area for investigation. For one thing, vowel formants can be difficult to measure reliably and validly, especially in a clinical situation. In addition, vowel formants are most easily detected when SFF is low, such as in a male voice. As SFF is raised, there are fewer harmonics per formant, and detection via spectral and Linear Predictive Coding (LPC) analyses becomes less reliable. Therefore, because most of our transfeminine clients want to target a non-male SFF, making reliable and consistent measures of formant frequencies is particularly difficult. Finally, unlike SFF, which has a clear perceptual correlation with the highness or lowness of perceived pitch, perceptual correlates for changes in vowel formant frequencies have received limited research attention. Even if we could measure vowel formant frequencies very accurately, would they line up with listener impressions of some subjective voice quality? The relationship at this time is not fully understood.

Those caveats in place, the existing literature does provide some support for the importance of changing vowel formant frequencies in voice modification. Mount and Salmon (1988) were the first to consider vowel formant frequencies in their case study of a single transfeminine subject who underwent 11 months of voice treatment. In addition to noting an increase in their client's SFF from 110 Hz to 205 Hz, they also found an increase from pre-test to post-test in their subject's vowel formants for the vowels /i/, /a/, and /u/, although only the second formants for the vowel /u/ extended into the female range. They noted that the subject reported that she was not consistently perceived as female by listeners until her formant frequencies increased. Gelfer and Schofield (2000) also measured both SFF and vowel formants. They found that their transfeminine subjects who were consistently perceived as female achieved SFFs of 164–199 Hz. Further, the second formant of /i/ was significantly higher for perceived-female subjects than it was for subjects perceived as male; however, when the perceived-female group was compared with the perceived-male group, *all* of the vowel formants in the perceived-female group were higher, though not significantly. Gelfer and Tice (2013) studied therapy outcomes for transfeminine subjects. They found that SFF increased from a mean of 119 Hz in the pre-test to 178 Hz in the immediate post-test (right after the conclusion of therapy). They also reported that compared with the pre-test, both the first and second formants of the vowel /i/ were higher in the immediate post-test period. It should be noted that in the pre-test, subjects were perceived as female by listeners only 2% of the time; in the immediate post-test, they were perceived as female 51% of the time. In summary, it appears that increases in vowel formant frequencies, especially the high front vowel /i/, are possible for a speaker to accomplish; and these elevated vowel

formants correlate with increased perception as female for transfeminine individuals, assuming that a fundamental frequency in the gender-fluid range is also achieved.

The most important evidence for the manipulation of vowel formants in working with the gender diverse population comes from Hillenbrand and Clark (2009). These researchers recorded 25 male and 25 female speakers each producing a sentence. The sentences were later digitally altered in a variety of ways: (a) both formant frequencies and the fundamental frequency were shifted to those appropriate for the opposite gender; (b) only the fundamental frequency was shifted to one appropriate for the opposite gender, and (c) only the formant frequencies were shifted to values appropriate for the opposite gender. In a fourth condition, the acoustic characteristics of the sentences were unchanged. Twenty-one listeners (speech-language pathology majors) were asked to rate each sample as being produced by a man or a woman. Results showed that when *both* fundamental frequency and formant frequencies were altered, listeners heard approximately 82% of the speech samples as being spoken by the opposite gender—that is, male speakers were perceived as females, and female speakers were perceived as males. However, when formant frequencies *only* were changed, the gender shift was much less marked: male speakers were perceived as females about 19% of the time, and female speakers were heard as males about 12% of the time. Somewhat better results were obtained when fundamental frequency *only* was changed: 34% of male speakers were perceived as females, and 19% of females were perceived as males.

The results of Hillenbrand and Clarke (2009) strongly suggest that formant frequencies and fundamental frequency must both be changed in concert with one another in order to bring about a shift in gender perception. The treatment studies cited above (Mount & Salmon, 1988; Gelfer & Tice, 2013) sought to change fundamental frequency directly, with changes in formant frequencies occurring indirectly. In both studies, increased voice feminization was perceptually confirmed.

A study by Carew, Dacakis, and Oates (2007) did just the opposite: focused primarily on changing formant frequencies through instruction and practice with forward versus backed tongue carriage, and lip spreading versus lip rounding, with changes in fundamental frequency occurring indirectly. These researchers found that all three formant frequencies tested, and the mean speaking fundamental frequency of the treated participants were significantly higher in the post-treatment period, compared with the pretreatment period. Perceptual judgments of the femininity of the participants' voices revealed less clear trends, but 7 out of 10 participants showed increased femininity scores. More research is needed to determine the efficacy of treatment focus (fundamental frequency vs. formant frequencies), but as predicted by Hillenbrand and Clark (2009), it appears that both parameters must be addressed to foster appropriate gender perception.

Formant Philosophy Applied to Transfeminine Communication Training

As with any speech and voice therapy or training, it is important to begin with strong theories that can be applied to assessment and treatment decisions. As has already been mentioned, the resonance aspect of the voice and speech is perhaps the most difficult to teach, due to a lack of a clear standard for what "feminine" resonance sounds like (most of us only know that "we know it when we hear it"), compounded by the difficulty in making objective measures of vowel formants in the clinical setting. However, on a perceptual and phonetic basis, a vowel or formant frequency paradigm provides the clinician with an approach that lends itself to manageable hierarchical organization. Extrapolating from the therapy techniques described by Carew et al. (2007), clinicians can organize therapy materials in a normal clinical hierarchy, emphasizing a combination of high-front spread vowels with voiceless consonant combinations as the easiest stimuli to produce with a feminine sound, progressing to low back rounded vowels as the most challenging, due to the inherent difficulty of increasing forward tongue carriage and lip spread on back rounded vowels.

How does the gender diverse client change formant frequencies of various vowels if formant frequencies reflect the size and configuration of the vocal tract? While such change might sound impossible, in fact it can be accomplished through changes in tongue height, tongue advancement, and mouth opening. For example, increased tongue height might raise the hyoid bone somewhat and thus reduce the length of the pharyngeal cavity, a factor in increasing the frequency of the first formant. A more fronted tongue position can reduce the size of the oral cavity, increasing the frequency of the second formant. A more open mouth or greater lip opening reduces acoustic impedance, increasing the frequency of all formants (Behrman, 2013). From a therapeutic standpoint, this would make front, spread vowels such as /i/ and /ɪ/ an excellent context in which to begin training feminine resonance patterns (though trial and error has proven that /i/ is a more consistently reliable context, perhaps since there is considerably more jaw drop for /ɪ/). The concept of a "frontal tone focus" and the sensations that accompany it also may invoke the desired articulatory changes.

In the singing world it is generally felt that overgeneralizing one vowel sound to all vowels will deaden the overall harmonic richness of a lyrical line (Miller, 1996). This may be the case, although "vowel bending" seems to be very helpful when stretching for notes out of a comfortable singing range. In the same way, the manipulation of vowels appears to be a successful strategy in feminizing speech tones, and will be further discussed in the therapy portion of the chapter.

Tone Color

Tone placement in singing is considered to be the relationship between fundamental frequency, vowel formants, and a "clustering of harmonic partials" (Benninger, Jacobson, & Johnson, 1994, p. 65). The "color" of the vowels moves from light to dark as they move from front to back (/i/, /ɪ/, /e/ /æ/ /ɑ/ /o/ /u/, /ʊ/). This shift in resonant color is often termed "chiaroscuro" (*light* and *dark*; literally *clear* and *obscured*) in the singing world; a term that has been coined from the style of the Baroque painter Caravaggio.

This "chiaroscuro," or light and dark, is one way to describe the sound of the feminine to masculine resonance tone shift (or masculine to feminine depending on whether the challenge is that of lightening or darkening). The feminine tone can be identified for the client as the "light" or more fronted, open production, presumably made with articulatory adjustments that facilitate an increase in vowel formant frequencies, while the masculine tone can be contrasted as "dark," a more posterior, closed production with lower formant frequencies.

It appears that using this term with clients heightens the awareness of vowel color and the ability to hear masculine versus feminine resonance. In addition, anecdotally, it appears to be the resonant quality that invites the comment "That is a woman's voice" versus "That voice certainly seems to be high enough to be a woman's, but still doesn't really sound like a woman; why?"

In order to change gender perception, articulatory changes in vowel production can be targeted in therapy. For example, overlaying an /i/ configuration across all vowels to brighten them will be discussed later in the chapter in the sections on therapy approaches to resonance. Conversely maximizing /u/ and /o/ for the transmasculine client to make the tones richer/deeper will also be discussed briefly as comparison (see also Chapter 9).

Resonant Voice Therapy

Proper formation of the oral cavity, where wave reflection takes place, produces a full-bodied, mature, authoritative, warm expressive tone; coordinating this action with proper use of the resonating areas adds brilliance, ringing, penetrating stentorian qualities. Wave reflection and resonance must feed each other; deny one and the other loses its luster.
—Lessac, 1967, p. 11

Resonance is an abstract term for many, and it is sometimes helpful to address the parameter of resonance for gender diverse clients in a broader context involving all aspects of speech production. As clients strive to improve their respiratory support for speech and phonatory production (a higher pitch with a light quality for the transfeminine client), the concept of a more fronted tone focus and articulatory placements seems to fit in quite naturally.

There are a number of voice programs that have been developed over the years to address bringing respiration, phonation, and resonance into balance. In particular, the Lessac-Madsen Resonant Voice Therapy (L-MRVT)[2] approach developed by Katherine Verdolini in 2000 and further formalized in 2008 (Verdolini, 2000; Verdolini Abbott, 2008), in combination with manipulating vowel context and production, can be extremely effective in training transfeminine clients to achieve a recognizably feminine resonance. It allows for a fusion of clinically based science and artistry, including: (a) a solid vocal health component, (b) specific sensory cues for what constitutes a correct trial, (c) clear goals for respiratory control, and (d) hierarchically tailored consonant-vowel transitions that help to provide the foundations for strong skill development and long-term maintenance of a feminine voice. It is also as close as possible to an evidence-based approach for this population (Awan, 2013). Resonant voice therapy originated in the theater arts tradition (Verdolini et al., 1995), predisposing the L-MRVT program perfectly to the inclusion of other arts-based approaches that clinicians may have at their disposal (e.g., theater and singing). As Stemple (2000) states, Resonant Voice Therapy is "more about discovery than trying." Ear and sensory training should be a major focus of therapy at the outset and throughout the process, to ensure a client's ability to accurately hear and feel subtle shifts in tone quality.

---

[2]The L-MRVT is designed as an eight-week training program with very specific targets and goals for each week. Clinicians who are interested in applying a version of this approach should take the time to learn it formally or study the rudiments of it, which can be found in Stemple's *Voice Therapy: Clinical Studies* (2000) and Verdolini's *Lessac Madsen Resonant Voice Therapy Clinician Manual* (2008).

Assessment of Resonance

As has been stated, resonance and tone focus are not easily measured instrumentally; therefore, the clinician must judge them subjectively, while assessing other voice and speech parameters objectively. For transfeminine clients, an equal-appearing scale might be used where 0 = masculine/posterior/chesty and 5 = feminine/fronted/upper larynx/head. The scale could be reversed for transmasculine clients. If the clinician has a sophisticated analysis program, it may be worth taking objective measures of formant frequency ranges at baseline for the vowels /i/, /a/, and /u/, both in isolated vowels and in appropriate sentences, where /i/, /a/, and /u/ occur in stressed words, such as "Put the blue spot on the key again" (Kempster, Garrett, Verdolini Abbott, Barkmeier-Kraemer, & Hillman, 2009). Pre-to post-test comparisons have the potential to provide useful data on client progress and, by extension, a basis for measuring client satisfaction, but in particular, increasing evidence-based data opportunities.

Dynamic Assessment

It is important for the clinician to probe the client's ability to shift resonance by presenting imitative stimuli such as two versions of /i/ at approximately 165 Hz or E3, or the lower end of the gender-acceptable range. A tuner or keyboard for baseline purposes may help. The clinician can produce an /i/ with a rounded (dark, or masculine, classical) vowel configuration, and then with the normal configuration for the /i/ with exaggerated lip spreading (a fronted or feminine early music singing-style configuration). A simple auditory discrimination test will demonstrate whether the client is able to hear the difference between the dark (more masculine) and the light (more feminine) sound. The client should then be asked to demonstrate this same distinction and report to the clinician how the sound and sensations were different. If the client is unable to hear and feel the distinctions, tactile cues or visual cues using a mirror can be helpful. It is essential that the client understand the distinction as early on in therapy as possible. This dynamic assessment will provide the clinician with excellent information regarding the client's learning strengths.

Training

Breath Support and Control

The clinician should be acutely aware at all times of the client's use of breath, both support and control. Many clients try to produce an /m/ hum by "pushing" the sound or even "pressing" it. Voice clinicians can use any number of approaches already in their clinical bag of tricks to address these issues. Clients should be reminded that the target sound is /mmm/, not the /hum/, which engages the tongue unnecessarily. However, if the client is truly unable to feel an easy /m/ hum with a free breath, and tension is visible in the neck area, the following "water trick" is a helpful antidote. The client should be instructed to take a small mouthful of water, hold it in the mouth by just closing the lips enough to prevent leakage, lean over with the forearms on the legs, and feel the weight of the water against the inside of the lips while producing "mmmm." This sensation of "liquid gravity" usually helps the client to release any tension that may have built up and to produce an easy /m/ hum with a free breath.

For clients who are unable at first to feel a satisfying deep breath, the following method suggested by Patsy Rodenburg (1992, 2000), voice coach to the Royal Shake-

speare Company, the National Theatre, and the Guildhall School of Music and Drama, is extremely helpful. Have the client lean forward in a sitting position with the forearms on the knees (the best analogy really is the "sitting on the toilet position"). Instruct the client to breathe in easily and then ask, "Where did you feel the muscles working as you breathed in?" Almost all clients will be amazed at how they experience the sensation of their belly expanding, as compared with their usual clavicular "grasp" at air. This same end can be achieved by gently holding on to the bottom of a chair or the edge of a table, or even pressing a hand gently against the thigh while speaking. The exercise anchors and prevents the lifting of the shoulders, and "holding" that is associated with clavicular breathing. For the client who is terminally stuck in clavicular breathing, gentle voicing while throwing a ball up in the air or against a wall will also end the cycle. Theatrical icons such as Cicely Berry (1973), as well as numerous others in the theatre and singing arts arena, also provide excellent problem-solving tools for reluctant easy-breathers. Many people, especially in the theatre vernacular, have found the work of Kristin Linklater (2006) to be extremely helpful. Her background will draw them toward methods and approaches that speak to them in the most meaningful way. Linklater's work and examples are discussed in detail in Chapter 15, more specifically geared toward performance.

L-MRVT Modified for the Gender Diverse Population

Vigilance in the area of vocal health cannot be stressed enough. Modification of any aspect of the voice requires this attention (Sataloff, 1998), and resonance is no exception. Conveniently, the L-MRVT program incorporates a vocal health component (water, steam, vaporizer in the bedroom if necessary, reflux and yelling/screaming precautions). The program is designed to promote optimal vocal fold adduction for healthy use, and in the case of the transfeminine client, promotes ease of transition from lower to higher frequencies and resonances.

High Front Vowels and Voiceless Consonants

Before beginning a modified L-MRVT hierarchy, it is helpful to accustom the client to the concept of vocal play—the discovery of the voice that was alluded to earlier in the chapter. When teaching resonance to the transfeminine client, it helps to think of the human body as a walking instrument. Vocal play on a series of high front vowels and voiceless consonants at a gender-acceptable (slightly above) pitch will provide the client with easy first-time stimuli that guarantee a light sound (e.g., /fi/, /ti/, /pi/, /si/). It helps to begin with meaningless sounds that have no emotion or naturalness attached to them. As will be discussed later in the chapter, changing the resonant quality of the voice can be, even though desired, an initial shock to the client.

Basic Training Gesture (m hum) to "Meet Me Peter and Beyond"

The L-MRVT program uses a "basic training gesture" (BTG) as the first step in the program hierarchy. The BTG progresses into a multisyllabic chant hierarchy and eventually into connected speech, and finally spontaneous conversation with the basic concept "peppered" throughout for maintenance of optimal vocal fold adduction and resonance (Verdolini, 2000; Verdolini Abbott, 2008). Following is a variation of the L-MRVT program adapted specifically for trans women and nonbinary clients. The usual clinical decisions

should be made with regard to numbers of stimuli and percent correct before progressing through various hierarchal steps. However, it is important to move the client along quickly enough to keep interest and confidence high, without over-challenging her/him. This approach can be easily modified for trans men using low, back/rounded, and protruded vowels.

Phase I

- Comprehensive stretches of the head and neck and trunk musculature to deactivate tension in muscles of phonation
- /M/ hum (literally "mmmm") at a comfortable gender-acceptable/feminine pitch (as has been established during the full voice assessment). The client should feel anterior oral vibrations (alveolar ridge is optimal) and the vocalization should feel good, easy, optimally "glowing" (Verdolini, 2000, L-MRVT workshop). Verdolini was the first to point out that the perfect sensation of vibration may occur on different pitches from day to day, or even hour to hour (Stemple, 2000). The clinician should not be shy about having the client try several different pitches (without radical shifts in semitone) if one is not working optimally at any particular moment.
- /mi/ chant, using a single pitch
- /mimi/—mild chant using a single pitch
- /mitmi/—easy, with very light contacts with normal speech intonation
- "meet me Peter"—mild chant using single pitch
- "meet me Peter"—with normalizing feminine intonation, but still very light contacts. Perfect articulation is not the goal here.
- "meet me Peter, meet me" with feminine intonation and easy, forward-focus resonance. The client should be listening for the light/dark traps as intonation shifts downward, and instructed to keep the

instrument (mouth) open after finishing a word for a best and natural diminution of sound, rather than an abrupt cut-off which forces a dark ending.

Combining L-MRVT with Other Approaches

Once the first phases of resonance have been taught and the client has a solid understanding of the capabilities of the "resonant instrument," therapy can progress. The therapist or trainer can feel comfortable employing the hierarchy that is familiar to all clinicians (words, phrases, sentences, reading, descriptions, short topic discussion, conversation, and so on), incorporating a myriad of stimuli available in the experienced clinician's mental and literal files, based on the client's needs and abilities. The above principles should be applied across the board. It is, however, worth drawing the clinician/trainer's attention to a few other creative ways to think about working on resonance.

Brightening and Lightening the Vowels: /i/ification

The influence of the high front vowel /i/ on a lighter tone has been alluded to earlier in the chapter. The application of an /i/ lip configuration across vowels, especially across the extended and more rounded and elongated vowels such as /u/, acts to artificially shorten the vocal tract due to lip-spreading for the /i/. This has the effect of slightly raising formant frequencies (Behrman, 2013), to produce a "lighter" sound. Peppered throughout speech, this helps to feminize the "darker" sounds during voice transition. It essentially showcases the treble tones and de-emphasizes the bass tones. Miller (1993) stated as much when he suggested that the "ring" in the voice can be

achieved by applying a front "timbre concept" to the back vowels as well. This is what clinicians today term "forward focus."

Within the context of training transfeminine clients in feminine resonance, Hirsch describes this as the /i/-ification of vowels across their spectra (Hirsch, 2006, 2017; Hirsch & Gelfer, 2012). It is essentially a resonance "work around." Asking the client to smile occasionally, with a look of surprised delight, when speaking can achieve the same goal, although presenting that maneuver as a panacea approach will not allow the client openness to a full range of emotional expression. Learning how to modify vowel production provides the client with a far more sophisticated set of skills with which to apply vocal color. The smiling/lip-spreading approach soon becomes modified to more of an internal smile sensation.

In order to help the client grow accustomed to the feeling of /i/-ifying, the clinician might generate word lists that focus on single syllable words employing the vowels beginning at the back of the mouth and moving to the front. The client should be instructed to think in terms of shaping an /i/ even when producing an /ʊ/ (e.g., *book* should be produced with a slight smile at first to superimpose the physiological gesture for /i/ over the /ʊ/ sound). It will become obvious if the modification has gone too far because the vowel will sound like a German umlaut (fünf). This is where the "discovery" that Stemple speaks of comes in.

Acoustic Assumptions: One Organized Approach to a Multitude of Resonance Challenges

During Hirsch's speech and hearing student years, she heard over and over again that "the physiological gesture gives rise to the acoustic output" (personal communication, Fred Minifie, multiple occasions, 1985–1989); a wonderfully grounding, logical, and true statement. What we do with the instrument creates the sound that we and the listener hear. This holds true for any instrument, vocal or otherwise. The sooner we can help clients to fully grasp this fact, the sooner they will be able to be in control of their instrument. As clients begin to understand better how to ask questions about why the voice sounds a certain way under certain conditions, they can be taught to use a set of physiologic solutions as an efficient way to make subtle changes that achieve a desired resonance. A simplified rubric of the acoustic results for certain articulatory gestures can dramatically help the client to diagnose specific resonance challenges, and can provide a framework for tangible problem solving.

Theories of anticipatory coarticulation, vocal tract configuration, and acoustic output were discussed in a 1977 *Journal of Phonetics* paper by Kent and Minifie (1977), and while this paper is now 41 years old, the acoustic tenets still hold true. The Lessac-Madsen Resonant Voice Therapy (L-MRVT) program previously discussed (Verdolini, 2000; Verdolini Abbott, 2008) combined with coarticulation, the Source-Filter Theory, and observations made during ensemble and solo performance are at the core of Hirsch's approach to resonance training when working with transgender and gender non-conforming clients. This approach is referred to as *Acoustic Assumptions* (Hirsch, 2017; Hirsch & Gelfer 2012). Hirsch has applied this approach, and the nuancing of the vocal instrument for both speech and performance voice, to train clients to help them find an individual sound depending on personal needs, style, and where they are on the gender spectrum. The rubric for the *Acoustic Assumptions* is detailed in Boxes 11–A and 11–B in the follow two pages.

Using the Acoustic Assumptions as a Guide

Let us analyze the word "great" using the information in Box 11–A as a guide. We know that the voiced glottal stop, /g/, has a darker resonant output than /k/, its unvoiced cognate. The second phoneme, /er/, is produced with a high degree of superior and lateral tongue tension with additional posterior tension, which tends to create a darker, cul-de-sac style of resonance. The mid front dipthong /eᴵ/ moves forward out of /gr/, causing a dramatic shift in the tone palette toward lightness, and the voiceless /t/ falls neatly at the end to provide the speaker an opportunity to finish the word "great" on a light note. If a client did have difficulty maintaining feminine resonance on the word "great," such an analysis of the phonemes of the word according to the acoustic assumptions in Box 11–A could help her understand her difficulty and improve the sound. In addition, the client has learned and mentally "logged" a new style of motor planning that carries across other similar sound challenges. The steps for this problem solving will be described later and are summarized in the text boxes.

In the case of "great," *anticipatory* coarticulation—the effect subsequent phonemes have on initial phonemes' production (Kent, 2009)—might be the key to a more feminine sound. A transfeminine client seeking voice modification might benefit from anticipation of the light conclusion of the word on /t/, in order to lighten the darker beginning of /gr/. In contrast, a transmasculine client aiming to modify his voice would focus more on maintaining the initial dark components of the word as he moves into the fronted, lighter phonemes. This phenomenon is known as *retentive* (or backward) coarticulation (Kent, 2009), and might be the key to a more masculine sound in the word "great." Internalizing a

Box 11–A. Acoustic Assumptions
A Framework for Problem Solving Resonance Challenges: Transfeminine

Learn these assumptions inside and out.

Voiced and Voiceless pairs (left set is voiced, right set is unvoiced/voiceless. Pairs move from front to back placement in the mouth)

b p	z s	th/th (the, thing)
d t	ʤ (jar) ch (chair)	zh/sh
v f	g k	

Voiced sounds are darker than voiceless. Articulate the voiced sound with a lighter touch to avoid a pronounced acoustic burst. Do not actually replace the sounds as this will affect your accent. To understand which sounds are voiced and which are not, you can check by feeling the Adam's Apple for vibrations (notch of thyroid cartilage) during voicing. Voiceless sounds produce no vibrations as long as they are produced on their own (i.e., no following sound).

m, n, ng (ing, bong, long): The nasal sounds are produced with a potentially very tight contact and constriction. This will produce a pressed, dark sound when they are released. Lighten or loosen the contact as much as possible so that the sound blends fluently with other sounds in close proximity. The acoustic burst will be deemphasized and the darkness of the nasality will diminish sooner. i.e. the contact between your tongue and the back of your top front teeth for /n/ should be light—don't push, for /m/ barely hold your lips together, and for /ng/ sense the slightest of contact between the back of the tongue and the soft palate, and do not squeeze at all.

Vowels and dipthongs in general produce a dark or low resonance, except for the ee /i/ (as in, Peter, feet) sound. Produce all vowels with an /i/ shape (light lip spreading) to lighten their tone. Do not stretch, just feel ee as a light lift. Eventually you will be able to feel this internally. Think /i/ when producing all vowels to bring the sound up and forward. A smile is an /i/ posture. It sounds sweeter because of the way the instrument and vocal tract filter the sound.

Liquids and Glides sounds /l/, er, (flow**er**) /y/ and /w/ are all produced with extreme tension of tongue or lips. Decrease the tension as much as you can without distorting the sound. Loosen the lips for the /w/ to produce it with less tone contrast. You might think /h/ after /w/(h) but do not actually articulate it. Produce the 'er' with a gentle mid-mouth feeling, rather fully pressing into the center of the palate.

A closed vocal instrument makes for a cave-like, dark sound, and abrupt blunt endings. Keeping the instrument (mouth) open, even beyond the end of a sentence keeps the sound alive and allows for a graceful diminution of resonant combinations. "Riding the vowel out" slightly might help, i.e. Haee (Hi), how aare, yoou?"(but remember to think ee!).

Order of Operations: 1. Read a phrase as though learning how to read; sound by sound. 2. Identify potential dark resonance areas. 3. Identify the solution, and 'code' it for change. 4. Articulate the phrase silently at a conversational rate applying the necessary physiological changes. 5. Record multiple drafts and adjust until satisfied with the new sound.

Box 11–B. Acoustic Assumptions
A Framework for Problem Solving Resonance Challenges: Transmasculine

Learn these assumptions inside and out. Reviewing them daily until you know them will help. Scan ahead to search out acoustic pitfalls, check your assumptions, and manipulate articulatory challenges accordingly to modify the tone of the sounds

Voiced and Voiceless pairs (left set is voiced, right set is unvoiced/voiceless. Pairs move from front to back placement in the mouth)

b p	z s	th/th
d t	ʤ (jar) ch (chair)	zh/sh
v f	g k	

Voiced sounds are darker than voiceless. Take advantage of the darker resonance of the voiced sound. Don't shy away from the heavy tone. Feel the buzz of the voicing. A little extra pressure on the contact (**b**ut, **th**at's **g**reat) will provide a louder, more pronounced contrast.

m, n, ng (ing, bong, long): the nasal sounds are produced with a potentially very tight contact and constriction. The more pressure build up, the darker the tone as the acoustic burst is released. Without pinching or holding the articulation unnaturally, take advantage of a little more pressure build to "add a dot of black to the colour of sound."

Vowels and dipthongs in general produce a dark or low resonance, except for the ee /i/ (as in, Peter, feet) sound. Produce all vowels with a slightly rounded or oval shape as much as possible to darken the tone. Focus the tone center and back. Where possible elongate the instrument slightly with a bit of lip protrusion to enhance a deeper tone—do not press the pitch lower, it will be unsupported and unhealthy. Relax the jaw—feel the space inside the mouth.

Liquids and Glides /l/, er, (flow**er**) /y/ and /w/ are all produced with extreme tension of tongue or lips. Maintaining a small degree of tension in this articulation will provide a darker acoustic burst on release due to greater pressure build up.

An open vocal instrument at the end of a sentence makes for a lighter tone, and a gradual diminution of harmonics. A slightly abrupt/blunt close will capture the darker tones from the instrument. Experiment with this—you will know when it's too much. "Sure, I'll try that/, whatever you say/!"

Order of Operations: 1. Read a phrase as though learning how to read; sound by sound. 2. Identify potential light resonance areas. 3. Identify the solution, and code it for change. 4. Articulate the phrase silently at a conversational rate applying the necessary physiological change. 5. Record multiple drafts and adjust until satisfied with the new sound.

few of the basic articulatory/acoustic relationships between phonemes provides the transgender or gender diverse client with an invaluable set of foundational problem-solving tools that can be applied across any word, sentence, or challenging longer phrases. Providing a systematic diagnostic and solution-based approach empowers the client to do individual analysis, allowing for a more secure maintenance of skills long after the therapeutic umbilicus has been cut. Clinicians should re-familiarize themselves with these assumptions should they choose to use this particular approach in training resonance.

Training Steps for Using the *Acoustic Assumptions.* The steps outlined below may seem cumbersome at first, but clients soon find themselves scanning ahead quickly if they are consistent and repetitive in their analysis. Almost immediately they report relief in knowing "what to do." Readers might refer to the *Assumptions* in Boxes 11–A and 11–B as they read the steps. Provide the client with the appropriate rubric for their gender identity and communication needs.

1. Instruct the client in basic anatomy and physiology of speech sounds and phonemes. Go through each phoneme category (as shown in the *Assumptions, Box 11-A and 11-B*) and explain potential resonance challenges and their possible solutions.
2. Develop a coding system for each solution (e.g., this author uses dv:devoicing/and an arrow down for modifying voiced tones and decreasing their tension or the buildup of pressure; an arrow down for decreasing tension, a "greater than" sign for keeping an open instrument, and an ee for producing an /i/ overlay across all vowels).
3. Use phrases of approximately four to six words that the client has developed from everyday life, have the client read each one slowly as though learning how to read, phoneme by phoneme. This will allow the client to feel the articulatory gesture of each phoneme. It helps if the phrases are typed large and with two to four spaces between lines.
4. Have the client identify the potential acoustic challenges in each phoneme (e.g., voiced sounds are darker than voiceless, nasals tend to have an abrupt acoustic burst, liquids tend to be tense and therefore may have an abrupt acoustic burst).
5. Have the client identify the solution that best suits the identified problem.
6. Have the client mark the code for that solution above each phoneme.
7. Have the client articulate the sentence silently at a normal pace, practicing the new articulatory gestures in order to *feel* the changes. Switching between the old and new way helps sometimes if the client cannot feel the difference automatically.
8. Have the client speak the sentence and record varying "edits" or "voice drafts." It is expected that the client will have to do this many times to fully grasp how to experiment with different solutions (i.e., changes in physiological gesture) to each problem. The more often the client does this, the faster and more intuitive the process becomes. Soon the client is scanning ahead quickly and solving acoustic problems before even stumbling across them. It is important that the client complete all steps for a phrase before moving on, rather than "coding" multiple phrases ahead of time.

Picking and Choosing

There are a number of excellent and interesting portions of the L-MRVT that can help in refining the client's understanding and appropriate use of feminine resonance. Three of them are especially useful for gender non-conforming clients. First, the "messa di voce" (crescendo and decrescendo) described in the program is marvelous for training volume variation while maintaining feminine resonance. The clinician is invited to research this further, but the basic concept is a chant on /mji/ (or /mi/) that begins as a pinpoint of sound, increases to a large sound, and returns to a pinpoint of sound. A helpful way to visualize this is by thinking of the sound as end-to-end triangles. Older clinicians might also remember the pinpoint of light when a television was first turned on. The concept of the messa di voce can be used for short meaningful utterances as well, such as "My name is _____" or "Hello, how are you?"

A second technique, the "mini" from the L-MRVT, which can be thought of as a pull-out (as within the fluency therapy context), might be incorporated into therapy tasks during the later stages in the hierarchy—at the level of spontaneous speech. If a client is repeatedly slipping into male resonance, she might stop and repeat what she just said using the techniques learned for feminine resonance (fronted tone focus, or light quality, for example) in order to reinforce correct production. The employment of the "mini" is a good approach for adding awareness and another tool for success, rather than panic. Minis can be pull-outs (or correct repetitions), but they might also include shifts in posture, a small hand gesture, fiddling with a ring and so forth. It is essentially a way to break the "vocal spell" and force a cognitive refocusing.

A third technique, the /m/ phoneme, can be used at the beginning of any word or phrase as a "vocal communicator" (Verdolini, 2000; Verdolini Abbott, 2008), or a way of "finding" feminine pitch and resonance prior to beginning an utterance. It can be used as an initial response such as "Mm, I'm not sure" or actually incorporated into a series of practice tasks as shown below. In this case, the client does a brief hum on a gender-acceptable or slightly higher frequency and then begins the phrase, e.g., "Mm, how are you?," "Mm, it's a lovely day," "Mm, even at night," and so forth.

As soon as possible, the client should be asked to develop and incorporate at least 20 to 30 personal phrases and sentences. The clinician should provide guidance regarding the most appropriate syllabic or word length based on current levels of success in therapy.

Interstitial words such as *if, and, um, so but, well* on a sustained 196 Hz or 208 Hz (3G or 3G#) can be helpful for maintaining resonance and pitch (e.g., "uuum, I think that sounds fine" or "aaand, if you wanted to have dinner later we could . . ."). Anecdotally, Hirsch has found that this is the only approach that appears to truly benefit from using a "money note."

Speaking a Foreign Language: Panic

How the individual feels may be reflected in the voice (Stemple, 2000). When clients begin work on shifting their resonance, they often experience a mixture of excitement and panic. "Oh my gosh, I don't sound at all like myself" is often the first response to hearing and feeling the true shift from a masculine to a feminine resonance. While there is intense joy expressed in finally achieving a sound that is recognizably in keeping with their gender identity, a look of loss and confusion usually creeps across clients' faces. It is not unusual for a client to go through a brief period of inhibition and back-peddling before continuing progress. It is the same look that appears on the face of a client learning to modify an accent. There is a lack of recognition, a fear of the unfamiliar, and a feeling of awkwardness expressed by the client.

This can be a fertile moment for the client and clinician. It is a moment when the client can begin to truly learn a new vocal personality, and begin to recognize the new sound more readily than the old one. For this reason, sometimes it helps to go back to the beginning and engage in meaningless vocalization. There has not been a client unwilling to begin true resonance work by engaging in "vocal play" before incorporating meaningful language.

For the more adventurous client, a strong foundation of understanding about the voice can be gleaned by experimenting with producing environmental sounds before trying to use them within meaningful language—a raindrop into a barrel, the "/pɔk/" of a cork as it leaves the bottle, the creak of a door (not the sound of the word *creak*, but the actual sound of the door), the sound of a newborn cry. This type of vocal play affords the client an opportunity to gain a deeper understanding of exactly how shifts in physiologic gesture affect the acoustic output. The client gains confidence in listening to herself making a variety of different sounds and becomes eager and enthusiastic about employing similar methods for shifting resonance. Therapy progress will soon be back on track.

Conclusions

Technical proficiency frees the singer [gender diverse client] from production concerns of the instrument so that artistic [emotional] communication may occur.
—Miller, 1993

Clinicians are not new to the concept that the physiologic gesture gives rise to the

acoustic output. Humans are no more than walking instruments capable of an enormously wide range of sounds. One has only to look to the capabilities of Tuvan or Mongolian throat singers (Lindestaad, Södersten, Merker, & Granqvist, 2001), or Indian harmonic choirs to understand that most of us limit ourselves to a rather narrow range of vocal possibilities. Given enough practice and patience, however, we are all (astoundingly) capable of producing two or three tones at once, even if we do fear having a vocal out-of-body experience. Even the best of us has to overcome certain inhibitions to access the full range of vocal mysteries, and no less the gender diverse client.

Resonance training is a creative challenge. It requires the extremes of what Stemple (2000) calls "eclectic voice therapy." As challenging as this aspect of voice and communication training with the gender diverse client can be, it is truly exciting and joyful. It calls upon the perfect marriage of art and science, and forces the clinician to reach deep into the clinical bag of tricks; to keep rifling and clattering around, until the proper blend of approaches is achieved.

Articulation and the Gender Diverse Population

Resonance and articulation are strongly connected, since both are supralaryngeal phenomena, which essentially use the same mechanism. Many of the concepts introduced in the consideration of resonance for the gender diverse client will be revisited in this section on articulatory modifications. While it is unlikely that articulatory changes alone can alter gender perception significantly, they may be able to contribute to the impression of the gender the speaker wishes to represent.

Theoretical Background Review

There is little recent evidence to demonstrate that articulatory variables strongly influence gender perception. However, there are anecdotal reports and observations documenting the concept that female articulation is more correct or precise than male articulation (Dacakis, Oates, & Douglas, 2012; Simpson, 2009).

Historically, interest in the area of gender differences in articulation dates back to the early 1950s, when multiple studies in sociolinguistics began to be published about observable gender differences in pronunciation. Oates and Dacakis (1983) summarized several of the original studies, which concluded that females tend to use more correct or standard articulation of speech sounds than men do. The most commonly cited examples refer to the fact that women are more likely than men to use the "standard realization of the verb ending /ing/ as opposed to the nonstandard /in/" (Oates & Dacakis, 1983, p. 144). This pattern was first noted by Smith in 1958 (as cited in Fashold, 1990), and has been reported with some regularity since then.

According to Gunzberger (1995), William Labov, who studied inner-city speech, "found a clear difference in the pronunciation of the voiceless fricative 'th' (as in 'thin'); women pronounced the sound in a 'correct' way; whereas, men often replaced 'th' by another sound, such as the 't' in 'tin.' This same pattern was also found with the voiced dental fricative 'th' (as in 'this')" (Gunzberger, 1995, p. 340). These findings have been corroborated by other research both in the United States and in Northern Ireland (Gunzberger, 1995). In addition, the postvocalic /r/ (such as seen in words like "far" and "care") tends to be more frequently pronounced by women than by men in the United States (Gunzberger, 1995), although

regional dialects can also contribute to /r/ variation.

So consistent have some of these gender-related speech findings been that one sociolinguist, Ralph Fasold, generalized about this tendency for male speakers "to use forms that are generally considered 'correct' less frequently than women speakers do" and coined the phrase "sociolinguistic gender pattern" to name this male tendency to "use socially disfavored variants of sociolinguistic variables, while women tend to avoid these in favor of socially more favored variants" (Fasold, 1990, p. 92). Various explanations for the "sociolinguistic gender pattern" have been offered over the years, many centering around the notion that women may use linguistic forms as a way of achieving social status, or that women may have needed to become more aware of this kind of signal in order to secure their social status linguistically (Fasold, 1990; Trudgill, 1983).

In a comprehensive review of the literature, Simpson (2009) reported on studies addressing the differences in vocal tract length and size between men and women, differences between vowel formant frequencies of men and women *not* attributable to vocal tract length and size, differences in articulatory speed and speed of tongue movements between male and female speakers, differences in voice onset time (VOT), and differences in vowel duration. Both anatomical/physiological variations and learned behavioral characteristics were considered to explain the reported findings. His conclusion, like the conclusions of so many researchers before him, was that regardless of the explanation of why things are the way they are, "The larger female vowel space, the longer duration of stressed vowels, the greater durational distinction between stressed and unstressed vowels, and less reduction of vowel qualities to [ə] can all be treated as phonetic correlates of speaking clearly. Alternatively, opposite patterns in male speakers can be seen as a tendency to speak less clearly" (Simpson, 2009, p. 636).

Only one study to date has attempted to experimentally determine whether or not the use of more precise articulatory patterns affects perceived gender of the speaker. In a symposium presentation, Free and Dacakis (2007) described a study in which they asked 20 transfeminine participants to read the Rainbow Passage twice, once with precise articulation, and a second time with omissions, reductions, and distortions of sounds. Listener participants (11 first-year students in speech-language pathology) were asked to identify whether the speakers were male or female, and to rate their perceived "gender representativeness" on a "very male–very female" scale. These and other details were reported by Dacakis et al. (2012), who also described the Free and Dacakis (2007) study in a "Current Opinions" review. Results revealed that 40% of the participants (8/20) were rated as female more often in the precise articulation condition as opposed to the imprecise articulation condition. It was also reported that 15 of the 20 speakers were rated more toward the female end of the continuum on the "very male–very female" scale when they used precise articulation (Dacakis et al., 2012).

Unfortunately, results of this study were confounded by the finding that the speech samples in the precise articulation condition were also produced with higher speaking fundamental frequencies (Free & Dacakis, 2007), so the effects of articulatory precision versus the effects of a higher speaking fundamental frequency could not be separated. In summary, the results of the study reported by Free and Dacakis (2007) suggest that articulatory precision can contribute to the perception of femininity in a transfeminine speaker but until the study

itself is submitted for peer review so that its methodology can be ascertained, the results can only be considered speculative.

The remainder of this section will focus on methods of improving articulatory precision for the transfeminine client. In particular, specific articulatory patterns that have potential salience in terms of transgender speech modification work will be highlighted.

Articulation Modification and the Transfeminine Client

As noted previously, there are a number of ways in which male and female speakers differ in terms of how they typically produce both vowel and consonant sounds. Once pointed out and demonstrated in therapy, these differences not only can become perceptually apparent and observable to clients, but they also are the kinds of differences that can be imitated and produced by a transfeminine client seeking to modify her own speech. Following are some key male-female articulation distinctions, with suggestions for those engaged in gender-related speech training/therapy.

Vowels

Easy Onsets

Initial vowel words are, by definition, produced with voice onset coming at the very beginning of the utterance. For the transfeminine individual, evaluation should determine if manner or quality of vocal onset is an interfering issue. In general, for any speaker, voice onset should be "easy," with smooth and gradual approximation of the vocal folds. For the transgender woman, however, it will be even more important to achieve a smooth or easy onset, in order to contribute to a perception of reduced speaking intensity and a slight increase in the perception of breathiness. These features have been noted to potentially "feminize" the voice (Davies et al., 2015).

To accomplish this, the client should be educated about the nature of hard versus easy glottal attacks, and be advised to avoid the abrupt and tight glottal contact that causes what we perceive to be a "hard attack." Prior to producing an easy onset, the client should be assisted in reducing or eliminating undue tension in the neck, shoulder, and chest area, as such tension is known to radiate to the larynx and interfere with smooth vocal fold vibration. Relaxation exercises may be appropriate to decrease shoulder, neck, and jaw tension especially, although general relaxation as a precursor to other exercises may be very beneficial for some clients as well.

Specific exercises to practice smooth or "easy" vowel onsets might include:

1. Saying initial /h/ or /sh/ words ("hello," "show," etc.). Because the vocal folds do not fully adduct when producing /h/ or /sh/, this exercise helps the client to get feedback and gain awareness of differences between hard and easy onsets. Eventually move from adding /h/ or /sh/ to the word beginning, to omitting /h/ and /sh/ while still trying to maintain the easy attack on the vowel (e.g., "hand"- "and," "hit"- "it," "shame"- "aim," "shake"- "ache," etc.).
2. After words, have the client produce short phrases or sentences heavily loaded with /h/ and /sh/ sounds (e.g., "Show Harry the hammer").
3. Move from single words to phrases to sentences containing initial vowel sounds (e.g., "Anna"— "Anna ate"— "Anna ate an

apple"). Have the client initially imagine whispering a silent /h/ before each word, if this helps to promote easy onsets.

Vowel Prolongation

As discussed above, women tend to elongate their vowels more than male speakers do. For the transfeminine client, exercises to practice and encourage increased vowel duration are warranted in many cases. Present words in which vowels appear in all positions (initial, medial, final) and have the client work on sustaining the vowel sounds. Move from words to phrases to sentence-length stimuli. Oral reading can be effective, as this activity allows the client to see and anticipate when vowels appear in the utterance. If using musical terminology to assist in explanations, the clinician might discuss with the client how sustaining vowels leads to more "legato" (reference to how musical tones can be produced in a connected, smoothly gliding manner) versus "staccato" prosody (marked by short, disconnected, separated, or distinct productions), while also having the effect of slightly lengthening overall speaking rate, which is a feminizing feature.

Consonants

Precision

As reported above, women tend to pronounce words with greater articulatory precision than men. It therefore can be an important goal with some transfeminine or gender non-conforming clients to address correctness and clarity of articulation. Through informal assessment during the initial consultation, the clinician needs to listen for any patterns of imprecision, as well as any consistent phonemic errors if these are present. If so, articulation therapy should be considered to remedy sounds in error. This therapy can be coordinated with easy onset of both voicing and consonant production for clients seeking to adopt a more feminine speaking style.

When appropriate, directed articulation exercises can be useful to increase the transfeminine or gender non-conforming client's awareness and self-monitoring skills for her own overall speech clarity. "Sloppy" or distorted phonemes should be targeted in order to improve production. This could be at single-word levels, if needed, to focus in on specific problematic sounds. Movement up the therapy hierarchy to sentences, oral reading. Structured and spontaneous running speech would then follow. Audio feedback may be useful in some cases to enhance the client's self-monitoring and awareness. The clinician can demonstrate improved articulatory precision for the client. Further, increased precision can be approached through decreased speech rate and utilization of syllable-by-syllable approach to utterances. Other exercises to increase precise use of the articulators include tongue-twisters (Glenn, Glenn, & Forman, 1998, p. 237), as well as production of word lists containing "difficult consonant clusters" (Pentz, 2014).

"Light" Contacts

Several speech-language pathologists have written about the effectiveness of teaching "light articulation" to trans women (Bryan-Smith, 1986; Chaloner, 1991; Spencer, 1988), to "lighten" the speech, giving an additional illusion of femininity. A focus on the production of light, forward articulation—tripping off the tongue—was suggested. Chaloner (1991) also recommended "light" articulation, advising that the client actively think

in terms of making "delicate" contacts with the articulators (lips, tongue, teeth), for example, when reading a given passage.

Linking or Blending Words

During running or connected speech, making smooth transitions from one word to the next has the effect of eliminating or decreasing opportunities for hard glottal attacks, as well as producing an overall more legato sound. The clinician should initially present to the client phrases and short sentences in which a final consonant sound precedes an initial vowel sound (e.g., "an apple," "if only," "circus elephant," "Bob's uncle"). Instruct the client to move smoothly from the first word into the second word by linking or blending the final consonant of the first word to the initial vowel of the next word, thereby eliminating the possibility for a hard glottal attack on the initial vowel word. When a consonant does not precede a vowel, insertion of a /w/ or /y/ sound (e.g., "I (y)-am" or "to (w)-Oklahoma") will have the same effect.

When the client has achieved the ability to successfully make blended transitions from consonant-to-vowel and vowel-to-vowel sounds, then she will be more ready to work on attaining flowing concordance for word transitions containing consonant-to-consonant sequences. To move from a word with a final consonant to a contiguous word with an initial consonant, the goal will be to produce "light" articulatory contacts, as described above. Bryan-Smith (1986) found that, when necessary, it can often be effective to have the client deliberately devoice voiced consonants, which has the effect of exposing the listener to less vocal quality. Chaloner (1991) also suggested helping the client to focus her speech forward in the face as much as possible, using the image of pushing the speech sounds forward to the lips when articulating.

Oral-Motor Aspects: Lip and Mouth Movements

A number of researchers have also noted that female speakers tend to use wider mouth opening (Andrews, 2006) and/or greater lip rounding (Oates & Dacakis, 1983) than men do. Unfortunately, sometimes in therapy, the goal of increased or more exaggerated mouth opening can overlap with pragmatic goals such as increased animation and expressiveness of facial expression. Work on increased lip rounding can also interfere with resonance work, given that slightly retracted and upturned lip corners can have the effect of shortening the vocal tract, thereby causing higher second formant frequencies in clients for whom this goal is salient. Thus, the goals of greater mouth opening and/or lip rounding should be introduced judiciously. When introducing these oral motor behaviors in therapy, and/or when making recommendations for home practice, the suggestion for the client to use a mirror can be a good one.

"Breathing Through" the Phonemes

Sometimes it is effective to suggest the use of a slightly breathy onset to articulation, which can have the effect of causing an overall softer utterance (Andrews, 2006). However, use of this approach will depend on the client's existing speech characteristics. Clients with a forceful, staccato speaking style may find work on slightly breathy speech onsets more helpful for voice feminization than clients who come to the voice change process with less abrupt speech onsets. Mount and

Salmon (1988), in their longitudinal case study, found success by having their transfeminine client initially work on achieving breathiness in initial /h/ words, and then later on in words beginning with vowels. The clinician can present exercises in which the client aims to emit "extra" exhaled breath while producing voiced consonants and vowels alike. Throughout this work, however, care needs to be taken to avoid making breathiness a goal in and of itself. Clients who have been working on breath support issues may not be good candidates for this approach, as it may interfere with the new breathing patterns that they are learning.

Additional Considerations

Actual therapy techniques to address articulation issues with gender diverse clients will oftentimes be very similar to methods used with any articulation client population. That is, the initial goal will be to heighten the client's awareness of each specific target phoneme to be modified, followed by development of self-monitoring and self-correction skills, followed by increased ability to correct the production in a structured context, and finally ending with habituation and carryover to outside the therapy setting. The main difference in methodology will be education of the client regarding gender-marking characteristics of his or her own articulation patterns, including increased awareness regarding the rationale behind selection of his or her specific target phonemes.

In therapy and/or when devising home practice programs, the following are some other general suggestions to consider when working primarily with transfeminine clients:

1. If using oral reading as a therapy stimulus, select materials with appropriate

content given the particular goals as well as the gender of your client. For example, if working on light articulatory contacts and easy onsets, select a passage with content that evokes a softness of imagery or emotion, as opposed to a passage in which, for instance, harsh or violent images or angry dialogue is being expressed. It can be useful with some transfeminine clients to select passages from fiction in which clients will be asked to read the lines of the female protagonist or another clearly feminine character.

2. Some clients benefit from suggestions to observe speakers of their target gender, for example, when seeing them on television, listening to the radio (e.g., call-in talk radio shows), or "people-watching" in public places. The clinician can guide clients to watch for specific target behaviors and to prepare to report back at their next appointment regarding what they observed. This technique is beneficial for all gender diverse clients.

3. Use of audio feedback is useful with some clients at certain stages of therapy. This activity can be especially appropriate for certain clients who may have long commutes to work, and who may be able to listen to stimulus materials in the car. Such an approach is useful for both trans women and trans men.

Conclusions

While articulatory differences between male and female speakers may be subtle, it is worthwhile to include assessment and treatment of articulation, as indicated, in an overall program of speech modification for gender diverse clients. In fact, there are many similarities between the work clients undertake on their resonance characteristics and the goals they adopt for articulatory modification. In both cases, the primary

focus is to modify production of speech sounds so that the client's gender identity can be more readily perceived by listeners. In the case of resonance characteristics, this work is mainly accomplished through subtle changes in vowel production to give the voice a different tone. In the case of articulation, clients primarily focus on consonant sounds, to alter the features we associate with gender. When the manipulation of vowels and consonants are bundled together, clients appear to be more readily able to achieve their voice and communication gender goals.

That said, with this particular client population, there will be no one specific feature or characteristic that alone will solve the problem of attaining gender-appropriate skills. Rather, the clinician must attend to all areas, verbal and non-verbal, segmental and non-segmental, in determining which combination of speech and communication behaviors will meet the goal of creating optimal change for each individual client.

During this process, clients need to be encouraged and educated that learning these skills must be accomplished by addressing each discrete area, one behavior at a time, at first. It is not possible to do it all at the same time. But eventually, once they have patiently learned each target feature, they can look forward to the time when they will be ready to "put it all together," hopefully realizing with delight that they are now communicating in a way that is appropriate to their chosen gender.

Vocal Intensity in Gender Identification

Vocal intensity, or volume, is influenced by both respiratory and laryngeal mechanisms. According to Ferrand (2012), "Intensity is regulated by the interaction between subglottal pressure generated by the respiratory system and glottal resistance generated by the laryngeal system" (p. 52). In general, males have greater lung volume than females (Behrman, 2013), a larger diaphragm (Suwatanapongched, Gierada, Slone, Pilgram, & Tuteur, 2003), and greater forced vital capacity, forced expiratory volume, and forced expiratory flow (Neder, Andreoni, Castelo-Filho, & Nery, 1999). It would not be surprising to find that these respiratory differences, coupled with the larger and more calcified male larynx and greater muscle mass of the laryngeal muscles in males (Behrman, 2013), may translate into increased vocal loudness in general in male speakers (Rendall et al., 2007). Indeed, studies of vocal loudness in cis-gendered speakers typically find a somewhat higher intensity level in the speech of males compared with females (see e.g., Gelfer & Young, 1997; Stathopoulos & Sapienza, 1993).

But what role does intensity play in gender identification? Does the intensity of a speaker's voice contribute to the perception that the speaker is male or female, or that their speech is masculine or feminine? Only a few studies address this issue. Andrews and Schmidt (1997) investigated the perceptual and acoustic characteristics of a group of male cross-dressers who provided speech samples in both their "male" mode of presentation and their "female" mode. For the perceptual analysis, ratings of all speech samples on 18 eight-point semantic differential scales were provided by 88 listeners. Acoustic analyses were also made of all speech samples. The investigators compared rating scale judgments of male and female modes for each speaker, to see what, if any, significant differences might be found between the two modes. They did the same for the acoustic measures. Not surprisingly, significant differences on the pitch perceptual rating scale (high-low) were seen for 10 out of 11 speakers, with female mode speech samples being rated higher in pitch

than male mode speech samples. In contrast, the loudness perceptual rating scale (loud-soft) showed significant differences for only 5 out of 11 speakers, with the female mode being rated softer. On a related scale, strong-weak, the speech samples in the male mode were rated as stronger for 7 out of 11 speakers.

Holmberg, Oates, Dacakis, and Grant (2010) also studied vocal intensity, as well as numerous other acoustic and aerodynamic characteristics of vocal production for 12 male speakers, 12 female speakers, and 25 transfeminine speakers. One of their many results was that the two transfeminine speakers who were rated as most female had somewhat lower intensity levels (75 dB and 76 dB) compared with the transfeminine speakers who were rated as most male (79 dB and 80 dB). On the strength of this finding, the authors concluded that "the use of low speech intensities could also contribute to a successful female voice" (p. 520).

Although the evidence regarding the role of vocal intensity in gender identification is scant, it might be interpreted in support of reducing vocal intensity for those who want to present as more feminine, and increasing vocal intensity for those who want to present as more masculine. On the other hand, those seeking an ambiguous gender presentation, who want neither male nor female characteristics to predominate in their voice, may want to vary intensity to express traits such as self-confidence or assertiveness. Thus, intensity goals for the gender diverse client will most likely need to be individualized, depending on the needs and wishes of the client.

Intervention

Once it is established that modification of vocal loudness is a recommended goal for voice therapy, it is important that the client understand and agree with the individual treatment objectives and rationales. Is the desired goal a decrease in overall loudness level, or an increase? Or perhaps the goal might be to focus on increased variability of loudness levels.

Management of loudness in a healthy gender diverse client (i.e., no organic abnormality in phonatory or respiratory functioning) will typically not be a primary goal, but rather one that overlaps with other goals. In rare cases where volume modification is seen as a high priority, intervention might begin by identifying the target or desired loudness level. As with any speech therapy goal, a critical first step will be to facilitate the client's self-awareness, in part through provision of auditory feedback. Toward this end, it can be useful to have the client listen to audio-recorded samples, and even compare their voice loudness with the clinician's, using questions such as, "Do you think your voice sounds louder, softer, or the same loudness as mine?" Part of this conversation might also include discussions to facilitate increased insight into the implications and ramifications of voice loudness on the client's desired target gender presentation. With improved ability to recognize their own typical intensity levels, work can begin on the self-monitoring, self-correction, or other indicated modification of habitual volume level, moving always from structured to less structured speech contexts (e.g., routine social phrases, picture description, sentence or paragraph production, response to questions, structured conversation, role-plays, spontaneous conversation).

Pragmatic Issues Related to Loudness Intervention

A beneficial therapy discussion might relate to the pragmatic issues surrounding vocal loudness. Particularly for transitioning

gender clients, it could be useful to explore various functional/social communication contexts to determine appropriate loudness levels, given the fact that the development of certain stylistic speech features is very much associated with cultural gender patterns and social learning. There may be questions as to what volume levels are considered appropriate for a man versus a woman, and vice versa. For example, what volume is suitable for quiet interactions with intimate family members, friends, or loved ones versus with a stranger in a public place (e.g., making inquiry at grocery store or gas station), versus what vocal intensity is appropriate for speaking at your particular place of employment? Socially, what is an acceptable conversation loudness level when interacting with someone one-on-one, versus speaking to others in a group social setting? What about speaking to a same-gender conversation partner versus interacting with someone of the opposite gender?

Loudness and Pitch Relationships

It is possible that work on speech intensity modification might go hand-in-hand with work on establishing a new pitch as well (see Chapter 10). There also could be therapy overlap in addressing the goals of loudness variation and intonation, for it is known that inflection does not only involve pitch; inflection can also involve variations in volume as well. Although not seen very often, sometimes a client will demonstrate little or no loudness variation. In this situation, perhaps the therapist could have the client listen to an audio recording of the client's own voice, requesting feedback regarding the recorded material. People who become aware of the monotony of their voices, and who are concerned about it, can usually develop loudness inflections with practice (Boone et al., 2014).

The Special Problem of Elevating Volume without Compromising Feminine Pitch or Tone

For transfeminine clients in certain circumstances, it may be that a gender-appropriate pitch does not necessarily produce the desired loudness level, and vice versa. In fact, the issue of maintaining a desired pitch level while needing to elevate volume has been known to pose a fairly common problem among some trans women, particularly in certain employment settings. For example, a transfeminine teacher or college professor may report that she has difficulty elevating her volume while simultaneously trying to maintain her desired feminine vocal pitch. She may complain that when trying to speak loudly enough to reach students seated at the back of a lecture hall, her voice may seem to deepen in pitch. Some clients, whose jobs require quite a bit of public speaking, may need to use external aids such as lapel microphones, in order to reduce potential vocal strain and promote increased vocal health practices. However, most clients would benefit from the awareness that pitch and volume can be controlled independently one from the other.

It can be useful to educate clients as to the underlying physiology and mechanisms of altering pitch and volume, followed by introducing breathing exercises to facilitate increased voice control through improved breath support. A useful exercise can be to have the transfeminine client find her desired pitch level and to practice sustaining /a/ at that level for several seconds. Then the client should inhale deeply and reproduce the same pitch at increased loudness levels, gaining awareness that it is entirely possible to achieve increased loudness without altering pitch. Any breathing exercise that produces increased subglottal air pressure, or that improves the force behind the air stream,

will lead to improved technique, whether it be abdominal-diaphragmatic breathing drills or practicing taking increased frequency of quick "replenishing" breaths between phrases and sentences. Clients should be encouraged to release and sustain breath, rather than force it out of their bodies. They also should be taught to develop a clear, focused idea of a specific vocal target toward the front of the mouth, or even outside of it. L-MRVT, as discussed earlier, is an excellent approach to consider in this instance.

In this regard, the distinction between the terms "loudness" and "projection" can become meaningful and relevant, for achieving good vocal projection is to achieve "a voice (that) is clear and carries naturally and effortlessly" (Myers & Finnegan, 2015). Clients seeking to project their voices without altering their pitch will become encouraged when they understand that projection is not necessarily synonymous with loudness. Even though it may be customary to use the word "loudness" to refer to increased vocal audibility, clarity, and distinctness in the context of public speaking, a well-projected soft voice can definitely have the power to reach the back of a large room.

According to Myers and Finnegan (2015), the key to projection is clear articulation, or even over articulation. In their study, eight actor participants read a passage under three different conditions: in their normal voice, with disordered articulation caused by use of a bite block, and with over articulation following instruction based on Lessac's articulation exercises. Both acoustic and perceptual analyses were performed on all samples. Results showed that there were only minimal non-significant differences in intensity measured in dB SPL between the three conditions; however, there were clear perceptual differences as perceived by 20 listeners. The over-articulated samples were judged as being the loudest 80% of the time, and judged as being the best projected 85% of the time. The researchers concluded that their study provided evidence "that the degree of articulation has a strong positive correlation to perceived loudness of the voice. When speakers used a style of over-articulation, their speech was perceived by listeners to be louder and better projected" (p. 390.e15). It is possible that for gender diverse clients wanting to project a female-appropriate voice despite their higher pitch or for those seeking a more forceful and projected voice to present their desired personality characteristics, increased articulatory precision may be the key to their success.

Conclusion

It is understandable that volume-related problems will be found among the gender diverse population, attributable not only to this population's unique gender concerns, but also to myriad other possible cultural, social, and personality factors that have the power to impact any speaker. For example, an individual who utilizes an inappropriately low volume could be perceived as possibly displaying a personal sense of insecurity, a lack of commitment, or fear of taking responsibility for having made a definitive statement (Martin & Darnley, 1992). A louder voice, on the other hand, is often associated with such characteristics as increased physical strength, and/or an increased sense of confidence or authority. Many gender diverse individuals are in the habit of trying to avoid calling attention to themselves, which might account for low volume. But then there will also be those individuals who may be in the habit of phonating at a slightly stronger intensity than

is optimal for their target gender. Thus, in cases where inappropriate volume presents as a salient matter, the gender diverse client may benefit not only from the more traditional types of speech therapy interventions described above, but also from insights that can be gained through therapeutic conversations about the various prosodic roles that volume plays in communication. Finally, attention to articulation in the quest for an appropriately projected voice may also be a treatment option.

Chapter Conclusion

It cannot be said too often: "The physiological gesture gives rise to the acoustic output" (personal communication, Fred Minifie, multiple occasions, 1985–1989). In this chapter, we have covered a number of topics that primarily relate to how the acoustic output of the vocal folds is modified by the supralaryngeal vocal tract. While intensity is a voice phenomenon, dependent on respiratory effort and vocal fold vibratory characteristics, both resonance and articulation are supralaryngeal phenomena. The interaction between the frequency and harmonic structure of vocal fold output and the size and shape of the vocal tract gives rise to both resonance and articulation. While both clients and clinicians typically have an intuitive understanding of how the output of vocal fold vibration can alter the gender perception of a voice, it is often less clear how the resonance characteristics of the vocal tract and articulatory movements of the tongue and lips can contribute to a listener's sense of speaker gender. This chapter has attempted to elucidate these relationships, and how supralaryngeal resonance can be harnessed artistically and clinically in the search to achieve a communication style that confidently reflects the client's gender identity.

References

Andrews, M. L. (2006). *Manual of voice treatment: pediatrics through geriatrics* (3rd ed.). Clifton Park, NY: Thomson/Delmar Learning.

Andrews, M. L., & Schmidt, C. P. (1997). Gender presentation: Perceptual and acoustical analyses of voice. *Journal of Voice, 11*(3), 307–313.

Awan, S. (2013). Both direct and indirect behavioral treatments are beneficial for the treatment of voice disorders in teachers. *Evidence-based Communication Assessment and Intervention, 7*(2), 57–62.

Azul, D., Nygren, U., Sodersten, M., & Neuschaefer-Rube, C. (2017). Transmasculine people's vocal function: A review of currently available evidence. *Journal of Voice, 31*(2), e261.

Behrman, A. (2013). *Speech and voice science* (2nd ed.). San Diego, CA: Plural Publishing, Inc.

Benninger, M. S., Jacobson, B. H., & Johnson, A. F. (1994). *Vocal arts medicine: The care and prevention of professional voice disorders*. New York, NY: Thieme Medical Publishers, Inc.

Berry, C. (1973). *Voice and the actor*. London, UK: Harrap.

Block, C. (2017). Making a case for transmasculine voice and communication training. *Perspectives of the ASHA Special Interest Groups SIG 3, 2*(1), 33–41.

Boone, D. R., McFarlane, S. C., Von Berg, S. L., & Zraick, R. (2014). *The voice and voice therapy* (9th ed.). Boston, MA: Pearson Education.

Bryan-Smith, P. (1986). Transsexual voice therapy. *Speech Therapy in Practice, 2*(3), 28–29.

Carew, L., Dacakis, G., & Oates, J. (2007). The effectiveness of oral resonance therapy on the perception of femininity of voice in male-to-female transsexuals. *Journal of Voice, 21*(5), 591–603.

Case, J. L. (1996). *Clinical management of voice disorders* (3rd ed.). Austin, TX: Pro-Ed.

Chaloner, J. (1991). The voice of the transsexual. In M. Fawcus (Ed.) *Voice disorders and their management*. London, UK: Chapman and Hall.

Chen, S. H., Hsiao, T. Y., Hsiao, L. C., Chung, Y. M., & Chiang, S. C. (2007). Outcome of resonant voice therapy for female teachers with voice disorders: Perceptual, physiological, acoustic, aerodynamic, and functional measurements. *Journal of Voice, 21*(2), 415–425.

Dacakis, G., Oates, J., & Douglas, J. (2012). Review/ Current Opinion: Beyond voice: Perceptions of gender in male-to-female transsexuals. *Current Opinions in Otolaryngology and Head and Neck Surgery, 20*, 165–170.

Davies, S., Papp, V. G., & Antoni, C. (2015). Voice and communication change for gender nonconforming individuals: Giving voice to the person inside. *International Journal of Transgenderism, 16*, 117–159.

Fasold, R. (1990). *Sociolinguistics of language*. Padstow, UK: TJ Press, Ltd.

Ferrand, C. T. (2012). *Voice disorders: Scope of theory and practice*. Boston, MA: Pearson Education, Inc.

Free, N., & Dacakis, G. (2007). Articulation and the perception of gender in male-to-female transsexuals. *International Journal of Transgenderism, 10*, 186–187.

Gelfer, M. P., & Schofield, K. J. (2000). Comparison of acoustic and perceptual measures of voice in male-to-female transsexuals perceived as female versus those perceived as male. *Journal of Voice, 14*(1), 22–33.

Gelfer, M. P., & Tice, R. M. (2013). Perceptual and acoustic outcomes of voice therapy for male-to-female transgender individuals immediately after therapy and 15 months later. *Journal of Voice, 27*(3), 335–347.

Gelfer, M. P., & Young, S. R. (1997). Comparisons of intensity measures and their stability in male and female speakers. *Journal of Voice, 11*, 178–186.

Glenn, E., Glenn, P., & Forman, S. (1998). *Your voice and articulation*. Boston, MA: Allyn and Bacon.

Gunzberger, D. (1995). Acoustic and perceptual implications of the transsexual voice. *Archives of Sexual Behavior, 24*(3), 339–348.

Hancock, A. B., & Garabedian, L. M. (2013). Transgender voice and communication treatment: A retrospective chart review of 25 cases. *International Journal of Language and Communication Disorders, 48*(1), 54–65.

Hillenbrand, J. M., & Clark, M. J. (2009). The role of f0 and formant frequencies in distinguishing the voices of men and women. *Attention, Perception and Psychophysics, 71*(5), 1150–1166.

Hirsch, S. (2006). Resonance. In R. K. Adler, S. Hirsch, & M. Mordaunt (Eds.), *Voice and communication therapy for the transgender/transsexual client: A comprehensive clinical guide* (pp. 209–224). San Diego, CA: Plural.

Hirsch, S. (2017). Combining voice, speech science and art approaches to resonant. Challenges in transgender voice and communication training.

Perspectives of the ASHA Special Interest Groups SIG 10 2(2), 73–82.

Hirsch, S., & Gelfer, M. P. (2012). Resonance. In R. K. Adler, S. Hirsch, & M. Mordaunt (Eds.), *Voice and communication therapy for the transgender/transsexual client: A comprehensive clinical guide* (2nd ed., pp. 225–247). San Diego, CA: Plural.

Holmberg, E. B., Oates, J., Dacakis, G., & Grant, C. (2010). Phonetograms, aerodynamic measurements, self-evaluations, and auditory perceptual ratings of male-to-female transsexual voice. *Journal of Voice, 24*(5), 511–522.

Kempster, G. B., Gerratt, B. R., Verdolini Abbot, K., Barkmeier-Kraemer, J., & Hillman, R. E. (2009). Consensus auditory-perceptual evaluation of voice: Development of a standardized clinical protocol. *American Journal of Speech-Language Pathology, 18*, 124–132.

Kent, R. (2009). Normal aspects of articulation. In J. Bernthal, N. Bankson, & P. Flipsen (Eds.), *Articulation and phonological disorders: Speech sound disorders in children* (6th ed., pp. 5–62). Boston, MA: Pearson.

Kent, R., & Minifie, F. (1977) Coarticulation in recent speech production models. *Journal of Phonetics, 5*, 115–133.

Lessac, A. (1967). *The use and training of the human voice: A practical approach to speech and voice dynamics*. New York, NY: DBS Publications.

Lindestaad, P.-A., Södersten, M., Merker, B., & Granqvist, S. (2001). Voice source characteristics in Mongolian "throat singing" studied with high-speed imaging technique, acoustic spectra and inverse filtering. *Journal of Voice, 15*(1), 78–85.

Linklater, K. (2006). *Freeing the natural voice: Imagery and art in the practice of voice and language*. London, UK Drama Publishers.

Martin, S., & Darnley, L. (1992). *The voice sourcebook*. Bicester, Oxon, UK: Winslow Press.

Miller, R. (1993). *Training tenor voices*. New York, NY: Schirmer.

Miller, R. (1996). *On the art of singing*. New York, NY: Oxford University Press.

Mount, K. H., & Salmon, S. J. (1988). Changing the vocal characteristics of a postoperative transsexual patient: A longitudinal study. *Journal of Communication Disorders, 21*, 229–238

Myers, B. R., & Finnegan, E. M. (2015). The effects of articulation on the perceived loudness of the projected voice. *Journal of Voice, 29*(3), 390.e9–390.e15.

Neder, J. A., Andreoni, S., Castelo-Filho, A., & Nery, L. E. (1999). Reference values for lung function tests. I. Static volumes. *Brazilian Journal of Medical and Biological Research, 32*, 703–717.

Oates, J., & Dacakis, G. (1983). Speech pathology considerations in the management of transsexualism: A review. *British Journal of Disorders of Communication, 18*(3), 139–151.

Pentz, A. L. (2014). *Sound stimuli handbook: Words, sentences and paragraphs for busy clinicians*. Austin, TX: Pro-Ed.

Raphael, L. J., Borden, G. J., & Harris, K. S. (2011) *Speech science primer: Physiology, acoustics, and perception of speech* (6th ed.). Philadelphia, PA: Lippincott, Williams and Wilkins.

Rendall, D., Vokey, J. R., & Nemeth, C. (2007). Lifting the curtain on the Wizard of Oz: Voice-based impressions of speaker size. *Journal of Experimental Psychology: Human Perception and Performance, 33*, 1208–1219.

Rodenburg, P. (1992) *The right to speak: Working with the voice*. New York, NY: Routledge.

Rodenburg, P (2000) *The actor speaks: Voice and the performer*. New York, NY: St. Martin's Press.

Roy, N., Weinrich, B., Gray, S. D., Tanner, K., Stemple, J. C., & Sapienza, C. M. (2003). Three treatments for teachers with voice disorders: A randomized clinical trial. *Journal of Speech-Language Hearing Research, 46*, 670–688.

Sataloff, R. T. (1998) *Vocal health and pedagogy*. San Diego, CA: Singular Publishing Group, Inc.

Schwartz, M. (1968). Identification of speaker sex from isolated, voiceless fricatives. *Journal of the Acoustical Society of America, 43*, 1178–1179.

Simpson, A. P. (2009). Phonetic differences between male and female speech. *Language and Linguistics Compass, 10*, 621–640.

Spencer, L. E. (1988). Speech characteristics of male-to-female transsexuals: A perceptual and acoustic study. *Folia Phoniatrica, 40*, 31–42.

Stathopoulos, E. T., & Sapienza, C. (1993). Respiratory and laryngeal function of women and men during vocal intensity variation. *Journal of Speech and Hearing Research, 36*, 64–75.

Stemple, J. (2000). *Voice therapy: Clinical studies* (2nd ed.). San Diego, CA: Singular Thompson Learning.

Stemple, J., Glaze, L. E., & Klaben, B. G. (2010). *Clinical voice pathology: Theory and management* (4th ed.). San Diego, CA: Plural Publishing.

Suwatanapongched, T., Gierada, D.S., Slone, R. M., Pilgram, T. K., & Tuteur, P. G. (2003). Variation in and shape in adults with normal pulmonary function. *Chest, 123*(6), 2019–2027.

Trudgill, P. (1983). *Sociolinguistics*. London, UK: Penguin Books

Verdolini, K. (2000). *LRVT training program*, Virginia Mason Hospital, Seattle, WA.

Verdolini Abbott, K. (2008) *Lessac Madsen resonant voice therapy clinician manual*. Oxfordshire, UK: Plural Publishing Inc.

Verdolini, K., Druker, D. G., Palmer, P. M., & Samawi, H. (1998). Laryngeal adduction in resonant voice. *Journal of Voice 12*(3), 315–327.

Verdolini-Marston, K., Burke, K., Lessac, A., Glaze, L., & Caldwell, E. (1995). Preliminary study of two methods of treatment for laryngeal nodules. *Journal of Voice, 9*(1), 74–85.

Wolfe, V., Ratusnik, D., Smith, F., & Northrop, G. (1990). Intonation and fundamental frequency in male-to-female transsexuals. *Journal of Speech and Hearing Disorders, 55*, 43–50.

Zemlin, W. R. (1998). *Speech and hearing science: Anatomy and physiology* (4th ed.). Needham Heights, MA: Allyn and Bacon.

12

Nonverbal Communication: Assessment and Training Considerations across the Gender and Cultural Spectrum

Sandy Hirsch and Joan Boonin

During the initial thirty seconds of an interaction, we draw an average of six to eight conclusions about a person before a single word is uttered.
—Audrey Nelson, Ph.D. with
Susan K. Golant, M.A., 2004,
*You Don't Say: Navigating Nonverbal
Communication Between the Sexes*

Introduction

Not only do we draw conclusions within 30 seconds of an interaction, we draw them from afar. Assumptions are made, and conclusions are drawn about people as we watch them walking down the street, sitting in a restaurant or even driving a car. In his fascinating work *Blink: The Power of Thinking Without Thinking* (2005), Malcolm Gladwell discusses the power of the mind to draw instantaneous and accurate conclusions about what is seen, even if the conclusion about what was seen is not really understood. In the book it is termed "thin slicing," and refers to the ability of the subconscious to "find patterns in situations and behavior based on very narrow slices of experience" (p. 23). Minute observations of human behavior provide an amalgam of clues that lead people to draw conclusions about gender and culture, mood and intention. In this same text (2005), he interviewed an ornithologist, whose explanation of bird identification is exactly how, it seems, the mind judges veracity: "Most of bird identification is based on a sort of subjective impression—the way a bird moves and little instantaneous appearances at different angles and sequences of different appearances, and as it turns its head and as it flies and as it turns around, you see sequences of different shapes and angles. . . . All that combines to create a unique impression of a bird that can't really be taken apart and described in words. . . . It's more natural and instinctive . . . you look at a bird, and it triggers little switches in your brain. It *looks* right. You know what it is at a glance" (p. 45).

Kachel, Steffens, and Niedlich (2016) remind us that Kagan (1964) suggested that "gender-role identity refers to a comparison of gender-related social norms and the gender-related characteristics of the individual (e.g., how a person actually looks compared to expected gender-typical appearances according to societal norms). Hence, for gender-role identity social comparisons as well as references to different gender-related aspects are emphasized (e.g., looks, behaviors, etc.), whereas gender-role adoption and preference are based on non-relative, absolute statements" (p. 3). In other words, the most important factor is an individual's own perception or interpretation of their gender identity. Azul (2015) takes this thinking a number of steps further when he suggests that "vocal gender is understood as the preliminary (not necessarily unanimous) result of a negotiation process between speaker and listener, and both the voice's gender and the nature of the negotiation process are assumed to vary with a change of conversation partners and cultural setting" (p. 76). It is precisely with this mindset that clinicians should also approach their nonverbal communication training with gender diverse clients: what are the client's personal spectrum wants, needs, and overall goals, and how does context influence them?

Human communication is deeply complex, made more so by the many modes of communication that we use. Part of human communication is verbal. To convey messages words are used, in either a spoken or a written form. In addition, nonverbal communication uses other means, such as facial expression, posture and gesture, and so forth to convey the message. In contrast to verbal communication, people are far less conscious of the nuances of nonverbal communication and the message that it conveys in different contexts. It is an integral part of how humans (and animals) convey meaning.

In the context of gender diverse voice and communication training, it would seem only logical then to give attention to aspects of nonverbal communication. In reality, however, nonverbal communication is still an often neglected, or at least a less well-defined, goal when providing services to gender diverse clients. No voice and communication program should be considered complete without at least tipping a hat to this very important aspect of communication (Andrews, 1999; Freidenberg, 2002; Hirsch, 2012; Oates & Dacakis, 1983; Van Borsel, De Cuypere, & den Berghe, 2001).

And yet, in spite of the obvious importance of this aspect of communication, we must be wary of what Wood and Fixmer-Oraiz (2015) term "essentializing." This is the reduction of something or a person to set characteristics "that are assumed to be central to its nature and present in every member of its category" (p. 18). Generalizations exist for a reason, but it should not be assumed that all people possess all essential qualities recognized by societal constructs. And while we have to accept for now that "gender is not a thing of the past" (Kachel, Stefens, & Niedlich, 2016), we must also acknowledge that how we define it is not static. It is different across cultures, and people's lives, and even over time. As Wood and Fixmer-Oraiz underscore, "even though what our society defines as feminine or masculine may seem natural to us, there is nothing necessary or innate about our particular meaning for any gender. . . . [W]e have more choice than we sometimes realize in how we enact gender in our lives" (p. 25). Clinicians and trainers might take to heart the mission statement made at the outset of every BC Trans Clinical Care Group (BCTCCG) meeting: "We agree to stay curious, knowing that the clients are the experts on their own lives. We aim to take a learner's approach to our work with trans and gender diverse peoples" (personal communication and permission from Marria Townsend, July 30, 2017). As clinicians and trainers we must be aware that clients may already be very sensitive and vulnerable to the possibility of failing, "being read," "being tagged," "being clocked," or simply not looking right, or moving "gracefully" enough in the case of trans women. Discussions today about nonverbal communication and how it fits into a person's gender identity, character, and social framework are becoming increasingly complex. However, the more people know, the more they can adapt to context. Addressing nonverbal communication will give clients tools to use, or reject, as they see fit over the course of their transition. Our job is to guide, not to dictate.

This chapter is intended as an overview of the different aspects of nonverbal communication, including aspects of written communication and a brief discussion of gender from a cross-cultural perspective. It is designed, not as an in-depth analysis, but rather as an overview of nonverbal communication, assessment, and some approaches to training. For some time now, in many Western societies ciswomen have been comfortably presenting in ways that span the gender spectrum. This has perhaps made it easier for trans men to relax into a fairly congruous nonverbal communication style. While male and female characteristics are discussed, and approaches for trans men woven into the chapter, the weight of information falls on guiding trans women during their transition.

Training Nonverbal Communication: Whose Responsibility?

Where does communication start and stop? It is within the American Speech-Language-Hearing Association speech-language clinical code of ethics to "educate and treat individuals about appropriate verbal, nonverbal, and voice characteristics (feminization or masculinization) that are congruent with their targeted gender identity" (2016, p. 11). An earlier iteration of the ethics stated that clinicians should engage in advocacy that "promotes and facilitates access to communication, including the reduction of societal, cultural, and linguistic barriers" (2016, p. 15).

Pragmatics, or social communication training, is a well-established aspect of speech-language pathologists' canon of training. We have embraced the training of nonverbal communication when working with patients suffering from right brain stroke or traumatic brain injury, and indeed for people with autism spectrum diagnoses. To be effective, this therapy should include such things as proxemics, facial expression, and body language. In the teenage or adult population this may include counseling and feedback in the area of clothing choices if they appear contextually illogical or at odds with a particular social setting. If a client with a head injury or a person on the autism spectrum is applying for a job, the clinician plays a significant role as a team member in providing feedback on interviewing skills and overall presentation, which may also include clothing choices. These aspects of nonverbal communication are included in the social skills curricula of many special education high school classes. Formerly, we simply termed these as areas of etiquette. This word is no longer considered descriptive for the purposes of therapy, and may even carry a negative social stigma. "Contextual appropriateness" serves as a less stigmatized term today.

Evidence-Based Support for Training Nonverbal Communication

To further support inclusion of nonverbal training when working with gender diverse voice and communication training, let us consider some of the research. Wood and Fixmer-Oraiz (2012) eloquently state that nonverbal communication supplements verbal or language-based communication. It "regulates interaction and conveys a relationship in interaction" (p. 124). Though few, there are a number of references within the related literature that suggest the inclusion of nonverbal training. Fisk (1974) and Edgerton (1974) both highlighted the importance of masculine-to-feminine (MtF, as described in the study) trans women developing consistently feminine social behaviors. Shaughnessy (1975), Oates and Dacakis (1983), Freidenberg (2002), and Hirsch (2003, 2006, 2012) also mentioned the need for nonverbal communication training within a gender diverse voice and communication training program.

There is scant research that points specifically to which nonverbal variables most influence the perception of gender. There does seem to be some agreement that both visual and auditory input combined most strongly paints a full gender picture (Hadjian et al., 1981). Van Borsel et al. (2001) published a helpful study taking the concept one step further, by comparing the perception of maleness/femaleness based on verbal alone, visual and verbal together, and visual only presentations. They concluded that perception of femaleness was strongest for visual only, weakest for auditory only, and comparable for audiovisual. Interestingly, when Van Borsel, de Pot, and De Cuypere (2009) replicated their study for transmasculine people, they found that there was not a correlation between physical appearance and perception of gender as with their earlier study. Evidence-based studies that include transgender clients are still lacking and would serve this area of communication well. Anecdotal evidence from clients who have changed their nonverbal communication behavior remains the

only real guide for the validity of this work. Those who have made nonverbal communication change a goal in therapy personally communicate increased confidence and a decrease in incidences of being misgendered.

What Does Nonverbal Communication Encompass?

Nonverbal communication can be defined in a number of different ways (Cicca, Step, & Turkstra, 2003; Harper, Wiens, & Matarazzo, 1978; Knapp, 1972). While some authors assume that all human behavior is potentially communicative, others would consider as communicative only those behaviors that are intentionally sent, or that function as such. In this chapter the term "nonverbal communication" will be used in the broadest possible sense, i.e., to mean any nonverbal behavior that may be interpreted as having meaning for a receiver, even if not intended as such by the sender. Since some (although few) clients initially have no idea of the communicative power of their biological gender habits, the latter definition is particularly pertinent to how the clinician places nonverbal communication goals within the gender diverse voice and communication context.

Nonverbal behaviors are various and fall into a number of distinct categories. The tomes of literature that address nonverbal communication have typically categorized them as follows:

- kinesics (related to body movements)
- haptics (touching behavior)
- proxemics (distance from other persons)
- oculesics (use of the eyes)
- olfaction (smell)
- physical appearance
- chronemics (the use of time)

- paralanguage or vocalics (vocal behavior other than words).[1]

In this chapter written communication is included in the list of nonverbal areas to consider.

Nonverbal Communication and Gender

It has been claimed that 65% to 90% of the meaning of a message is transmitted nonverbally (Birdwhistell, 1970; Fromkin & Rodman, 1983). Moreover, just like verbal communication, nonverbal communication shows some clear differences between men and women (Oates & Dacakis, 1997). According to Deborah Tannen in *Gender and Discourse* (1994), girls and boys establish differences in how they use nonverbal communication as early as second grade (7 years old). In a study that she conducted on second, sixth, and tenth graders, as well as 25-year-olds, Tannen recognized that her female subjects sat closer together, faced each other, maintained eye contact and touched each other (this study was conducted in the US). Boys sat at an angle, looked at their surroundings and seemed restless. Wood and Fixmer-Oraiz (2015) point out different manners in which men and women regulate conversation. They suggest that women often use nonverbal communication as an invitation into a conversation, such as with a smile, or looking at someone who has not yet spoken. Men, by contrast, might avoid eye con-

tact in order to ensure that they do not lose "the stage" (Wood & Fixmer-Oraiz, p. 124). Equally, women tend to cede space in a conversation, whereas, men tend to establish their space and keep it. This surely begs the question of why this might be.

An Anthropological Perspective: What Is Our Motivation?

When working with clients on nonverbal communication, Hirsch has found it helpful in initial discussions on the topic to initiate a conversation about why people might behave differently along the gender or indeed cultural spectrum. This appears to be particularly helpful for clients who at first express some ambivalence about this area of communication but ultimately end up wanting to delve deeper into it. Following is a brief look at the literature that may lay the foundations for such a discussion.

It is said that women all over the world tend to be more accurate in their interpretation of nonverbal cues and more responsive to nonverbal cues than men (Nelson & Golant, 2004; Petrevu, 2001; Tannen, 1990). It may serve women well to be more in tune with nonverbal cues. It allows them access to information that is vital for forming close bonds quickly. When considered within an anthropological paradigm, men appear to have been more motivated by the fight-or-flight response, whereas women have seemed more motivated by a tend-and-befriend response (Taylor et al., 2000). In brief, it may not be particularly helpful for men to give away their emotional secrets. They have needed to protect their personal interests so as to own the best cave, or fell the largest Mammoth as one way of advertising themselves as the best possible mate

---

[1]There are a number of definitions of paralanguage, some of which are synonymous with the wider term "nonverbal communication" or "body language" and some of which mean nonverbal vocalizations that signal some meaning. The subtlety with which they are analyzed (http://en.wikipedia.org/wiki/Paralinguistics retrieved December 17, 2017) would require a separate chapter, and will therefore not be discussed in this one.

(Dahl, 1998).[2] Women, on the other hand, have needed as many allies as possible so as to protect themselves and their children from harm (Taylor et al., 2000). It certainly would not be logical or intelligent for them to run away and abandon the brood. This fundamental difference plays itself out repeatedly every day all over the world. And yet, there are primitive cultures that contradict this basic generalization about the motivations of men and women. Margaret Mead in *Sex and Temperament in Three Primitive Societies* (1963) discussed what she termed "gender flexing," a progressive term for the time. She reported that in New Guinea the Arapesh peoples display feminine traits equally among men and women. They are ubiquitously a passive and peaceful, almost deferential people. The Mundugumour tribe socializes men and women alike to be aggressive and competitive. Women wean their young early, and nurture little (p. 283). In Nepal men are more nurturing than women, and the women do heavy labor as well as the nurturing of the children. There are exceptions to every generalization.

Differences in cultural behavior can stem from a myriad of sources (climate, religion, ancient folklore, etc.), all of which this chapter cannot hope to encompass. For one detailed perspective on possible origins of cultural and gender diversity, the reader is encouraged to take advantage of a fascinating paper by Stephan Dahl entitled *Communications and Culture Transformation* (Dahl, 1998)[3] in which he eloquently elucidates the many influences that are brought to bear on cultural habit. Suffice to say, it

is incumbent on everyone to remain inquisitive and attuned to the differences in race, culture, and gender that contribute to the rich stew that is called the human race; "cross-cultural [and transgender] communication cannot-be carried on successfully unless [the logic of the culture] is understood" (Park, 1979, p. 94).

Cultural Idiosynracies: Differences in Motivation

There are a number of idiosyncratic nonverbal behaviors that may be viewed as an amalgam of all of the above categories and are unique to certain cultures. In Mexico, for example, it is very rude to rap on a bathroom door in the "tum ta da dum dum, dum dum rhythm" (Axtell, 1998). For the purposes of this chapter, these idiosyncrasies will be discussed under the heading of "Culturally Specific Customs and Codes." Some of them will be relevant to the gender discussion, and others are mentioned simply as a way to point up the need to thoughtfully consider all of the parameters of working with peoples from one culture over another, whether within a gender diverse paradigm or otherwise.

To make life a little more complicated, though interesting, movements can convey opposing meanings from culture to culture. Those used frequently in one culture may be highly offensive in another (Dahl, 1998). For instance, as Dahl points out, Asian cultures may not show any kinesics at all, whereas southern European cultures use them generously. In France, social context may determine the character of kinesics. In professional settings body language is restrained; in social settings gestures are easy and open (Axtell, 1998). The microanalysis of movement can become absurd, but it is important to start with some broad understandings

---

[2] http://dahl.at/wordpress/research-publications/inter cultural-communication/communications-and-culture -transformation/ shared with Hirsch by the author August 26, 2011.

[3] http://dahl.at/wordpress/research-publications/inter cultural-communication/communications-and-culture -transformation/ shared with Hirsch by the author August 26th, 2011.

to use as points of reference, so that communication can be logical and congruous. Rather like two people dancing together, it is only fun or meaningful if they are both dancing to the same music. In other words, clients may need to learn that what they are communicating is what they intended.

Nonverbal Communication Deconstructed: It's in the Details

Kinesics

Kinesics may otherwise be known as body language, or more broadly nonverbal behavior as it relates to movement. This section describes aspects of communication that can be broken down into the following areas:

- haptics (touching behavior)
- proxemics (distance from other persons)
- gesture
- overall movement behaviors

Other areas of nonverbal communication that will be discussed are facial expression and oculesics (eye contact). "Paralanguage" is also widely used as an umbrella term.

Anatomy and Movement

While men and women vary in size from culture to culture, human anatomy, aside from cultural generalizations for height, etc., does not. A brief examination of a drawing of a nude or a painting of a naked man and/or woman will show that by and large the female anatomy forms the shape of an S and the male anatomy is closer to an A. Interestingly, this universality is acted out in the Czech Republic, where the gestures for woman and man are two inside out "S"s

(hourglass shapes), and an upside down triangle, respectively (Archer, 1997). Boticelli's *Venus Rising from the Clamshell* and Michelangelo's *David* are excellent examples in art of "S" and "A" shapes for men and women. Museums are full of examples of these female and male shapes, and should be considered as fertile study ground for clinicians and clients alike.

In keeping with the "S" shape, there are numerous references in the literature to female movement being fluid (Glass, 1992; Laing, 1989) while men's movements are more metered and controlled. Glass (1992) helpfully delineated some of the more obvious differences between male and female body language that may on the whole be applied cross-culturally within the habitual continuum of any given culture.

Taking Slices from Top-to-Toe

Kinesics can be viewed from the standpoint of body parts (arms, legs, etc.) or the body as a whole. It may be helpful for the clinician to think in terms of large body movements (e.g., trunk, shoulders and overall physicality) and individual body part movements (e.g., arms, hands, fingers, legs, and feet). Though generalizations are just that, it does help to have a broad sense of some of the obvious markers of male and female movement. Particularly relevant to this chapter is how movements translate cross-culturally. On the whole, the information stands across cultures, and the gender differences themselves may be considered intra-culturally. As Julius Fast said in his seminal work in 1970, "A study of body language is a study of the mixture of all body movements from those that apply in one culture to those that cut across all cultural barriers" (p. 16). For instance, it is generally recognized that cultures from cold, northern climes are more restrained in movement and gesture in general. This is logical given what people do to keep warm. They fold in on themselves; tuck hands into legs, or under arms, and hunch over against the wind. Southern, warmer climes breed more relaxed cultures with less inhibition about movement. Again, anyone who has spent a hot season anywhere will have experienced the easy languid sensations that come with living in the heat. Irrespective of temperature, Eastern cultures tend to be more restrained in their movements compared with Western cultures (Dahl, 1998). And some cultures are known for their movements. Think, for instance, of the popular saying that Italians talk with their hands.

Below are some broad brushstrokes regarding the movement of men and women (Glass, 1992; Hirsch, 2012; Laing, 1989).

■ Head movements: Women move the head more as part of communication, often mirroring the movements of a conversational partner (Nelson & Golant, 2004), or in response to information from distant speakers such as lecturers. Men tend to listen with the head in static position. Head tilts are a universal sign of acquiescence that are exhibited cross-culturally and even among other species (Nelson & Golant, 2004, as cited in Burgoon, Guerrero, & Floyd, 2016).

■ Trunk movements: Female movements and posture tend to be counterbalanced, emphasizing the S shape (Archer, 1997, and art universally), and using the entire body from head to toe. The trunk does not move as much as that of women. Women tend to lean in while communicating, while men maintain a more backward position while listening (Glass, 1992). Men tend to move their body position more frequently than women, who keep overall body movements more contained (i.e., they don't spread themselves wide). This distinction should not be confused with gender differences in gestural behavior.

■ Arm movements: Women take up less space, with arm movements being closer to the body; men use wider arm gestures and leave larger spaces between the arms and the body.

■ Hands and fingers: Women are expressive and painterly with their hands, with open fluid fingers and curved motions. Men use linear horizontal or vertical gestures with fingers closed. Women break at the wrist, men find this very difficult (anecdotal from training experiences). Women tend to have a slightly weaker handshake than men— this being particularly noted in the amount of pressure exerted with the thumb on the top of the receiver's hand.

■ Hip movement: Women use swinging, undulating motions. Men move on a more linear plane.

■ Gait: Woman's gait is shorter and narrower than a man's gait. Difference in stance and gait width is logical given obvious anatomical differences between men and women.

■ Leg and foot movements: Women's feet move expressively, often independently of the rest of the body, using "cat tail"-like figure-eight motions especially when seated. Men tend to tap feet or wiggle (Glass, 1992). Certainly it is very common to hear people all over the world talk about "wiggly boys." In Spain, it is unladylike to cross the legs (Axtell, 1998). Japanese women generally do not cross their legs, and sit on them or tuck them off to the side (Axtell, 1998). In Scotland men cross legs at the knee, women at the ankles (Axtell, 1998).

Differences in Gestural Style between Women and Men

Women tend to use more defensive movements and gestures when uncomfortable with men. They cross their legs, wiggle their feet, fold their arms, shift posture, and use adaptors such as playing with a pen or pulling up their socks (Sommer, 1969). It is unclear whether these women studied were from the United States only or from a variety of cultures. In some cultures, such as Ecuador's, it is impolite for women to fidget at all. As with movement, female gestures tend to be more fluid than those of men, with movements being both toward and away from the body. Male gestures tend more to be away from the body and to stop abruptly. Burgoon et al. (2016) noted that women tend to use more of a palms-up and shoulder shrug to imply uncertainty, whereas men tend to use more of a pointing gesture to show dominance. Judy Pearson concludes that the differences in male and female gestures are so evident that genders may be distinguished by gestures alone (1984).

To every generalization there is a contradiction: other studies indicate that women use fewer and more restrained gestures than men. Hanna and Wilson (1998) reported that women use fewer gestures when they are with other women but more gestures when they are with men. Nelson and Golant (2004) suggest that men may control their nonverbal behaviors in order not to give away their power (p. 27). Despite these conflicting reports, there is general agreement that women's gestures are more fluid and generally toward the body, while men's gestures are farther away from the body (Glass, 1992).

Facial Expression

Yond Cassius has a lean and hungry look.
—*Julius Caesar*, Act 1, Sc 2,
William Shakespeare, 1599

Facial expression has been studied in depth for many years. Such importance is placed on the power of facial expression in conveying both superficial and inner meaning that the U.S. government has a special division that focuses specifically on training people in how to read faces. Even a very "flat," "unexpressive" face is an open book to the perceptive observer (Gladwell, 2005). The power of facial expression should not be ignored with regard to communication training with gender diverse people. During an authenticity training session for trans women taught by Hirsch in 2002, she noted that one of her clients who had appeared 100% female throughout the weekend began suddenly to appear male during the last 15–20 minutes of the session. An earnest, set look had crept into this participant's facial expression, as well as her voice sounding deeper. She looked as though she had already left the training session mentally and had returned in her mind to her job, which she does as a man. Through an email exchange over the course of the next two days, the participant confirmed that this was in fact exactly what had happened. Her facial expression had perfectly articulated her inner story.

Basic Gender Differences in Facial Expression

LaFrance, Hecht, and Noyes (1994), as cited in Burgoon et al. (2016), describe the expressivity demand theory, which states that sex, relationship, context, and situation influence different levels of expressiveness. It is important to assess gender differences through this lens. As stated earlier, context must lead. Nelson and Golant (2004) reported that women communicate with all of their senses, which equips them well to pick up the details in communication and to listen empathically. It is reported that women are more skilled both at sending and interpreting facial expression than are men. Furthermore, women use more facial expressions in general and in particular smile more than men (Soojin, 2000). Multiple references in the literature suggest that women use facial expression and both send and receive expressive messages more than their male counterparts. They suggest that the facial expressions of women are more welcoming and friendly, whereas those of men are more reserved. Glass (1992) corroborates too that women's facial expressions are generally warmer and that they provide more feedback than men with their facial expressions. Men, it appears, provide less feedback through facial expression or reaction during communication (Glass, 1992). Nelson and Golant (1992) described men's facial expressions as being "masked" in order not to give away their power (p. 29).

Oculesics

Oculesics refers to the study of nonverbal communication as it relates to the eyes and eyebrows, including eye movement in general, gaze, as well as eye contact with another person. In general, it is thought that the higher a person is in hierarchy socially, the more eye contact they are allowed to make (Nelson & Golant, 2004).

Basic Gender Differences in Oculesics

Nelson and Golant (2004) suggest that men use eye contact to establish dominance, whereas women use it to check in, or in submission. It appears that women establish more eye contact during conversations than men (Burgoon, Buller, & Woodall, 1996). Women are more comfortable giving eye

contact than men (Argyle & Ingham, 1972; Ivy & Backlund, 1994), though they are less likely to stare, and will break eye contact more frequently. Argyle and Ingham (1972) also reported that women with men make less eye contact than any other "sex dyad." A downward glance is considered a sign of modesty in women, or remorse in a child (Nelson & Golant, 2004). Wide eyes are a sign of naiveté, while raised upper lids are a sign of displeasure, and eyes rolled back a sign of impatience or fatigue (Nelson & Golant, 2004).

Haptics and Gender Differences

"Haptics" is the term that refers to touching behavior. Haptic behavior indicates a degree of intimacy (Heslin, 1974, retrieved August, 2005). A consideration of haptics should not only include a discussion of *when* to touch, but also *where* to touch. During conversation, people touch one another as a form of sympathy, acquiescence, to stress a point, in humor, and so on. They may reach out and touch an elbow, a hand, a shoulder, and in more intimate relationships a leg or face. There is enormous variability, however, in the acceptance of touch between cultures and between genders. In Latin cultures, for example, there is a great deal of touching during conversation. In other cultures, touching is strictly limited to greeting and departure. Axtell (1998) described this distinction as contact versus no-contact cultures.

A review of some of the literature on haptics (Nelson & Golant, 2004) revealed that women are touched more than men and are touched mostly by men. Women tend to associate touch with warmth and expression, and are touched more gently. They initiate more hugging and touching that expresses support, affection, and comfort. Men, on the other hand, are touched less than women, initiate touch toward women more, and are touched more harshly. They tend to use touch to direct, assert power, or express sexual interest, and women touch both genders more frequently.

Proxemics and Gender Differences

"Proxemics" refers to the distance between people during communication—in other words, the way personal space is structured between men and women, or from culture to culture. A study of proxemics should, by definition, be considered in tandem with a study on haptics, since one significantly influences the other.

It has been Hirsch's observation that gender diverse clients, in particular trans women, tend to overcompensate for distance during interactions. Based on an understanding that women are more comfortable than men with being close, clients will rapidly close a gap without regard for levels of familiarity in a relationship. Clinicians should make their clients aware of "contextual appropriateness" before training feminine closeness generically.

Women tend to approach others closer and prefer side-by-side interaction. Their spatial zones are drawn closer. Women friends lean against each other during conversation, they may walk arm-in-arm, and in general are not intimidated by closeness with each other. This is not as true for women with men, depending on the nature of the relationship. Men apparently use more personal space and prefer face-to-face conversation (albeit with a posture of distance). They are more likely to invade others' personal space, especially that of women. Personal observation would suggest that women also certainly communicate face-to-face a great deal, especially when deep in intimate conversation over a table.

Qualifications to Consider for Teaching Nonverbal Aspects of Communication

As with any area of communication therapy, it is important to have the skill set necessary for teaching (ASHA Code of Ethics [revised] ASHA supplement, 23, pp. 13–15, Principle of Ethics II, Rules of Ethics: B). Training in a theater and performance background, as well as training in movement as part of theater training, can help to meet such skill criteria. Theater, yoga, or Pilates and myriad other ancillary topics should not be ignored as a means to learning the skills necessary for developing a creative nonverbal communication program. Understanding some of the fundamentals of behaviorism and anthropology is also a helpful prerequisite.

Failing the ability to add this training to an already full quiver, there are some excellent resources available to help clinicians understand some of the fundamentals of theater work. Some of these are offered in the bibliography, though they are not by any means exhaustive. Making use of the professional intelligence of friends and colleagues who have experience in the performing arts and "body work" is also a helpful way to gain invaluable knowledge quickly and at no cost. It should go without saying that any knowledge gained be used within an ethical framework for the clinician. Only materials that do not require special training should be borrowed across disciplines.

Setting the Stage for Training: Observing Differences across Gender

It is helpful to have researchers such as Tannen and Glass, Burgoon and Nelson, as well as countless others who have taken some of the guesswork out of otherwise endless and seemingly random attempts at quantification. It is essential, however, that if clinicians are to do justice to their clients' goal of reaching an honest and personal presentation of their gender identity, they engage in active personal research to keep information current and contextually or culturally applicable. Personal observations kept in a log can be referred to and integrated into training (e.g., a woman at the hairdresser who continually moves her foot back and forth in a figure-eight motion like a cat's tail).

Real life is where clinicians will find the richest palette of behaviors to reference for clients and they should encourage clients to make similar formal observations in a journal. Spending time in a number of different contexts to make observations about how men and women behave will over time help to create a large dictionary of behaviors for reference. As with any therapeutic goal, it is critical that the clinician understand how to perform the tasks to meet that goal. Clinicians must therefore practice moving and behaving in a manner that is congruent with their opposite gender. Isolating and examining small movements and/or unique behaviors is a manageable way to begin this practice.

Books, magazines, movies, and photographs offer a wealth of opportunities to play the "spot the difference" game with clients. There are a number of films that provide marvelous opportunities for detailed study of feminine nonverbal communication char-

acteristics. In particular, *Strangers in Good Company* (Cynthia Scott, 1990) is highly recommended. The cast is all women and of very diverse types, ages, cultures, and backgrounds. It provides a special look into the behaviors of everyday women, rather than picture-perfect or "model"-style women.

It is important that clients are guided to look to the type of woman or man that they feel themselves to be, so that observations can be integrated in a congruous way. If they pick and choose characteristics randomly (a walk here, a gesture there, a flick of the hair somewhere else), they run the risk of developing a patchwork presentation. This looks superimposed, rather than being authentically integrated into an honest and realistic representation of who they are. In addition, a random approach may add to any internal confusion they may already feel, rather than help to gel a unique personality.

Assessment

Tools

As yet, there are no established standardized tools used for assessing nonverbal communication with the transgender population. As was mentioned earlier, the continuum of masculine to feminine behaviors is very long, and influenced by multiple factors ranging from culture, race, socioeconomic status, and even the climate of an area. Some of these cultural differences were discussed earlier in this chapter. In assessing clients, it is therefore necessary to base results on both observational and research-based generalizations such as have been described above.

Tools for assessment are simple and beautifully inexpensive, and can be found in most clinics or private practice offices. The clinician will need:

- Eyes, ears, and a note pad
- Intake and Assessment forms/data collection forms
- Video recorder and digital camera if possible

Taking a Thorough History

Clinicians should take a thorough history during the initial assessment and never stop watching and taking notes. It is important to ask *lots* of questions during the intake session. The clinician should gain a solid sense of personal interests and *who* the client is individually, rather than simply whether she is behaving in a male or female manner. Using a previously established chart of behaviors (organized top-to-toe as described below) for data collection, the clinician should try not to be distracted by the obvious, rather should pay attention to small, interesting details such as how the client scratches her head, how glasses get adjusted, or how a folder gets placed on the desk or table. It is helpful to hone the ability to keep eye contact while doing multiple top-to-toe scans throughout the intake session. Where possible, the clinician might try and create situations that will push the client into "habitual" or genetic gender behavior. This will serve as an excellent measure of behaviors in multiple contexts outside of the clinic. It has been this clinician's experience that transfeminine clients usually fall into more male behavior patterns when pushed to discuss factual or intellectual topics. Conversely, transmasculine clients have a tendency to present in a more feminine manner when discussing emotionally based subjects. One trans woman pointed out during an authenticity training weekend that during discussions about gender confirmation surgery (GCS) the transfeminine clients invariably end up discussing method, instrumentation, and price, as compared with the transmasculine clients, who talk about how they feel or felt about going through surgery.

Establishing a Baseline

Regardless of whether we are training transfeminine or transmasculine clients, it is important to begin with a generic working list of what to observe. It is helpful to organize areas in a top-to-toe system as follows:

Upper Body

- Head: Posture, movement, and facial expressiveness, eyes; movement and expression; eye contact
- Shoulders: positioning and movement
- Trunk: positioning; overall proximity to conversational partner—forward or back. Posture/stance
- Arms: posture and movement
- Hands: quality and quantity of movement and gesture (e.g., distal versus proximal, unilateral versus bilateral). Orientation of back of hands and palms (e.g., facing in or out)

Lower Body

- Hips
- Legs
- Feet

The continuum of maleness and femaleness is very wide and in certain cultures almost blended. We therefore do not have a standardized way of taking data on nonverbal behaviors. Nor are we likely to find one, given the enormous range of human behavior. We can, however, create an equal appearing scale of 0–5 for maleness/femaleness (refer to Chapter 7). We can also create a more general male/female judgment scale. Is the overall impression of head, hands, shoulders, etc. male or female? An equal-appearing scale in combination with a general and subjective judgment or assessment is going to give us and the client a fairly accurate measure of how the outside world may perceive him/her/them. As noted in the introduction to this chapter, the brain makes a split-second judgment, and this is based on a rapid tally of individual parts and the whole. If the overall impression is one versus the other, it is probably accurate. If the client disagrees, it is the clinician's job to figure out how to help him/her make a shift and feel convinced and satisfied by the end result.

Starting the Data Collection Clock

A fresh and unprepared presentation is going to provide a clinician with the most honest assessment of "real life" behavior. Since a "comprehensive body/voice" approach has already been discussed with the client, it should not come as any surprise when the clinician begins taking notes on nonverbal markers early on in the first meeting. As mentioned above, a top-to-toe approach helps to organize the assessment. It is helpful to take on the mindset of a spy, or a detective. In working with gender diverse clients it is not only important to ask the question "Is this male/female behavior?," but "Does what I see make sense overall?" A famous English, female spy was captured in occupied France by the Germans during WWII. In her book called *I Looked Right* (Denham, 1956) she tells how in a habitual moment she forgot that looking right before crossing could only mean that she

was British, Australian, or a New Zealander. Someone paying attention noticed the incongruity of her behavior and put two and two together very quickly. The assiduous clinician must similarly spy shamelessly all the time. Depending on the specific clinical setting, clinicians may or may not have the luxury of observing the client getting out of the car or walking up the street and into the clinic. If this is logistically possible, the clinician should take full advantage of these opportunities; they provide invaluable information. Equally important is observing the client walk back to the car, get into it, and drive away. Even how the car door is closed can provide an important piece to the complex puzzle.

Training: Approaches and Techniques

Many approaches discussed below can be applied across the gender spectrum. Trans men seem less concerned with their nonverbal behavior than trans women, so the majority of exercises discussed are applicable to the latter. Where applicable, exercises for trans men are discussed.

Teaching nonverbal communication skills may feel like a mercurial task, but the clinician should take comfort in knowing that all of the nonverbal areas can be approached using the same basic framework. The following format can be applied across all nonverbal areas:

- Establish an acceptable range of femininity or masculinity with the client that matches personality and lifestyle.
- Assign three 30-minute observation periods a week.
- Suggest that the client keep a journal and a gesture, movement, and clothing "vocabulary book."

- Take selfies and short videos to monitor change.
- Video selfies while talking help to integrate facial expression and voice/speech with gender identity.
- Teach from a standpoint of deconstruction and reconstruction (i.e., analyze and break down existing behaviors, and then rebuild new ones).
- Establish a schedule of repetitive imitation exercises for both small motor and large motor movements.

It is important that the clinician frequently reinforce the client's integration of voice and gender image. To achieve congruity, each client should be aware of his or her personal unique features and characteristics. Much of this information will have been gleaned at the intake level, in communication with the client's psychologist if necessary, by using pictures and photographs, discussion of literary models of feminine or masculine voice, and possibly writing exercises. The ultimate goal is a congruous blend of verbal and nonverbal communication. Once the working ground rules have been established, the clinician can begin teaching to each area of attention from top to toe.

Head: Posture and Movement

Glass (1992) points out that women tend to mirror each other's head movements during conversation. Men tend to remain static. A little observation on the clinician's part will quickly establish the details of each client's movement patterns, as well as noticing some broad generalizations.

Warm-up exercises are essential to train greater flexibility of movement. Head exercises that encourage the client to move in concert with a conversational partner

are excellent. Following are some exercises that might be considered:

- imitative mirror exercises with the clinician during "silent conversation"
- imitative conversational movements of female characters on television or film
- videotape and analysis of female friends in conversation or a woman in conversation with a male friend
- practicing inner conversations with head movements, a very easy and powerful way to develop feminine head movements.

Facial Expression

In this author's opinion, working on facial expression is the easiest of the nonverbal areas to teach. If we think within a Parkinsonian or head injury paradigm, the fog begins to lift slightly. The client can be trained to do regular warm up and stretching exercises to hypersensitize the face. The upper and lower face should be targeted separately and then together. The more the client is able to hone muscular isolation exercises, the better. A mirror is critical at the initial stages of training, since most clients have little or no idea about how mobile or immobile their own face is, or can be. Certain muscular cues can be established early on so that the mirror can be phased out relatively quickly, since the majority of clients do not enjoy spending a lot of time in front of the therapy room mirror!

Shoulders

Clinicians might encourage slow, small, isolated shoulder movements to train bilateral shoulder control and the ability to move parts of the body separately and in concert with one another. This can be established early on even during deactivation of muscle tension exercises for resonance work. Using observation exercises, have the client practice isolated movements to develop varying lines of motion more characteristic of women than men. For trans men, shoulder exercises that encourage the sensation of the span of the upper back will help to establish a masculine stretch and flex. Standing with hands on table wide apart or feeling the full spread of hands on hips, etc. helps to retrain muscle memory.

Arms, Elbows, and Wrists

As a general rule, it is good practice for trans-feminine clients to increase their awareness of the amount of space that is left open between the arms and the trunk and the fingers and the thumb. Closing these spaces slightly will create the illusion of "smaller." Trans men might be encouraged to open their "wings," and to increase the space between the body and inner arm. Putting the hands up on the arms of a chair with the elbows out quickly provides that sensation of increased space.

Women's movements tend to follow more of a figure-eight or circular series of movements, as opposed to men, whose movements tend to be more linear and finite (Glass, 1992; Laing, 1989). The objective has to be to train fluid, graceful movements. This can be done using chiffon scarves, furling ribbon, or any objects or materials that encourage fluidity and follow-through. The materials can be thrown in the air and caught fluidly as they gently fall, moved in a figure-eight motion with one hand, or passed gracefully from person to person if in group therapy. In addition, resistance exercises through water are beneficial. Suggest the client practice running a hand slowly back and forth through bath water

to practice "breaking at the wrist" in one motion. The following isolation exercises are helpful in training the feminine-specific hand/wrist relationship.

- Extend the arm out, leaving a gentle bend at the elbow. Let the hand hang limply at the wrist. Slowly rotate the wrist outward until gravity allows it to flip and the hand is now lying palm up with the fingers relaxed and curling slightly inward above the palm.
- Hold the forearm up at 90 degrees with the hand relaxed at the wrist like an upside-down L. Slowly begin moving the hand and forearm back and forth in snake-like motion to practice the wrist break. The movement should look as though you are drawing things out of the air in the slow snake-like motion.

If one plays with one's hands in this fashion, one will discover many variations on the arm/hand/snake theme. It is very difficult for cis men to develop this particular movement with natural fluidity and may require more practice than seems reasonable to any hardworking client. Clients should be counseled to bite off small pieces, and come back to them over and over again throughout any given week. For trans men, exercises that focus on reducing the "break at the wrist" and increasing flat plain movements will decrease overall fluidity and increase more concrete movements.

Hands

The previous water resistance exercise will also work well to enhance awareness of fluid finger motion. Activities that encourage detailed fine motor movement, such as individually sorting beads or picking up peanuts individually, increase awareness of the finger tips and deemphasize the use of the palm of the hand. Prestidigitation exercises similar to practicing scales on the piano will help with isolated finger use. Picking up thin objects with the thumb and index finger will develop more habitual distal attention than proximal attention.

One of the most noticeable gender physical differences is hand size. While it is obviously not possible for the client to reduce the size, it is possible to make suggestions that will influence the perception of size. If the client develops the habit of keeping thumb and middle finger gently in contact, the space between thumb and indicator will close enough to cup the hand just gently, and give the perception that the hand is smaller than it really is. It is important, however, not to encourage specific "holding," rather to encourage finger/thumb sensitivity.

In the case of trans men, developing more palm-based, flat-planed hand movements in order to move the focus proximally will open the hands wider. Picking up "bunches" of things instead of individual pieces will discourage the finer motor movements and encourage a gross motor approach. Holding on to a medium-sized ball with a bit of weight to it will encourage a shift in fine to gross motor memory.

Trunk

Increasing awareness of trunk movement requires perhaps the least amount of specific attention during nonverbal communication training. If the client is able to develop a congruous flow of feminine movement in the other areas of posture and movement, then by its very nature the trunk will come along as well. That being said, it is helpful to cue the client to move as though being led by strings from the clavicle toward the horizon. If the clinician has done yoga, this description may seem familiar. If not, it is helpful to practice focusing from the clavicle before teaching this approach.

Have the client stand at the opposite end of the room from you. Attach imaginary strings to the client's clavicle, and slowly draw her toward you holding the imaginary strings. Instruct the client to walk toward you looking at you, or an imaginary person walking past. This exercise helps to dramatically change overall posture, trains looking up rather than down and plants the seed of the trunk "going along for the ride" instead of leading with the shoulders and the upper body in general. The shift in "point of departure" becomes evident almost immediately and gives the client a strong foundation in how to marry other movements to this new approach to carriage.

The Walk: General Considerations

We have observed and the literature corroborates that the following generalizations hold fairly true for the female walk.

- Gait is narrower than for men.
- Stride is shorter than for men.
- Rate is slower.
- The foot follows through along the ground almost as though on a conveyor belt.
- The leg lags behind longer than for men.
- Hips move gently from side to side in concert with stride.
- Footfall is quieter due to a gentler landing and less emphasis on the heel falling to the ground when the walker is in stocking feet (personal observation). For an interesting perspective regarding differences in male and female footfall and biomechanics the clinician is invited to go

to an interesting study by Cutting (1978) in addition to numerous fascinating studies on human biomechanics to be found at: http://people.psych.cornell.edu/~jec7 /biological_motion (retrieved August 19, 2017).

The Walk: Training

In Hirsch's more than 25 years of working with gender diverse people, she has never encountered a trans man who wanted to work on walking. This appears to be an area of nonverbal communication that transitions very naturally for trans men and will therefore not be fully addressed in this section. Colleagues have commented that occasionally their transmasculine clients, like trans women, exaggerate what they feel to be a more binary walk for their gender identity. As with all of nonverbal communication, a case by case approach is appropriate.

In considering "the walk," clinicians should take context, individual personality, and body type into consideration. This was intimated in the introduction. Not all women are perfectly feminine by Western society's standards, and it would be unfair and unrealistic to set those goals for everyone. It is important that clients understand this as well. We ALL sometimes forget to fully appreciate our individuality when bludgeoned by what society considers an ideal! Many women today think of themselves on the "tomboy" end of feminine, with sprees out into the classically feminine realm when inspired to do so for professional or particular social occasions, or if that is their personality.

The annoying truth is that cis women can afford to blur the gender margin. A myriad of tags and characteristics allow for this flexibility. Clinicians are charged with the challenge of helping our clients achieve

both feminine and personal honesty that is in line with their gender identity. So in teaching "the walk" we have to balance goals toward being perceived as feminine, at the same time as reminding the client that woman A is the kind of woman who will hop on and off a curb, while woman B has never done it in her life—this author included!

Nonverbal Communication Bag of Tricks

It helps to regularly add one or two tools to the bag of tricks used in teaching nonverbal communication. The following is a list of helpful tools and should by no means be considered exhaustive.

■ Theraball™: There are three or four different sizes of Theraball—the height of the client will determine which ball to use. Have the client sit on the ball with feet planted firmly on the ground using the "sitz bones" (ischial tuberosities) as the guide for sitting posture. This helps tremendously for shifting awareness from sitting back "in the bucket" (more male) to rising up out of the pelvic girdle (more female). Instruct the client to rotate the hips in circular motions transferring the weight from one buttock to the other. Using the Theraball in this fashion gives the client a strong starting point for developing more of an undulating hip movement while walking, and moving in general.

■ Theraband™: This is excellent for giving the trans feminine client a sensation of swinging the hips. Clinicians should practice this first on a friend and vice versa, to make sure that the exercise can be performed safely and comfortably. Place the Theraband on the client's posterior and around the hips. Ask the client to lean back slightly into the band and test for resistance. If necessary, use a thicker or thinner band depending on size and weight. With the knees slightly bent, and the feet apart about 8 inches, the client should gently lean back into the band as if casually leaning back against a counter. When the clinician has a firm sense of the client's balance, "play" the Theraband back and forth in a flat steering wheel motion to move the client's hips, as if teaching "the Twist." Instruct the client to relax and to let you do the work. She should not be doing any work at all, and should not be leaning forward in anticipation. The shoulders and arms should just "go along for the ride."

- Stretchy rubber tubing: Wonderful for shortening and narrowing gait. The client should step into a circle of tied tubing and place it just above the knees. Practicing walking in this fashion provides good kinesthetic sensation for a shorter, narrower, slower gait.
- Balance cushion (Dyna-Disc™, is very helpful, but there are other similar products): Excellent for developing feminine posture and establishing leading from the clavicle. Also great for developing gluteal muscles important in developing a feminine walk. Have the client stand on the balance cushion in stocking feet and practice centering the balance, with and without the eyes open.
- Art Mannequin: Used for showing different postures and gestures. The clinician can demonstrate positioning, or the client can use the mannequin to demonstrate understanding of nonverbal posture and gestures, or to ask questions.
- Wooden dowel or broom handle (learned from Denae Doyle, movement specialist

for transgender clients, Esprit Conference, Port Angeles, WA, 2003): Used for measuring appropriate length of gait. Have the client place the dowel on the shoulders behind the head. With outstretched arms over the dowel, the wrists should rest on top of either ends of the dowel, with the hands hanging forward. The client should then swing the dowel slowly forward on one side, while the ipsilateral leg swings forward. The distance that the leg can swing forward with the body rotated at approximately 45 degrees is approximately the appropriate feminine gait length for that person.

Miscellaneous Exercises

Mirrored Movement

Mirrored movement exercises are helpful for anyone on the gender spectrum. They increase awareness of gross and fine motor movements, and can be a fun way for people to use their friends or partners as models of movement.

If you are working with a group, or if you are comfortable doing this yourself, the following mirror exercise is marvelous for developing a peripheral sense of isolated movements. Stand facing the client at about 3 feet distance. Choose a "leader" and a "follower." The leader initiates easy gross movements slowly enough for the partner to mimic exactly. Partners must maintain eye contact at all times, and only peripheral vision and sense as they guide for imitation. Participants may use the whole body but it is crucial that each movement be clearly enough defined for the follower to actually follow. Movements may vary between gross motor and small motor. Continue in this manner for a couple of minutes and then switch leader/follower.

Translating Gestures

Translating gestures is also a focused way to train self-efficacy and awareness in shifting the gendered nature of gestures. This exercise needs to wait until the client is very comfortable with working at a microcosmic level, and experimenting with a variety of movement styles. Have clients choose a short movement sequence. Have them think very carefully about the male and female version of the movement, and slowly move from the male version to the female version or vice versa—in other words translating the movement from one gender to the other. This takes some practice but, again, develops an acute sense of subtle and obvious differences.

Doing Nothing/Sitting Still

There is a temptation when faced with a situation that requires not much at all, to "overdo." This is especially true if people feel inhibited, conspicuous, or uncomfortable for some reason. Overdoing may be playing with the hair all of the time, fussing with the hands, doing something random with objects from a purse, looking around to see if others are looking around, etc. Gender diverse clients fall easily into this trap due to a desire to ensure that they are perceived in their gender identity. The truth is that honesty and naturalness come from within, not without. There is nothing that we do without good reason, and much of the time we live an active mental life, with no apparent outward physicality. Waiting for the doctor or sitting at a train station are perfect examples of this.

Doing nothing is driven solely by who we are physically, mentally, and emotionally—personal context is everything. People who seem insincere usually are insincere; and not through any affectation, they are just nervous about playing it right.

Doing nothing does not require a great deal of attention within a nonverbal communication program, but a few practice scenarios will help a client enormously along the path of relaxing into quiet spontaneity and authenticity. Below are some examples of scenarios that are helpful for practicing inner versus outer processes.

- Waiting for an old friend at a train station
- Sitting at a doctor's office
- Looking at pieces of art at a museum
- Waiting in line to be served at a café
- Watching a movie
- Sitting on a park bench
- Waiting for the bus

This is by no means an exhaustive list; the clinician can easily come up with 5 or 10 more ideas. Have clients enact the scenario for no more than one to two minutes. If possible, videotape them, and then ask for and provide feedback regarding what was seen (and unseen, so to speak). This is an excellent exercise for the client to practice alone at home—it is an exercise in self-awareness and trust. For the advanced client it is also an exercise in listening to the fluency of the inner voice: is it masculine or feminine? We know that we are fluent in a foreign language when we begin to dream in that language, or when the foreign word pops up before the word in our mother tongue. It is an exciting moment when this happens, and it is a joy when clients come to a session bubbling over with glee at no longer being able to draw clearly upon their "man" or "woman."

Clothing Considerations

Anecdotally, few clients these days ask for input or help with clothing. This is an area that requires extreme sensitivity. Many people are in an experimental phase in terms of their style of clothing, and care must be taken to support them wholeheartedly, while providing constructive feedback. Context and personal choice should lead: gender-fluid clients are going to have very different goals than binary clients. They may want to present in recognizably female clothing while identifying in a non-binary gender. If a client does not ask for input regarding clothing, it is recommended that clinicians do not initiate a discussion about it. On occasion, however, a client may openly ask, "I'm still being misgendered and I can't figure out why. Do you have any suggestions?" If the clinician feels that there are aspects of clothing that may be muddying gender perception, this could be considered as an invitation to comment.

Cis women have long had the freedom to dress in clothes that span the gender spectrum. Making a clothing switch to more of a binary gender appearance is not a long journey for most trans men. In Hirsch's experience, clothing considerations are noticeably less of a pressing issue for them. It is unusual for trans men to have a desire to dress in a recognizably feminine manner. As such there appears to be less room for ambiguity or uncertainty in the visual perception of gender.

Transfeminine clients, on the other hand, have a more complicated task due to the very fact that cis women wear a very wide range of gender-neutral/masculine clothes. Trans women (sometimes frustratingly!) tend to have to make choices closer to the feminine than the neutral margin in order to increase the likelihood of a consistent perception of femininity. Incongruities can sometimes "throw" a perception. It may be a small detail such as specifically masculine shoes, or white, male, athletic socks, or a T-shirt with sleeves that stop right at the most prominent part of a bicep. If a client comes with concerns about having been misgendered, finding the incongruity or detail that detracts from gender identity requires close observation, and sometimes, "it just looks [incongruous], you know it when you see it" (Gladwell, p. 45).

Finally, clothing should not be assessed so much on a basis of femininity or masculinity, but on the basis of whether the whole picture makes sense—in other words, is there contextual logic? With that in mind, a clinician might simply make a note on the assessment form as to whether clothing choices make sense/don't make sense, are congruous/incongruous, are or are not contextually logical, and whether a client specifically stated a need or goal in that area of presentation.

For those clients who are most comfortable and happy in a binary role, the following story may be helpful. The client may want to assess clothing choices based on the three criteria of age, personality, and context (including daily plans, weather, environment, etc.). A story sometimes helps to underscore the impact of an approach. A very perceptive and hardworking transfeminine client of Hirsch's came into a session one day saying, "I figured out how to check my clothing!" She had realized that if she asked herself the questions "Where am I going? How old am I? and What time of day is it?" she could make an honest assessment of whether she had chosen her clothes for the day appropriately. If the answers to her questions were in alignment for her with the choices that she had made, she felt confident moving into her day. When clients ask us, "How do you think I look today?" perhaps we can help them answer their own question without judgment: "Where are you going? Who are you? How old are you? What time of day is it?." We are here to serve, we are not here to judge.

Written Communication and the Gender Diverse Client

Over the past two decades, growing interest and research in gender-related writing differences continue to be evidenced in scholarly work by educators, sociolinguists, gender theorists, and many who study aspects of computer-mediated communication. This literature, examples of which will be referenced below, has contributed much to the body of work that we may find beneficial in our work with transgender clients.

It is acknowledged throughout the literature that the attempt to study or make generalizations about gender and writing can be fraught with complexity, even to the point where some critics question the validity of such research—for example, claiming that differences found in written interactions are mainly associated with context as opposed to the genders of the writers. Nonetheless, in our work with certain clients, it may be useful to review and discuss suggested gender-related differences in written communication. Even though we as therapists are mindful that some of the salient gender-marking features identified in the literature may be arguable by research critics (e.g., on the grounds that they were perhaps imperfectly measured or interpreted, or that they represent stereotypes), we know that some clients will nonetheless wish to be educated regarding key male-female writing differences. As

with any gender-related marker that may be pertinent to our client, it is the therapist's role to educate him or her, if this is an area of concern or interest. After that, it then becomes the individual client's decision as to whether or not she wishes to practice working on internalizing and incorporating a given target behavior.

A Review of the Literature

A review of the literature on gender differences in written expression reveals that there has been a range of genres that have been investigated. For the purpose of this chapter, it seems useful to present remarkable findings from studies of male-female differences found in:

■ Fiction and Non-Fiction Textual Analysis
■ Email and Written Correspondence
■ Computer-Mediated Communication
■ Instant Messaging/Texting
■ Blogging

Fiction and Non-Fiction Textual Analysis

To date, one of the most comprehensive and reliable studies of gender and written language is the 2003 investigation titled "Gender, Genre, and Writing Style in Formal Written Texts" (Argamon et al., 2003). This project involved analyzing a sample of 604 fiction and non-fiction documents (which included 25 million words) from the British National Corpus. The results of the study confirmed many previously held popular perceptions while also adding to the literature, with key findings as follows:

■ Gender-related differences exist in both *lexical* and *syntactic* features of formal writing.

- Female writing contains a significantly greater usage of features that previous researchers have characterized as "involved."
- Male writing contains greater use of features that have been characterized as "informational."

Specifically, it was found that female writers used pronouns to a significantly greater degree than did the male authors, in both fiction and non-fiction (Argamon et al., 2003). The pronouns primarily used by females were the personal pronouns *I, you,* and *she*. The use of these pronouns was seen as having the effect of encoding a relationship between the writer and the reader (especially the first person singular and second person pronouns). That is, documents containing features that show interaction between the speaker/writer and the listener/reader, such as first and second person pronouns, can be interpreted as evidencing greater author "involvement."

With regard to men's writing, which was characterized as more "informational," Argamon et al. (2003) pointed to male authors' significantly greater tendency to use "determiners" or "specifiers"—*a, the, that,* and *these*—as well as specific numbers (*one, two, three*) and "quantifiers" ("*more," "some,*" etc.). These kinds of words basically serve to make reference to concrete facts involving objects, places, or time, while also reducing the "involvedness" of the text. Interestingly, and by contrast, the pronoun *it*, which is never personal, was used in equal amounts by males and females. Thus, through computational analysis of numerous texts across a wide range of genres, Argamon et al. (2003) were able to put forth the suggestion that female writers are more inclined to make connections with readers, while male authors prefer to inform their readers.

Another sizable study, titled *Gender Differences in Language Use: An Analysis of 14,000 Text Samples* (Newman et al., 2008), used standardized categories to analyze a database of 14,000 text files from 70 separate studies. The authors explored gender differences in language using their own computerized text analysis tool known as Linguistic Inventory and Word Count (LIWC). LIWC "analyzes text samples on a word-by-word basis and compares each to a dictionary of over 2,000 words divided into 74 categories." Certain categories, such as articles, were grammatical in nature. Other categories, developed by independent judges, were thematic in nature. These judges would read the samples and decide the thematic categories under which each word should go. For example, the word "happy" would be assigned to the category labeled "Positive Emotion Words."

It should be noted that Newman et al.'s study used an extremely diverse corpus, including data from studies that were conducted over a 22-year period (1980–2002) and included samples of fiction going back as far as the seventeenth century, as well as a small sample of text (7%) that was transcribed from speech. Based on the fact that the authors did indicate in their article that their findings were essentially consistent across different contexts, however, this writer finds their conclusions interesting, instructive, and worthy of inclusion here. Following is a summary of selected remarkable findings:

Women:

- Used more words related to psychological and social processes.
- Were more apt to discuss people and what they were doing.
- Used more words to express thoughts, emotions, senses, other people, negations, and verbs in present and past tense.
- Were more inclined to communicate internal processes, including doubts.

Men:

- More often used language to label external events, objects, and processes.
- Referred more to object properties and impersonal topics.
- Used more words to discuss occupation, money, and sport.
- Used more technical linguistic features such as numbers, articles, prepositions, and long words.
- More often added swear words for emphasis.

Although these findings were generally consistent across different contexts, the gender differences were more evident on tasks that placed fewer constraints on language use, i.e., tasks that were more open-ended in nature.

Email and Written Correspondence

The elements of *style* and *content* in both emails and written letters to male and female friends have been topics of research. The *style* categories identified in one relevant study (Colley et al., 2004) focused on "formality, excitability, nonessentials and relational devices." These selected features were in part based on previous research findings that revealed more emotional features in women's writing (e.g., markers of excitability such as exclamation points, capitalization, intensifying adverbs such as "really"), and nonessentials (e.g., brackets, dashes, parentheses, trailing dots or other such embellishments) that may be indicative of a weaker or less direct language style (Rubin & Greene, 1992).

The *content* categories were derived from the data themselves and included activity categories (e.g., sport, holidays, work, shopping), relationships categories (e.g., family, specific same-sex friends, specific opposite-sex friends), and personal disclosure categories, including descriptions of specific incidents, positive emotions, and negative emotions.

Through analyzing the emails and letters sent by men and women to friends on the topic of how they had spent their summer (Colley et al., 2004), remarkable findings were:

- Word counts of all communications revealed that women wrote longer messages than the men.
- In terms of content, women focused more on "personal and domestic topics" than did men; women more often mentioned family, shopping, a specific incident, and positive emotion.
- Sport was mentioned by both women and men, and found in both letters and emails. However, sport was more often mentioned in communications to male recipients.
- Stylistically, women's writing was more "relational" and "expressive" than men's. Specifically, more women than men "made initial personal inquiries and gave affectionate signatures." However, when a woman was the recipient of a man's letter or email, more men wrote affectionate signatures and mentioned future contact.
- In the more informal emails, it was found that women used more humor and multiple exclamation marks when writing to their female friends.
- Men used more offensive language (e.g., swear words) while women used more emotionality (e.g., multiple exclamation marks, positive intensifiers such as "really" and "soooo") in their written communication.

Computer-Mediated Communication

While the above studies addressed one-on-one written and email communication between friends and acquaintances, there has also been tremendous growth in public email such as seen in message boards, mailing lists, and chat rooms. Ways in which public email of any form differs from email between friends centers around these facts: (a) Electronic mail discussion groups consist of groups of people who for the most part are strangers to one another; (b) the groups can be of any size, from several people to tens of thousands of people; (c) the aim of these groups is typically to allow communicators to offer information, advice, opinions, or other kinds of comments on specific identified topics.

As we have become more accustomed to this form of computer-mediated conversation, we recognize that many email messages are written in a way that so resembles spoken language that we now sometimes refer to the act of writing email messages back and forth as "holding a conversation online" (Shea, 1994, p. 35).

Various observers and researchers have weighed in on gender-related differences found in these kinds of computer-mediated communication forums. Following are observations and findings that may be of interest to transgendered individuals who seek to modify the style of their own online contributions:

■ Men in online groups tend to limit the interaction, while women are more apt to engage and prolong the contact. "Men come online to give information or give an answer. . . . Women add a question, tweak a thread, or make things more complicated" (Dr. David Silver, Assistant Professor at the University of Washington and the Director of the online Resource Center for Cyber Culture Studies, as quoted in Cohen, 2001).

■ On the other hand, sometimes the perceived anonymity of email can lead some otherwise shy or reluctant communicators to open up and divulge more information or share emotions that they might not do in a face-to-face interaction. Using email can create a "beneficial distance" at times when verbal communication might feel "too rich." "For many men, email may take some of the emotional charge off loaded situations" (Dr. Susan Herring, Associate Professor of Information Science and Linguistics at Indiana University, as quoted in Cohen, 2001).

■ Susan Herring also has written about how, in online communications, women are much more likely to produce polite language, offer suggestions and support , use emoticons and representations of laughter ("lol,," "haha," etc.), as well as ask questions (Cohen, 2001).

■ Men, on the other hand, tend to make strong assertions, are more apt to openly disagree with others, use sarcasm and even profanity and insults (Cohen, 2001).

Instant Messaging (IM) and Texting

Instant messaging (IM) and texting are forms of real-time text-based communication between two or more people using personal computers, tablets and cell phones, or other such devices. Sometimes people refer to IM as "online chat," as it occurs in real time. However, although some forms of "online chat" can occur among strangers in a multi-user environment, instant messaging is based on a list of connections between known users who make contact through the use of their "Buddy List," "Contact List," or "Friend List." Although IM-ing and texting are written communication, they occur more immediately and are more direct than email. As a result, they often resemble speech more than they do writing.

In research investigating gender differences in the instant messaging behavior of college students (Baron, 2004), it was found that:

- Messages between women tended to be more formal, that is, with fewer contractions and better punctuation, than that between men.
- Women used a "more schooled, standard writing style."
- Women were more likely to use emoticons.
- Whereas average turn length was similar across genders, the longest single turns in female-female (FF) conversations were longer than those in male-male (MM) conversations.
- The average FF conversation was longer, both in number of turns and in overall time than the average MM conversation.
- Men used contractions, i.e., chose contracted forms 77% of the time, while women used contracted forms only 57% of the time.
- It took women on average 41 seconds and nearly 10 exchanges to close a conversation, which suggested similarity to the prolonged goodbyes that characterize women's face-to-face interaction.
- Men ended their IM sessions more than twice as quickly as did the women (Baron, 2004; Schirber, 2005). Overall, however, Baron's impression is that "the female IM looks more like a written genre, while the male IM looks more like a spoken genre" (Schirber, 2005).

Blogging

A blog is a website that contains an online personal journal with reflections, comments, and often hyperlinks provided by the writer. Although blogs are usually maintained by an individual, many blogs are interactive, allowing visitors to leave comments or messages. Since a blog contains

text, this online resource now provides language researchers with a wealth of new data to explore.

Argamon, Koppel, Pennebaker, and Schler (2007), and Schler, Koppel, Argamon, and Pennebaker (2005) used millions of words from the blogosphere to study blog language and how people use it on a large scale. Utilizing text drawn from a corpus of 71,000 blogs from blogger.com, the authors examined the effects of age and gender on writing style and topic. To analyze their data, the authors identified 2 different kinds of distinguishing features: *style-related features* and *content-related features*. Key findings follow:

- Women used more pronouns, assent/negation words, and "blog words," which included written expressions that have been developed specifically for internet communication (e.g., lol, haha). Female bloggers also were found to discuss their personal lives—and use a more personal writing style—than were males (Schler et al., 2005).
- Men used more articles, more prepositions, and more hyperlinks (or links), which are references to other documents or websites that the reader can directly follow. Male bloggers of all ages were found to blog more about politics, technology, and money than were their female cohorts (Schler et al., 2005).
- The authors concluded that these findings were supportive of the hypothesis that female writing tends to emphasize "involvedness," while male writing tends to emphasize information (Schler et al., p. 2).

Another interesting finding from this study is: "Regardless of gender, writing style grows increasingly 'male' with age; pronouns and assent/negation become scarcer, while prepositions and determiners become more frequent. Blog words are a clear hallmark of youth, while the use of hyperlinks increase with age" (Schler et al., p. 4). The focus of their 2007 study was to examine the blog corpus for content-based features, revealing:

- Male bloggers more frequently used the factors titled *Religion, Politics, Business,* and *Internet* (Argamon et al., 2007).
- Female bloggers more frequently used the factors *Conversation, At Home, Fun, Romance,* and *Swearing* (Argamon et al, 2007).

Implications for Intervention

When a writer of any gender, age, or culture puts pen to paper or types out words using a keyboard, he or she makes numerous choices and selections from a variety of stylistic elements that can range from characteristics of *form* (e.g., sentence length, syntax, morphology, punctuation), to *content* (e.g., vocabulary/lexical choices), to *pragmatics* (e.g., topic selection, dialect, voice). The result is written output that may contain clues as to his or her social identity, including gender.

As clinicians who are trained to analyze communication output not only from the speech/voice perceptual perspective, but also from the perspective of linguistic form, semantic content, and social pragmatics, speech-language pathologists potentially have much to offer transgender clients who are interested in analyzing and modifying their writing. Some therapeutic interventions may include the following:

1. We can provide educational materials to our clients—for example, by offering lists or summaries of salient male-female differences found in the literature (e.g., as outlined in this chapter).

2. We can provide exercises and activities aimed at increasing a writer's awareness of stylistic choices he/she has been making, and then working with the client to explore more gender-authentic ways of expressing the same basic content.

3. It can be useful for clients to keep a journal.

4. Some individuals find it beneficial to maintain a little notebook of phrases, expressions, or vocabulary that they may wish to begin to integrate into their writing.

5. Writing exercises can be presented using a hierarchy similar to that used in the treatment of verbal/spoken language. For instance, activities may begin with basic object or picture description, and progress to activities such as scene description, answering short questions that transmit basic information, and ultimately move to tasks that involve higher-level complex or abstract expression of ideas and opinions. Based on a client's needs and interests, writing activities can also involve writing personal or professional notes, letters, or memoranda.

6. Clinicians may wish to suggest to their transgender clients specific authors who tend to write with a strong feminine or masculine voice. Serious writers among our clientele may also be interested in studying more detailed findings such as those available in the larger text analysis articles cited in this chapter.

7. It may be important to help some transgender clients understand the boundaries and conventions of intimacy in their written communication. When signing off at the end of a letter, for example, some clients may need help to understand the potential inappropriateness of

such phrases as "hugs and kisses" unless the writer is actually writing to an intimate relation.

8. Finally, some clients might be interested in knowing about the "Gender Guesser." Gender Guesser is a program developed by researchers Moshe Koppel of Bar-Ilan University in Israel, and Shlomo Argamon of Illinois Institute of Technology, to predict the gender of an author. The Gender Guesser program uses a simplified version of the algorithm developed by these researchers and accessible at http://www.hackerfactor.com/GenderGuesser.php#Analyze (retrieved August 19, 2017). The Gender Guesser is based on an earlier program, no longer available, called Gender Genie.

Measuring Outcomes: Does Nonverbal Training Make a Difference?

Measuring the outcomes of nonverbal training is very difficult. There is little to no research available and no standardized tests that can be used to be certain of beneficial outcomes. As with so much clinical work in development, we often have to rely on the quality of life changes and personal feedback from our clients. It also brings us back to the importance of setting clear personal goals at the outset of voice and communication training. What has changed, how are clients being perceived, and in what contexts do they experience a difference in how people interpret their gender identity?

Anecdotally nonverbal communication training appears to make a difference. Testimonials from transfeminine clients are evidence to this fact. A survey of clients, albeit small, who have taken Hirsch's two-day

training "Turning Your Insides Out" act as evidence. The question "Do you feel you have gained in confidence living as a woman?" gleaned the following results, where 0 = low rating and 5 = highest rating: 43% rating of 5; 50% rating of 4; and 7% (1 person) a rating of 2. This individual stated that she was still very frightened generally. A year later she contacted the clinician to say that over time she had fully processed the information from the workshop and felt that she had gained enormously from its content. She is living happily and confidently in her gender identity.

Client feedback and levels of satisfaction do not always mirror the impressions or judgments of the casual observer, but does this matter in the end if the client feels complete, congruous, happy and personally honest? This is an important and huge question that is being discussed daily as we move farther into a broader understanding of gender. While the word "authenticity" is losing favor, it might still be mulled within the context of the Oxford English Dictionary definition: "original, first-hand, prototypical; real, actual, genuine; self-originated, belonging to [oneself]." It is within the context of this last definition of authenticity that the clinician should consider measuring the true success of outcomes.

The fine-tuning of nonverbal communication and overall authenticity "self-origination" can continue as a lifelong pursuit, but at some point the client needs to simply live life and stop questioning the validity of certain choices that he or she has made. By the same token, clinicians need to recognize when the nonverbal behaviors of a client are true enough, congruous enough, and "passable" enough. It can be challenging to stop commenting, to stop trying to perfect the whole picture. Gender diverse clients sometimes seek what they consider to be "perfection," and it is our job as clinicians to guide them to satisfaction and peace.

Summary

We are living in a time when gender stereotypes are being critically questioned socially, politically, and in the workplace; and rightly so. The work we do with gender diverse clients needs to be viewed through a number of lenses, not least of all the following: the client is the expert about their own sense of gender, and we must lead all teaching with context. As has been stated in a number of ways throughout this chapter, if clients have expressed the desire or need to work on nonverbal communication, the more they know, the more they can adapt to context. It is critical that clinicians do the necessary homework that allows them to be culturally sensitive and relevant to the task at hand; the challenges of teaching nonverbal communication skills to the gender diverse client are many and obvious. It might be easy to ignore them, or comment randomly and casually on nonverbal communication areas in the hopes that things will just develop independently of therapy. However, in reality, they usually do not. If clients have expressed an interest in developing different nonverbal behaviors, clinicians must take the charge of teaching them creatively and with an open mind. We must be alert to their own possible rigidity, and be bold and creative in our attempts to find exercises and examples that resonate with each client individually. The importance of the work might be underscored by this final testimonial from one of Hirsch's clients: "Authenticity [training], which includes everything from hand and facial movements, to voice, and ways of thinking, has made a huge difference in my confidence and ability to live more fully in my chosen gender."

References and Sources of Further Interest

Adler, R., Hirsch, S., & Mordaunt, M. (2006). *Voice and communication therapy for the transgender/transsexual client: A comprehensive clinical guide.* San Diego, CA: Plural Publishing Inc.

Adler, R., Hirsch, S., & Mordaunt, M. (2012). *Voice and communication therapy for the transgender/transsexual client: A comprehensive clinical guide* (2nd ed.). San Diego, CA: Plural Publishing Inc.

American Speech-Language-Hearing Association (2016). Scope of practice in speech-language pathology. Rockville, MD. Retrieved February 15, 2016, from https://www.asha.org/uploadedFiles/SP2016-00343.pdf.

Andrews, M. L. (1999). *Manual of voice treatment: Pediatrics through geriatrics* (2nd ed.). San Diego, CA: Singular Publishing Group.

Andrews, M. L., & Schmidt, C. (1997). Gender presentation: Perceptual and acoustical analyses of voice. *Journal of Voice*, 11, 307–313.

Archer, D. (Producer), & Silver, J. (Director) (2001). *Gender and communication: Male-female differences in language and nonverbal behavior* [Videorecording]. Berkeley, CA: Berkeley Media LLC.

Argamon, S., Koppel, M., Fine, J., & Shimoni, A. (2003). Gender, genre, and writing style in formal written texts. *Text, 23*(3), 221–246.

Argamon, S., Koppel, M., Pennebaker, J., & Schler, J. (2007). Mining the blogosphere: Age, gender, and the varieties of self-expression. *First Monday*, http://firstmonday.org./issues/issue12_9/argamon/index.html

Argyle, M., & Ingham, R. (1972). Gaze, mutual gaze and proximity. *Semiotica, 6*, 32–49.

Axtell, R. E. (1998). *The do's and taboos of body language around the world.* New York, NY: John Wiley and Sons, Inc.

Azul, D. (2015). On the varied and complex factors affecting gender diverse people's vocal situations: Implications for clinical practice. *SIG 3 Perspectives on Voice and Voice Disorders, 25*(2), 75–86.

Baron, N. (2004). See you online: Gender issues in college student use of instant messaging. *Journal of Language and Social Psychology, 23*(4), 397–423.

Benninger, M. S., Jacobson, B. H., & Johnson, A. F. (1993). *Vocal arts medicine: The care and prevention of professional voice disorders*. New York, NY: Thieme Medical Publishers.

Berry, C. (1973). *Voice and the actor*. London, UK: Harrap.

Birdwhistell, R. L. (1970). *Kinesics and context: Essays on body motion communication*. Philadelphia, PA: University of Pennsylvania Press. Bottom of Form.

Black, A. B. (2002). *The perceivable auditory difference between male and female footsteps. independent research*. Retrieved July 7, 2011, from http://www-cs-students.stanford.edu/~jblack/footsteps.pdf.

Borisoff, D., McIlwain, C., Kotchemidova, C., & Brown, R. Nonverbal communication and culture [Videorecording]. Produced by Odyssey Productions LLC. New York, NY, Distributed by Insight Media [2005].

Boylan, J. F. (2002). *She's not there*. New York, NY: Broadway Books.

Braddick, M. J. (Ed.) (2009). *The politics of gesture: Historical perspectives*. Oxford, UK and New York, NY: Oxford Journals, Oxford University Press.

Briton, N. J., & Hall, J. A. (1995). Beliefs about male and female nonverbal communicaton. *Sex Roles, 32*, 79–90.

Burgoon, J. K., Buller, D. B., & Woodall, W. G. (Eds.) (1996). *Nonverbal communication: The unspoken dialogue* (2nd ed.). New York, NY: Harper and Row.

Burgoon, J. K., Guerrero, L. K., & Floyd, K. (2016). *Nonverbal communication*. New York, NY: Routledge.

Canary, D. J., & Dindia, K. (Eds.). (1998). *Sex differences and similarities in communication: Critical essays and empirical investigations of sex and gender in interaction*. Mahwah, NJ: Lawrence Erlbaum and Associates.

Cicca, A. H., Step, M., & Turkstra, L. (2003). Show me what you mean: Nonverbal communication theory and application. *ASHA Leader, 34*, 4–5.

Coates, J. (1993). *Women, men, and language* (2nd ed.). Harlow, UK: Longman Group.

Cohen, J. (2001). He-mails, she-mails: Where sender meets gender. *New York Times*, May 17.

Colley, A., & Todd, Z. (2002). Gender-linked differences in the style and content of e-mails to friends. *Journal of Language and Social Psychology, 21*(4), 380–392. http://jls.sagepub.com/content/21/4/380.

Colley, A., Todd, Z., Bland, M., Holmes, M., Khanon, N., & Pike, H. (2004). Style and content in e-mails and letters to male and female friends. *Journal of Language and Social Psychology, 23*(3), 369–378. http://jls.sagepub.com/content/23/3/369.

Cutting, J. E. (1978). Generation of synthetic male and female walkers through manipulation of a biomechanical invariant. *Perception, 7*, 393–403.

Dahl, S. (1998). *Communications and culture transformation*. http://dahl.at/wordpress/research-publications/intercultural-communication/communications-and-culture-transformation (shared with Hirsch via email from author, August 26, 2011).

Davis, M., & Skupien, J. (Eds.) (1982). *Body movement and nonverbal communication: An annotated bibliography*. Bloomington, IN: Indiana University Press.

Denham, E. (1956). *I looked right*. Garden City, NY: Doubleday.

Doyle, D. (2003). *Feminine movement*. Esprit Gala Conference Presentation, Port Angeles, WA.

Edgerton, M. T. (1974). The surgical treatment of transsexuals. *Clinical Plastic Surgery, 1*(2), 285–323.

Ekman, P. (1999). Facial expressions. In T. Dalgleish & T. Power (Eds.), *The handbook of cognition and emotion* (pp. 301–320). Sussex, UK: John Wiley & Sons, Ltd.

Ettner, R. (1996). *Confessions of a gender defender*. Chicago, IL: Spectrum Press.

Fast, J. (1970). *Body language*. New York, NY: M. Evans and Company, Inc.

Fisk, N. (1974). Gender dysphoria syndrome. *Western Journal of Medicine, 120*(5), 386–391.

Freidenberg, C. B. (2002). Working with male-to-female transgendered clients: Clinical considerations. *Contemporary Issues in Communication Science Disorders, 29*, 43–58.

Fromkin, V., & Rodman, J. (1983). *An introduction to language*. New York, NY: CBS College Publishing.

Geary, D. C., & Flinn, M. V. (2002). Sex differences in behavioural and hormonal response to social threat: Commentary on Taylor et al. *Psychological Review, 109*(4), 745–750.

Gladwell, M. (2005). *Blink: The power of thinking without thinking*. New York, NY: Little Brown and Company.

Glass, L. (1992). *He says, she says: Closing the communication gap between the sexes*. New York, NY: G.P. Putnam and Sons.

Goman, C. K. (2008). *The nonverbal advantage: Secrets and science of body language at work* San Francisco, CA: Berrett-Koehler Publishers, Inc.

Goodman, E., & O'Brien, P. (2000). *I know just what you mean: The power of friendship in women's lives*. New York, NY: Simon and Schuster.

Hadjian, S., Allred, J., & Mahaffrey, R. (1981). *Objective and subjective measures of a male transsexual versus females*. ASHA conference presentation, Los Angeles, CA.

Hanna, M. S., & Wilson, G. L. (1998). *Communicating in business and professional settings* (4th ed.). New York, NY: McGraw-Hill Companies, Inc.

Harper, R. G., Wiens, A. N., & Mararazzo, J. D. (1978). *Non-verbal communication: The state of the art*. New York, NY: Wiley.

Harrigan, J. A., Rosenthal, R., & Scherer, K. R. (Eds.) (2005). *The new handbook of methods in nonverbal behavior research*. Oxford, UK and New York, NY: Oxford University Press.

Hirsch, S. (2003). *Approaches to nonverbal communication in male-to-female voice feminization treatment*. Presentation at the Annual Convention of the American Speech-Language-Hearing Association, Chicago, IL.

Ivy, D. K., & Backlund, P. (1994). *Exploring genderspeak*. New York, NY: McGraw-Hill Companies.

Jarrard, M. E., & Randall, P. R. (1982). *Women speaking: An annotated bibliography of verbal and nonverbal communication (1970–1980)*. New York, NY: Garland.

Kachel, S., Steffens, M. C., & Niedlich, C. (2016). Traditional masculinity and femininity: Validation of a new scale assessing gender roles. *Frontiers in Psychology*, 7, 956. http://doi.org/10.3389/fpsyg.2016.00956.

Kates, G. (1995). *Monsieur d'Eon is a woman: A tale of political intrigue and sexual masquerade*. New York, NY: Basic Books, Harper Collins.

Key, M. R. (1975). *Male, female language*. Metuchen, NJ: Scarecrow Press.

Knapp, M. (1972). *Nonverbal communication in human interaction*. New York, NY: Holt, Rinehart & Winston.

Knowles, E. (1999). *The Oxford dictionary of quotations* (5th ed.). Oxford, UK: Oxford University Press.

Laing, A. (1989). *Speaking as a woman*. King of Prussia, PA: Creative Design Services.

Lehmann-Haupt, C. (1999). In women's groups, back to 'girl talk'. Sunday *New York Times*, April 11.

Leigh, L. (2001). *Out and about: The emancipated cross-dresser*. Phoenix, AZ: Double Star Press.

Lessac, A. (1967). *The use and training of the human voice: A practical approach to speech and voice dynamics*. New York, NY: DBS Publications, Inc.

Mason, J. (Editor and Publisher) (1979). *The family of woman: A world-wide photographic perception of female life and being*. New York, NY: Grosset & Dunlap.

Mayo, C., & Henley N. M. (1981). *Gender and nonverbal behavior*. New York, NY: Springer-Verlag.

McCloskey, D. N. (1999). *Crossing: A memoir*. Chicago, IL and London, UK: University of Chicago Press.

Mead, M. (1963). *Sex and temperament in three primitive societies*. New York, NY: Harper-Collins.

Mordaunt, M., & Osborne, J. (1999). *Voice therapy for transgendered clients: A clinical and consumer perspective*. Presentation at the Annual Convention of the American Speech-Language-Hearing Association, San Francisco, CA.

Nelson, A., & Damken Brown, C. (2012). *The gender communication handbook: Conquering collisions between men and women*. San Francisco, CA: Pfeiffer.

Nelson, A., & Golant, S. K. (2004). *You don't say: Navigating nonverbal communication between the sexes*. New York, NY: Prentice-Hall.

Neville Miller, A. (2011). Men and women's communication is different—sometimes. *Communication Currents*, 6, 1. Retrieved September 2011, from http://www.natcom.org/CommCurrents Article.aspx?id=2147484130.

Newman, M., Groom, C., Handelman, L., & Pennebaker, J. (2008). Gender differences in language use: An analysis of 14,000 text samples. *Discourse Processes*, 45(3), 211–236.

Oates, J. M., & Dacakis, G. (1983). Speech pathology considerations in the management of transsexualism—a review. *British Journal of Disorders of Communication, 18*(3), 139–151.

Oates, J. M., & Dacakis, G. (1997). Voice change in transsexuals. *Venereology—the Interdisciplinary International Journal of Sexual Health, 10*(3), 178–187.

O'Connell, P. (2003). Gender genie. *New York Times: Online Diary*, September 11, p. 4.

Paludi, M. A. (Ed.) (2004). *Praeger guide to the psychology of gender*. Westport, CT: Praeger Publishers.

Park, Myung-Seok. (1979). *Communication styles in two different cultures: Korean and American*. Seoul, South Korea: Han Shin Publishing Co.

Pearson, J. (1984). *Gender and communication*. Dubuque, Iowa: William C. Brown.

Putrevu, S. (2001). Exploring the origins and information processing differences between men and women. *Academy of Marketing Science Review, 2001*(10) Available: http://www.amsreview.org/articles/putrevu10-2001.pdf.

Roen, D. H., Peguesse, C., & Abordonado, V. (1995). Gender and language variation in written communication. In D. L. Rubin (Ed.), *Composing social identity in written language* (pp. 113–127). Hillsdale, NJ: Lawrence Erlbaum Associates.

Rowe, A. A. (1996). *Where have all the smart women gone?* Seattle, WA: Hara Publishing.

Rubin, D. L. (1995). Introducing social identity. In D. L. Rubin (Ed.). *Composing social identity in written language* (pp. 16–26). Hillsdale, NJ: Lawrence Erlbaum Associates.

Rubin, D. L., & Greene, K. (1992). Gender typical style in written discourse. *Research in the Teaching of English, 26*, 7–40.

Sagant, E. (1999). *Creating a feminine carriage: Figure, posture, walk and gestures*. Oakland, CA: Elaine Sagant.

Schirber, M. (2005, March 1). Study: Instant messaging is surprisingly formal :-) LiveScience. http://livescience.com/technology/050301_internet_language.html.

Schler, J., Koppel, M., Argamon, S., & Pennebaker, J. (2005). Effects of age and gender on blogging. *American Association for Artificial Intelligence* (www.aaai.org).

Scott, C. (1990). *Strangers in good company*. National Film Board of Canada, Studio 3.

Shakespeare, W., Peter Alexander (Ed.) (1954). *A Midsummer Night's Dream*. The Tudor Edition of The Complete Works.

Shaughnessy, P. (1975). *A case report of voice, speech and body language in transsexual female*. ASHA conference presentation.

Shea, V. (1994). *Net etiquette*, San Francisco, CA: Albion Books.

Soojin, S. O. (2000). *Explanation for the gender differences in expressing emotions*. Retrieved February 19, 2018, from http://ccat.sas.upenn.edu/plc/communication/soojin.htm.

Sommer, R. (1969). *Personal space: The behavioral basis of design*. Englewood Cllffs, NJ: Prentice-Hall.

Spencer, L. E. (1988). Speech characteristics of male-to-female transsexuals: A perceptual and acoustic study. *Folia Phoniat, 40*(1), 31–42.

Stanislavski, C. (1949). *Building a character*. New York, NY: Theatre Arts Books.

Tannen, D. (1990). *You just don't understand*. New York, NY: Ballantine Books.

Tannen, D. (1994). *Gender and discourse*. New York, NY: Oxford University Press.

Taylor, S. E., Klein, L. C., Lewis, B. P., Gruenewald, T. L., Gurung, R. A. R., & Updegraff, J. A. (2000). Behavioral responses to stress in females: Tend-and-befriend, not fight-or-flight. *Psychological Review, 107*(3), 411–429.

Taylor, S.E., Lewis, B.P., Greunewald, T.L., Gurung, R.A.R., Udegraff, J.A., & Klein, L.C. (2002). Sex differences in behavioral response to threat: Reply to Geary and Flinn (2002). *Psychological Review, 109*(4). 751–753.

Van Borsel, J, De Cuypere, G., & den Berghe, H. (2001). Physical appearance and voice in male to female transsexuals. *Journal of Voice. 15*(4), 570–575.

Van Borsel, J., De Pot, K., & De Cuypere, G. (2009). Voice and physical appearance in female-to-male transsexuals. *Journal of Voice, 23*(4), 494–497.

Vargas, M. F. (1986). *Louder than words: An introduction to non-verbal communication*. Ames IA: Iowa State University Press.

Wharton, T. (2009). *Pragmatics and non-verbal communication*. Cambridge, UK and New York, NY: Cambridge University Press.

Wikipedia. *Crossdressing*. Retrieved May 28, 2005, from http://en.wikipedia.org/wiki/Cross-dressing.

Wood, J,T., & Fixmer-Oraiz, N, (2015). *Gendered lives: Communication, gender and culture* (12th ed.). Boston, MA: Cenage Learning.

Woolf, V. (1929). *A room of one's own*. London, UK: Granada Publishing, Ltd.

13

Group Voice and Communication Training

Daniel M. Kayajian, Jack Pickering, and Michelle Mordaunt

Introduction

Group therapy in speech-language pathology and audiology has been described in the professional literature for decades. In fact, a brief database search uncovered articles on group intervention from the late 1940s (e.g., Backus & Dunn, 1947). Since that time, research has investigated the application of group therapy for a number of communication disorders, including, but not limited to, stuttering, aphasia, voice disorders, traumatic brain injury, autism, and speech sound disorders (Arnott et al., 2014; Bilgehan, 2015; Caughter & Dunsmuir, 2017; Dahlberg et al., 2007; Law et al., 2012; Nickels, 2016; Sherratt & Simmons-Mackie, 2016; Simberg et al., 2006; Skelton & Richard, 2016). While there is a paucity of research evidence supporting group training in transgender voice and communication, groups have existed for some time and approaches to group training have been described in the professional literature.

Luterman (2008) recognizes two types of groups in speech-language pathology: communication therapy groups and counseling groups. It would be reasonable to imagine that many groups serve both func-tions simultaneously. According to Luterman (2008), a group's goals include:

- Content (in our case related to voice and speech)
- Affect release (the ability to express feelings in a safe environment)
- Personal growth (group members grow, take on leadership, support others)

In regard to leadership, Holland and Nelson (2014) provide two important points that must be recognized for group training to be successful: (a) our leadership as group facilitator is important in the group's success; and (b) group training is a chance for group members to demonstrate and practice leadership skills, which enhance self-confidence, promote advocacy (self-advocacy and perhaps beyond), and facilitate personal growth. The nature of this leadership can be different for each group member, but the potential for successful growth within a group context can be significant. Flasher and Fogle (2012) point out that it can be a challenge for a clinician to lead a group; we have to be present in the moment and attentive to the group dynamic. It is also important to recognize that groups evolve over time. Luterman (2008) describes the development that often takes place in a group context. He identifies the following phases of group development:

1. The Group at Inception: At this time, consider how we introduce ourselves and ask group members to introduce themselves; for our clients who are transgender that means their name and pronoun(s). Confrontation is not usually needed, but observation of resistance and discomfort are important.
2. The Working Group: This is the part of the group where you have cohesiveness, occasional conflict, and a redefinition of leadership. Content is valuable during this stage, and trust is developed. An effective group handles conflict that arises.
3. The Terminating Group: This is sometimes not easy for us to manage, but important. Terminating a group can result in a grief response. We can find it difficult to build termination into our group planning, in part because we do not have good data on how long is long enough; and how much training, group and/or individual, is necessary.

While group therapy is often applied in our discipline and others, speech-language pathologists have limited exposure to, and are given little information about, group therapy in clinical training. With this in mind, some of the primary benefits and challenges that confront practicing clinicians working in a group context will be described.

Group Therapy Benefits and Challenges

In his discussion of "Curative factors of groups," Luterman (2008) suggests that counseling groups provide the following benefits for group participants:

- Instillation of hope: Hope comes from seeing others succeed.
- Universality: This instills the sense that you are not alone.
- Imparting information: Group members bring information as much as the group leader.
- Altruism: Group members help each other as part of a community.
- Interpersonal learning: The group is a safe vehicle for enhancing interactional skills.
- Group cohesiveness: A shared trust is developed as the group becomes a "team."
- Catharsis: The group is a place to release stress and negative feelings.
- Existential issues: Personal growth comes from the exploration of one's "existence."

There are other benefits of group training as well. For example, groups provide a context for conversation and functional interaction, so practice is meaningful to the group members. Logistically, health care constraints in the United States make group therapy appealing. Finally, there is a growing appreciation for the positive impact of group therapy on addressing chronic psychosocial issues for those with communication disorders or differences (depression, social anxiety, etc.). Holland and Nelson (2014) say that groups are: (a) places where communication practice can be completed, including skills that may be learned in individual sessions, (b) opportunities to practice positive psychology exercises (for example, gratitude and advocacy), and (c) a way for clients to "come to grips" with how life has changed—adjusting to a new normal.

While group training can work well and has the potential to facilitate voice and communication change, there are also challenges. For example, it is often difficult to address individual needs and communication styles in a group setting. Furthermore, providing activities that engage all members of a group can be difficult, particularly if the level of experience among group members is different. Clinicians need to be aware that group training can occasionally lead to conflict among group participants, and there may be topics initiated that may extend beyond our professional purview. Knowing that clients may be seeing a mental health counselor is important, and collaborating with the counselor provides positive support. The following section describes some creative components of group training: activities, strategies, and ideas that may enhance the group process and ultimately facilitate positive change in voice and communication for people who are transgender.

Creative Components for Group Training

Mindfulness and gratitude. Mindfulness and gratitude are effective and creative ways to deliver an integrative approach to voice and communication modification in a group setting. Mindfulness is the ability to maintain awareness and engage in the present moment without attachment or judgment (Shapiro & Carlson, 2009). It is an activity that cultivates intention, promoting flexibility and self-exploration including self-esteem, attitudes, and feelings as related to voice and communication in this instance. Mindfulness also improves attention, or the awareness of what we are experiencing, and can affect attitude, since it is done without judgment, in a positive, accepting, and non-reactive way. Kabat-Zinn (2003) tells us that mindfulness helps us set the stage for what is possible.

Mindfulness has been increasingly researched over the past several years, given the interest in and application of mindfulness-based interventions. This is particularly true among mental health providers and other helping professionals. Currently there is solid evidence that mindfulness can be effectively utilized to treat both mental and physical health issues (Shapiro & Carlson, 2009). For the general population, mindfulness has also been shown to reduce rumination (Chambers et al., 2008), reduce stress (Hofmann et al., 2010), improve the ability to focus and attend (Moore & Malinowski, 2009), improve empathy (Shapiro, Schwartz, & Bonner, 1998), and enhance compassion (Shapiro, Astin, Bishop, & Cordova, 2005).

It has been our experience at The College of St. Rose that beginning group sessions with mindfulness breathing and relaxation prepares both the clients and the clinicians mentally and physically focuses their attention on diaphragmatic breathing, upper/lower body tension and posture. The guided mindfulness exercises may also include body scan (increasing kinesthetic awareness), movement (heightening proprioception), and mindful listening (enhancing focus and attentiveness). Mindfulness exercises are led by clinicians, though clients may also lead, providing a unique communication opportunity.

Group training at Saint Rose is ended in a similar fashion with a shared expression of gratitude. Acts of gratitude have been found to strengthen relationships, promote positivity, and increase happiness (Seligman, 2012). "Gratitude helps people refocus on what they have instead of what they lack" (Harvard Mental Health Letter, 2011). Clinicians generally lead gratitude exercises, which may include a verbal or written expression of gratitude by the clients for someone/something they are grateful for. Written exercises, like completing thank you notes, may be shared by group members at their own discretion but provide a concrete representation of the participants' feelings of gratitude, among clients and clinicians alike.

Mentoring, modeling, and interaction. Group training also provides opportunities for mentoring, modeling, and dynamic interactions. As an example, icebreakers and functional role-playing (McCready et al., 2011) can be effective ways to facilitate communication among clients and clinicians in a non-threatening, supportive environment. This can provide a context for conversational activities and role-playing where clients can focus on their specific voice and communication goals, even if they are different across group members. This context also creates opportunities for group members to give supportive and reflective feedback. Clients may take the role of mentor and/or serve as a model for newer group members. At the same time, the clinician serves as a supportive communication partner, communication model for the group members, and a source for constructive feedback. In a college or university setting, classroom presentations are also effective for providing creative communication opportunities for clients who may present information solely or in collaboration with their clinician on topics relevant to voice and communication. Here, clients can practice generalization of their voice and communication skills, which fosters peer support and community building.

Group training also promotes growth within the broader gender diverse community by building and strengthening social connections fostered by the varied communication opportunities. This in turn helps group members learn from each other regarding various aspects of their transition that then extends outside the group into the larger transgender community. Here, group members find additional supports, if necessary, or may take on an advocacy role within the broader transgender community.

Mission statement and guidelines. Developing a mission statement for group training can be beneficial to establish and communicate structure, purpose, and organization for the group. It creates an opportunity to set expectations and lay the framework for the group's goals, ethics, and culture. Creating the statement and guidelines with the group members and having ongoing discussions about the principles as part of the group facilitates leadership and buy-in, which can help the group members feel ownership. In February 2012, at The College of St. Rose, a mission statement and guiding principles were crafted in collaboration with the group members and a mental health counselor who specializes in transgender health. The mission statement and guiding principles follow.

Mission Statement

The Voice and Communication Modification Program at The College of St. Rose is committed to supporting transgender women and men to achieve their authentic voice in a safe, nurturing environment. Group members, student clinicians, and program supervisors will work together to establish a positive culture that celebrates diversity, facilitates personal growth, and promotes effective voice and communication change.

Guiding Principles for the Voice and Communication Program

- Respect: We are respectful to ourselves and others who take part in the program.
- Confidentiality: We will respect and maintain confidentiality and privacy of each member of the group.
- Step up/Step back: We give supportive attention to the person who is speaking and provide everyone with the opportunity to share.
- Responsibility/Commitment: We share the responsibility for making the group work.
- "I" statements: We use "I" rather than "you" statements to promote acceptance and accountability.

- Feedback: We are solution focused, providing positive, constructive feedback which is welcomed and welcoming.
- Goals: We will stay true to our individual goals as well as the goals of the group.

Approaches to Group Training for People Who Are Transgender

Anecdotal evidence suggests that group voice and communication training, like individual services, for transgender individuals, is growing and can be an effective means of facilitating voice and communication change. At the present time, descriptions of group training are limited in the professional literature, and there is a paucity of research supporting its application (Adler, Hirsch, & Mordaunt, 2012; Davies, 2006; Davies, Papp, & Antoni, 2015; Mordaunt, 2012; Oates & Dacakis, 2015; Pickering & Kayajian, 2009). Despite the limited empirical evidence, Kayajian's survey research with transgender individuals over a decade ago indicated a preference for both individual and group intervention to modify voice and communication (2005). Examples of group training for people who are transgender are described below.

Group Training Prior to and After Individual Training

Mordaunt (2012) included descriptions of group training in the second edition of this book. She outlined the application of groups both prior to and after individual intervention. Group training prior to individual services may serve to increase the client's awareness of voice and communication training. Careful intake information is gathered, providing an opportunity to learn about your group members (readiness, expectations, etc.) and start the important process of developing rapport (see Chapter 7 for additional information on intake). The primary objectives of the group training *prior* to individual sessions are to: (a) increase client knowledge and awareness of voice and communication feminization therapy practices; (b) introduce specific voice and feminization techniques for home practice (or masculinization for trans men); and (c) determine client understanding of and commitment to the individual therapy process. Furthermore, this type of group training provides a means to introduce group members to the clinician's approach so as to reduce confusion and misunderstandings once the person begins individual voice and communication training.

It was suggested that group training prior to individual training consist of the following target areas:

- Client education, breathing, and relaxation techniques
- Resonance techniques
- Pitch and pitch range
- Intonation and lexical features
- Nonverbal communication
- Self-assessment

Mordaunt suggests eight weekly sessions in order to cover the information, implement a schedule for practice, and introduce (not master) voice and communication strategies. Video feedback is introduced and short, staged conversations are videotaped and evaluated. Toward the end of the group, clinicians work with group members to recognize improvements made and use journaling to reflect on their experiences in conversation outside the group.

Group training *after* individual training is not always necessary, but there can be enormous benefits for some individuals after successful completion of individual voice and communication sessions. According to Mordaunt (2012), the primary objectives of the group training *after* individual training are to: (a) increase the client's ability to generalize learned skills to daily living; (b) provide ongoing support as the client continues to make adjustments to her voice and communication; and (c) encourage the client to challenge herself to continue to improve communication skills.

The skill and number of group participants can vary, and the length of sessions, duration of each group, and topics of discussion can be designed to address the specific needs of the group members. Sessions of 60 to 90 minutes for four to six weeks may be ideal for this type of group. Target areas will include generalization of skills, client self-awareness, client self-assessment, and support. Techniques used for generalization include increasing the duration for using a particular technique or strategy, sharing conversation with specific communication partners, implementing skills in a variety of settings, and using "trigger" or key phrases to encourage use of strategies or techniques. The manner by which the generalization strategies are introduced and implemented will be dictated by the clinician in collaboration with the group members.

Like the pre-individual group training, videotaping and journaling can be applied to support generalization in groups after individual training. Some clients will utilize this group to gain support as they spend increased time applying their voice and communication strategies outside of training sessions. Specific situational challenges can be established that allow the group members to increase their conversational opportunities outside the group context.

Hybrid Group and Individual Training

Changing Keys is a program described by Davies and Goldberg (2006) that provides voice and communication training with both individual and group components. As described in the authors' earlier publication, individual sessions are accompanied by six two-hour group sessions that meet on a weekly basis. Four activities are built into the group sessions: (a) an update on the previous week's practice and accomplishments, (b) vocal training that focuses on resonant voice, (c) exercises about specific aspects of voice and communication, and (d) informational discussion of topics relevant to transgender voice and communication (Davies & Goldberg, 2006).

In a recent document, "Principles of *Changing Keys*," Davies (2016) states that *Changing Keys* is designed to provide free and accessible services to transgender women throughout British Columbia, Canada. Practicing speech-language pathologists and students are invited to take part in the program after meeting specific criteria, which provides a context for individual attention during group activities. As such, clinicians serve as important facilitators throughout the program.

Careful assessment is done before and after the program sessions, providing the ability to individualize services, even in the group setting. Refresher sessions are offered a few months after the program or during ongoing drop-in sessions. During the program (referred to as a course), participants in groups of six people focus on voice, with emphasis on evidence-based practice strategies to modify speaking pitch, pitch range, intonation, resonance, voice placement, voice quality, and articulatory contact. The program's manual provides information that each group participant can read beforehand, so there is increased practice time within the group. Most of the "class time" in *Changing Keys* is used to provide individual voice and speech training with the support of the facilitating clinicians. The group format offers opportunities for short discussion of issues, which provides valuable practice for each member of the group. Finally, home practice is integrated into the program to habituate voice change (Davies, 2016).

The transgender voice and communication modification at The College of Saint Rose, like *Changing Keys*, has group and individual components (Pickering, 2015; Pickering & Kayajian, 2009, 2014). The group meets for two hours each Monday evening in the college's speech and hearing center. In the fall and spring semesters, 12 meetings are held; in the summer, 9 meetings take place. Data gathered over the first five years of the program indicated that approximately 75% of the clients spent approximately one year (three semesters) as members of the program (Pickering & Kayajian, 2014). The Saint Rose program incorporates both individual and group components with the help of graduate students studying speech-language pathology.

Intake information and baseline data are gathered in the beginning of a group member's experience in the program and then every four to six months. The program's first group members helped create the intake questions so that the forms would be sensitive to the individual's needs and concerns. As noted above, graduate student clinicians (five to seven per semester) serve as supportive communication partners and coaches within the program.

The program follows a specific series of activities each evening:

- Mindfulness/relaxation/awareness
- Vocal health and vocal warm-up
- Group communication skill development
- Individual intervention
- Gratitude

As mentioned in an earlier section, the focus of mindfulness activities is often on breathing and upper body tension, but self-esteem, feelings, and attitudes are also explored. The evening ends with shared grat-

itude and an opportunity to provide feedback from a collective, positive perspective (Holland & Nelson, 2014). Activities used to facilitate voice modification during group warm-up are based on evidence-based practice approaches in voice disorders: Vocal Function Exercises (VFEs; Stemple, Glaze, & Klaben, 2010) and Resonant Voice Therapy (Verdolini-Marston, Burke, Lessac, Glaze, & Caldwell, 1995). These approaches, adapted for transgender individuals, are described in Behrman and Haskell (2013). Aspects of straw phonation have recently been added to facilitate a clear voice, forward resonance, and decreased effort (Kapsner-Smith, Hunter, Kirkham, Cox, & Titze, 2015). Straw phonation provides an alternative approach to facilitating forward resonance and a clearer, less effortful voice.

As these techniques are implemented, clients are exposed to and practice target frequencies that are consistent with an adult cisfemale voice (notes F3–A3; 175–220 Hz). Tablet technology and apps that respond to fundamental frequency (electronic pianos, guitar tuners, etc.) are applied to support the group member's change in pitch. Vocal warm-up is a critical part of each session, and expectations for the group members may be different and may change as the semester progresses.

In addition to a focus on voice and resonance, the program targets other aspects of communication in both group and individual parts of the session. Clients and clinicians collaborate on group lessons that focus on a variety of communication components, including pitch and inflection, resonance, articulation, loudness and projection, nonverbal communication, language, and nonverbal vocalization (like coughing or laughing). Ice breakers are sometimes incorporated into the group portion of the session to facilitate communication. After a group lesson, the individualized portion of the program is implemented, where each client's individual goals are addressed with the help of a student clinician. This individual component takes up approximately 45 minutes of each two-hour session.

At WPATH's 2014 Biennial Symposium, a series of "lessons learned" over the first 5 years of the Saint Rose program were described (Pickering & Kayajian, 2014). Demographically, the 56 group participants were an average age of 46.37 years (range: 18–75 years). More recently, the group has included more young adults and some adolescents. The mean number of semesters attended was 2.73 (approximately 10 months). Student-based research suggests that the activities of the group are capable of changing listener perception of gender, specifically pitch and inflection, resonance/tone, loudness, and nonverbal communication.

The group context was shown to improve self-esteem as judged by the clients and listeners, although there was occasionally a perceptual mismatch between client-speakers and clinician-listeners. Furthermore, case studies indicated that voice change (increased fundamental frequency and pitch) was attainable, and VFEs and biofeedback appeared to support the change. In addition to voice, clients identified other important aspects of communication that facilitated improved communication, including nonverbal communication, projection, and resonance (Baker, 2010).

Transfer and maintenance of voice change have been elusive for some people in the program, even with encouragement to practice on a daily basis. As a result, classroom visits are implemented to provide a context for voice and communication practice, as well as self-advocacy. During the class visits, group participants tell their stories and help students in the class learn about the transgender experience. Cultural competence was noted to improve when the transgender individuals shared their stories with others.

Finally, the group context appeared to be effective according to feedback generated by the program clients, and the students' role of clinician-counselor is an important one (Baker, 2010; Pickering & Kayajian, 2014).

Summary and Conclusion

What can we glean from this investigation of group training for people who are transgender and seeking services in voice and communication modification?

1. Group training provides an opportunity to share information and provide support for participants involved in transgender voice and communication modification.
2. Group training encourages collaboration, self-advocacy, and leadership for both group members and facilitators.
3. Group training can take many forms and can be an alternative or complement to individual training.
4. Group training provides a context for applying evidence-based practice in voice training and can be enhanced with careful, ongoing assessment.
5. Group training provides a context for applying creative activities that facilitate community building and conversation in a naturalistic environment.
6. Group training allows students and practicing speech-language pathologists to share in the provision of voice and communication training.

For those who are transgender or gender non-conforming, groups are often viewed as classes or courses that are provided to support voice and communication modification. For practicing clinicians, they are a context for service provision, research, and in some cases clinical education. A less formal approach to the group training described above is the application of workshops or open houses that may: (a) introduce transgender individuals to appropriate and effective voice and communication services, (b) be a helpful means of supplementing individual training, or (c) facilitate the maintenance of skills learned in group sessions (Block, 2015).

As the research increases in transgender voice and communication training, there is likely to be an increase in the application and study of group training as a potential option for intervention. This is reflected in recent presentations at the ASHA Convention and the biennial WPATH Symposium (e.g., Waller & Penzell, 2016). Issues of access and client need may make group training programs increasingly appealing, and the benefits of group intervention, alone or as part of a larger training program, should be considered by clinicians providing services to those who are transgender. This would be the case for all people who are gender non-conforming, not just those transitioning from male to female.

References

Adler, R. K., Hirsch, S., & Mordaunt, M. (2012). *Voice and communication therapy for the transgender/transsexual client: A comprehensive clinical guide* (2nd ed.). San Diego, CA: Plural Publishing, Inc.

Arnott, S., Onslow, M, O'Brien, S., Packman, S., Jones, M., & Block, S. (2014). Group Lidcombe Program treatment for early stuttering: A randomized controlled trial. *Journal of Speech, Language, and Hearing Research, 57*(5) 1606–1618.

Backus, O. L., & Dunn, H. M. (1947). Intensive group therapy in speech rehabilitation. *Journal of Speech Disorders, 12*(1), 36–60.

Baker, L. (2010). *The effect of voice feminization therapy on listener and client perceptions of gender and vocal communication for MtF transsexuals*. Unpublished master's thesis, The College of Saint Rose, Albany, NY.

Behrman, A., & Haskell, J. (2013). *Exercises for voice therapy* (2nd ed.). San Diego, CA: Plural Publishing.

Bilgehan, E. (2015). The use of music interventions to improve social skills in adolescents with autism spectrum disorders in integrated group music therapy sessions. *Procedia—Social and Behavioral Sciences, 197*(25), 207–213.

Block, C. (2015, February). *Diagnostic and training considerations for transgender speakers*. A presentation at the Mid-South Conference on Communication Disorders, Memphis TN.

Caughter, S., & Dunsmuir, S. (2017). An exploration of the mechanisms of change following an integrated group intervention for stuttering, as perceived by school-aged children who stutter (CWS). *Journal of Fluency Disorders, 51*(1), 8–23.

Chambers, R., Chuen Lee Yo, B., & Allen, N. B. (2008). The impact of intensive mindfulness training on attentional control, cognitive style, and affect. *Cognitive Therapy and Research Volume, 32* (3), 303–322.

Dahlberg, C. A., Cusick, C. P., Hawley, L. A., Newman, J. K., Morey, C. E., Harrison-Felix, C. L., & Whiteneck, G. G. (2007). Treatment efficacy of social communication skills training after traumatic brain injury: A randomized treatment and deferred treatment controlled trial. *Archives of Physical Medicine and Rehabilitation, 88*(12), 1561–1573.

Davies, S. (2016, November). *Principles of Changing Keys*. Vancouver, British Columbia: Author.

Davies, S., & Goldberg, J. M. (2006). Clinical aspects of transgender speech feminization and masculinization. *International Journal of Transgenderism, 9*(3–4), 167–196.

Davies, S., Papp, V., & Antoni, C. (2015). Voice and communication change for gender nonconforming individuals: Giving voice to the person inside. *International Journal of Transgenderism, 16*(3), 117–159.

Flasher, L. V., & Fogle, P. T. (2012). *Counseling skills for speech-language pathologists and audiologists* (2nd ed.). Clifton Park, NY: Delmar-Cengage Learning.

Harvard Mental Health Letter (2011, November). In praise of gratitude. *Harvard Health Publishing, Harvard Medical School*. Retrieved from https://www.health.harvard.edu/newsletter_article/in-praise-of-gratitude

Hofmann, S., Sawyer, A. T., Witt, A. A., & Oh, D. (2010). The effect of mindfulness-based therapy on anxiety and depression: A meta-analytic review.

Journal of Consulting and Clinical Psychology American Psychological Association 78 (2), 169–183.

Holland A. L., & Nelson, R. L. (2014). *Counseling on communication disorders: A wellness perspective* (2nd ed.). San Diego, CA: Plural Publishing.

Kabat-Zinn, J. (2003). Mindfulness-based interventions in context: Past, present, future. *Clinical Psychology: Science and Practice, 10*, 122–156.

Kapsner-Smith, M. R., Hunter, E. J., Kirkham, K., Cox, K., & Titze, I. R. (2015). A randomized controlled trial of two semi-occluded vocal tract voice therapy protocols. *Journal of Speech, Language, Hearing Research, 58*(3), 535–549.

Kayajian, D. (2005). *The perceptions of individuals who are male-to-female transsexuals/transgendered regarding voice, voice feminization, and non-verbal communication.* Unpublished master's thesis, The College of Saint Rose, Albany, NY.

Law, T, Lee, Y. S., Fiona, L., Ho, A. C., Vlantis, A. C., van Hasselt, A. C., & Tong, M. C. (2012). The effectiveness of group voice therapy: A group climate perspective. *Journal of Voice, 26*(2), 41–48.

Luterman, D. M. (2008). *Counseling persons with communication disorders and their families* (5th ed.). Austin, TX: Pro-Ed Inc.

McCready, V. Campbell, M., Crutchley, S., & Edwards, C. (2011). Doris: Becoming who you are: A voice and communication group program for a male to female transgender client. In S. Chabon & E. Cohn (Eds.), *The communication disorder casebook: Learning by example* (pp. 518–532). Upper Saddle River, NJ: Pearson Education, Inc.

Moore, A., & Malinkowski, P. (2009). Meditation, mindfulness and cognitive flexibility. *Conscious Cognition, 18*(1), 176–186.

Mordaunt, M. (2012). Group therapy. In R. Adler, S. Hirsch, & M. Mordaunt (Eds.), *Voice and communication therapy for the transgender/transsexual client: A comprehensive clinical guide* (2nd ed.). San Diego, CA: Plural Publishing, Inc.

Nickels, L. McDonald, B., & Mason, C. (2016). The impact of group therapy on word retrieval in people with chronic aphasia. *NeuroRehabilitation, 39*(1), 81–95.

Oates, J., & Dacakis, G. (2015). Transgender voice and communication: Research evidence underpinning voice intervention for male-to-female transsexual women. *SIG 3 Perspectives on Voice and Voice Disorders, 25*(2), 48–58.

Pickering, J. (2015). Transgender voice and communication: Introduction and international context. *SIG 3, Perspectives on Voice and Voice Disorders,* 25(1), 25–31.

Pickering, J., & Kayajian, D. (2009). Voice program assists transgender community. *ASHA Leader, 14*(3), 18–20.

Pickering, J. E., & Kayajian, D. (February, 2014). *Group voice and communication intervention: The first five years.* 2014 World Professional Association for Transgender Health Biennial Symposium, Bangkok, Thailand.

Seligman, M. (2012). *Flourish: A visionary new understanding of happiness and well-being.* New York, NY: Free Press.

Shapiro, S. L., Astin, J. A., Bishop, S. R., & Cordova, M. (2005). Mindfulness-based stress reduction for health care professionals: Results from a randomized trial. *International Journal of Stress Management, 12*, 164–176.

Shapiro, S. L., & Carlson, L. E. (2009). *The art and science of mindfulness integrating mindfulness into psychology and the helping professions.* Washington, DC: American Psychological Association.

Shapiro, S. L., Schwartz, G. E., & Bonner, G. (1998). Effects of mindfulness-based stress reduction on medical and premedical students. *Journal of Behavioral Medicine, 21*, 581–599.

Sherratt, S., & Simmons-Mackie, N. (2016). Shared humour in aphasia groups: "They should be called cheer groups." *Aphasiology, 30*(9), 1039–1057.

Simberg, S., Sala, E., Tuomainen, J., Sellman, J., & Rönnemaa, A. (2006). The effectiveness of group therapy for students with mild voice disorders: A controlled clinical trial. *Journal of Voice, 20*(1), 97–109.

Skelton, S. L., & Richard, J. T. (2016). Application of a motor learning treatment for speech sound disorders in small groups. *Perceptual and Motor Skills, 122*(3), 840–854.

Stemple, J. C., Glaze L. E., & Klaben, B. (2010). *Clinical voice pathology: Theory and management* (4th ed.). San Diego, CA: Plural Publishing.

Verdolini-Marston, K., Burke, M. K., Lessac, A., Glaze, L., & Caldwell, E. (1995). Preliminary study of two methods of treatment for laryngeal nodules. *Journal of Voice, 9*, 74–85.

Waller, N., & Penzell, S. (2016, November). *Be heard for who you are: A seven-week voice/communication program for transgender pediatric clients.* A presentation at the 2016 Annual Convention of the American Speech-Language-Hearing Association, Philadelphia, PA.

14

The Singing Voice

Anita L. Kozan and Sandra C. Hammond

Introduction

The conditioning of the singing voice of the individual who is making a life-changing transition is every bit as thrilling as it is demanding. The person's vocal range is shifting downward for the transmasculine individual, while the transfeminine individual is focusing on developing a higher range. Transgender people are literally, as well as figuratively, finding their "outer voice" with which to speak and sing, just as they are finally getting to express their "inner voice," the voice of their true identity as a human being. The most important guideline here is that there are no "right or wrongs" in what range or ranges in which the singer chooses to sing. That is as much a right of the individual and as personal a decision as is the decision to transition. Our work as clinicians who specialize in the care of the singing voice is to help the singer use their voice in the healthiest manner possible.

The focus on health care for transgender and gender non-conforming individuals has grown exponentially since this book's second edition was published in 2012. Speech-language clinicians, teachers of singing, choral directors, movement experts, psychologists, social workers, nurses, and physicians have begun or continue to

seek expertise in their chosen fields that supports the care of their transfeminine and transmasculine clients, students, and patients. Care of the voice now shares the stage at conferences focused on individuals across the gender spectrum. Websites, blogs, YouTube videos, and instructional methods including those using telecommunications are beginning to burgeon, with some focus on the singing voice as well as on the speaking voice. The World Professional Association for Transgender Health (WPATH) has expanded the Standards of Care (SOC) for Voice and Communication Therapy for transgender and gender non-conforming individuals. The SOC 7th Version asserts that speech-language pathologists who meet the educational and experiential guidelines are the primary providers of service. "Other professionals, such as vocal coaches, theatre professionals, singing teachers, and movement experts may play a valuable adjunct role. Such professionals will ideally have experience working with, or be actively collaborating with, speech-language pathologists." (WPATH SOC, V.7, 2015, p. 52). Fortunately, these collaborations are happening with greater frequency and regularity. Equally, select experienced speech-language clinicians who are also singers have applied singing techniques to the speaking voice as well as to the singing voice. Likewise, select classically trained and experienced teachers of singing, most notably Alexandros Constansis, have experimented with their own voices as they began to transition and then researched the application of principles to voice care for their students. Constansis (2009) applied his paradigm carefully to each transmasculine subject who participated in his research. His training as a classical singer and teacher brought knowledge to his work that is congruent with the knowledge that speech-language clinicians use when working on voice and speech disorders. In speech, language, and voice therapy, the principle of generalization, while frowned upon in the academic setting without research on each individual or group (Gerald Siegel, personal communication, June 14, 1995), is the stock-in-trade of speech-language clinicians who must rely on their experience of what does and does not work, as well as on knowledge of relevant research findings. This fact of clinical life is recognized and supported by the WPATH Standards of Care for speech-language pathologists. Indeed, the entire contents of the SOC (p. 2) are described as "flexible clinical guidelines." Clinical work in speech and communication science offers opportunities for pioneering observations in our fields by testing various therapy techniques and then communicating the observations to others who can consider whether or not to study them in a controlled research paradigm.

This chapter focuses on the research, observations, and experiences of the authors and highlights the work of a select group of transgender, gender non-conforming, and cisgender professionals whose practice includes the singing voice. It is our intention to highlight the importance of WPATH's Standards of Care for Voice and Communication Therapy and to present opportunities for greater understanding and inclusion of work on the singing voice in achieving healthy speaking and singing abilities, for transgender and gender non-binary individuals. Just as speech and language pathologists recognize, respect, and use our clients' preferred terms, the authors support WPATH's recognition and inclusion of teachers of singing and work on singing voice exercises in voice and communication care for all individuals who could benefit. Kozan (2016) reported that over 50% of the transfeminine, transmasculine, and gender non-binary individuals seen in her private practice engaged in some form of singing, ranging from singing alone in the car or shower to being paid to sing for an audience. Indeed, the acceptance of Holden Madagame, a trans man, into the UK's Glyndebourne Academy for continued development of his tenor voice for operatic singing, is an indication of the importance of the singing voice in the overall scope of voice and communication therapy for transgender clients. The authors look to WPATH to continue to enhance the Standards of Care for Voice and Communication Therapy, Assessment and Treatment Considerations with this addition: Treatment may also involve the use of singing voice exercises and interval training schedules to help clients preserve and develop the singing voice as well as improve the quality of the speaking voice (Kozan, 2012).

Music bypasses the cortex and goes directly to the limbic system, where it triggers emotion and memory. In a matter of moments, we can be moved to ecstasy or to tears (Jourdain, 1997). The beauty of the singing voice provides another channel for reaching out and connecting with others, as well as a way to connect deeply within ourselves. Helping transgender or gender non-conforming singers develop voices that they are proud to call their own is a humbling experience. To help with the birth of a voice . . . to hear the voice's song . . . few accomplishments are so truly thrilling. The power of music is indisputable.

Philosophy of Professional Voice

Qualifications of the Speech-Language Clinician

Not every speech and language pathologist will have the qualifications described below but perhaps will be the best qualified among the professionals available to work with transgender clients. Each professional is guided by conscience and by ethical standards when making decisions about what services can be offered. Advising the client about a lack of skill or experience but taking an "I'll give it a try" attitude is not good enough. The clinician must have sufficient knowledge not only to "do no harm" but also to know how to "do good," to skillfully judge and shape vocal behaviors, and to re-direct or withdraw any vocal task or exercise that is uncomfortable or unproductive for the client.

Clinicians who provide service to transgender people with specific focus on development or rehabilitation of the singing voice will best serve clients when they meet the WPATH Standards of Care for speech-language clinicians and:

■ possess knowledge and experience as singers
■ sing in tune, with and without the aid of accompaniment
■ read music, both treble and bass clef
■ understand the keyboard and use a tablature or notation system to document the client's vocal range
■ identify, describe, and demonstrate differences in vocal resonance, within their vocal range
■ understand the concept of passaggio
■ demonstrate vocal exercises, easy onset of vowels technique, and singing vocalises

Some clients are best served by a team of specialists: a speech-language clinician who specializes in the singing voice, an otolaryngologist who specializes in voice, and a teacher of singing who is skilled in working with individuals who are just learning to sing, as well as working with individuals who need to re-condition the voice or to condition a new range in the voice. The speaking voice trainer might be the fourth team member, using singing voice exercises to improve the quality of the speaking voice. The client will benefit when each member of the team brings experience and sensitivity to the individual client's needs, along with communication skills that enhance working with the other professionals as well as with the client. The American Speech-Language-Hearing Association (ASHA) convened an Ad Hoc Joint Committee together with the National Association of Teachers of Singing and the Voice and Speech Trainers Association and published a technical report entitled *The Role of the Speech-Language Pathologist, the Teacher of Singing, and the Speaking Voice Trainer in Voice Habilitation* (2005). The three organizations recognized "that the etiology of a voice disorder may be related to either improper singing or to improper speaking technique" (p. 1). They agreed on "the importance of interdisciplinary management of speakers and singers with voice problems and disorders" (p. 1). The group agreed that "multiple specialization" among speech and language pathologists, otolaryngologists, teachers of singing, and voice and speech trainers "is rare and that in most cases, the management team will need to consist of at least three individuals" (p. 2). The group concluded that each professional needed to acquire knowledge in the fields of the other professions in order to function successfully as part of the management team. This document supersedes ASHA's earlier publication on Voice and Communication Therapy for Transgender/

Transsexual Clients (1997–2001), which did not mention the possible role of the speech and language pathologist with the singing voice (ASHA Technical Report, 2005).

The increased interest among graduate students and clinical fellows in providing voice and communication therapy for transgender clients has led to a concern among the speech-language pathologists supervising those students. Barbara F. Worth, B.Mus., M.S., CCC-SLP is the Senior Voice Therapist at The Voice Center, Beth Israel Hospital, Harvard Medical School, specializing in care of transgender individuals, professional voice users, and singers, with 85–90% of her caseload focused on voice care for transgender clients. Worth recommended that all speech-language pathology students and interested clinicians need to have a knowledge base and experience with evaluation and treatment of basic voice disorders before focusing on voice care for transfeminine and transmasculine clients (B. Worth, personal communication, November 17, 2016). The WPATH SOC V.7 (p. 52), for speech-language clinicians, could be amended to list this criterion first: Specialized training and competence in the assessment and treatment of voice disorders in the general population (Kozan, 2016, 2017).

Professional Relationship with Clients

All clinicians develop a manner in which they interact with their clients. Kozan prefers to develop a collegial relationship with each individual. The initial evaluation provides an opportunity to describe how we will work together. This is the most common discussion of the topic with patients seen in a medical setting:

"I look at the work that we are undertaking as a journey that we will take together.

Yes, I am the doctor and you are the patient. But, I also work from the philosophy that you are the teacher and I am the student. I bring you all of my years of knowledge and experience and I will do everything possible to help you develop your voice in the healthiest manner possible. I don't know how far we will be able to go, but I will help you go as far as is possible. I ask you to bring up your observations about your voice and your experiences concerning anything and everything that could possibly have an effect on your voice. I look at our work as if we were putting a giant puzzle together. Each piece of information could provide another piece to the puzzle. Nothing is too insignificant to bring up in our discussions. It might lead to an insight or a brainstorm that helps us figure out another piece to the puzzle and takes us in a whole new direction with healing your voice."

"Each time we meet, I will write recommendations for the specific goals that I want you to concentrate on until our next appointment. Your goals will reflect your observations on your progress. The next time that we meet, we will start the therapy session by reviewing the progress you've made on your goals, then discuss your observations, work on specific tasks, and finally upgrade and set new goals."

Evaluation Considerations

Philosophy

Rehabilitation of the speaking voice normally precedes rehabilitation of the singing voice, or is carried out concurrently with someone who is singing professionally. The best of circumstances will allow for the singer to refrain from singing anything other than what the clinician has recommended. The transgender singer might have an injured speaking voice but a healthy singing technique, with the speaking voice injury adversely affecting the quality of the singing voice. Other singers might be experiencing difficulty only with their singing voice. However, this can occur before, during, or after their transition. If you have determined that the client's speaking voice is being produced in a healthy manner, the focus can be solely on the singing voice. Therapy for the transmasculine singer who is exploring a new vocal range previously unavailable to him focuses on conditioning the voice. Therapy for a singer who has injured his voice focuses on re-conditioning his voice. If the transgender singer has had a lengthy period of vocal rest from singing because of a vocal injury, his voice is viewed as being de-conditioned and the re-conditioning process must be done with even greater care.

Therapy for the transfeminine client involves exploring and conditioning a range of the voice that may have been used only rarely in the past. Again, work on the speaking voice will be important in demonstrating what might be possible for the singer, as well as beginning the conditioning process. For some transgender clients, work on singing provides the gateway to finding a healthy vocal range for their speaking voice. Women who have worked on developing their singing voice prior to transition might wish to continue to study with the same teacher of singing while they expand their range. Some women choose to sing in a range that includes lower notes than the range used for their speaking voice. Other women want to develop a range that will be perceived as clearly female. Some versatile (and talented) singers will pick their "part" in choral works depending upon their available range, singing an octave higher or lower, or singing with the baritones, tenors, or altos, as their range allows. These decisions belong to the singer. The role of the clinician is to help the singer develop a healthy vocal technique. The joy of being able to sing, wherever the range might be, will be its own reward.

Singer's History

The human voice is an instrument that can never be "put away in its case." Whatever we do with our entire body, day and night, has the potential for affecting the voice. Care of the voice is an art and a science. At the time of the evaluation, information about training, performances, rehearsal and performance conditions, and use of warm-up and cool-down exercises might be particularly relevant. The first meeting with the singer also presents an opportunity to ask what first name and pronouns to use when addressing the singer. The person's given name might still be used legally, but the singer should be given the opportunity to choose. Ask if there is any other information that the singer wants to share that will make your communication more comfortable for the singer.

Vocal Tasks

A formal voice evaluation for the singer can consist of as many or as few vocal tasks as are deemed necessary and appropriate for the individual client. The reader is referred to Sataloff (1997) for a detailed review of what might be included. Formal voice evaluations can include standard measures such as a prolonged /a/ ("ah") on any pitch that is comfortable for the client, held out as long as the person is able. This is the one time the clinician should ask the client to forcefully exhale to the very end of the breath. Perceptual judgments are made on the uniformity and clarity of voice quality, pitch stability, and voice volume. Repetitions of the /a/ task might be requested at different pitches or loudness levels. Observations of breath support can be made. A comparison of productions of voiceless /s/ with voiced /z/ gives some indication of glottal efficiency, as will comparing /z/ with /a/. Observations of vocal tremor in /a/ and /z/ can be compared with production of /s/. Hard glottal attacks or easy onsets on /a/ can be observed. The trained singer will be asked to sing the voiced phonemes in a "straight" tone, without vibrato, if possible, in the event that vibrato is spontaneously produced at all. Kozan uses these tasks for basic information about the singer's approach to the tasks as well as the results and does not quantify the results.

Glissandi

Glissandi, slides across pitches, are demonstrated for imitation or requested for production. The singer produces:

- a descending glissando from mid-range to the lowest end of the vocal range,
- an ascending glissando from the lowest end to the mid-range,
- an ascending glissando from the mid-range to the highest end of the range,
- a descending glissando from the highest end to the mid-range,
- a descending glissando from the highest end all the way to the lowest end.

The singer should not force the pitch to either end of the range and is asked to sing softly on all tasks. Observations are made of consistency in quality, changes in quality across the passaggio and between the registers, prevalence of vocal fry/glottal

fry in the lowest end of the pitch range or in the mid-range due to lack of breath release, and changes in quality in the higher range of the voice. The ability to freely slide across pitches indicates good flexibility of the larynx and freedom from "muscling" the sound. If a singer has trouble descending the scale, it can suggest some difficulty with the normal relaxation of vocal fold tension for pitch lowering. If the singer has trouble ascending the scale, it can suggest some difficulty with the normal increase in tension, and might suggest that there is some weakness in one or both vocal folds.

Vocal Range

A piano, electronic keyboard, or one of many free or inexpensive smartphone apps will be useful in documenting the singer's vocal range and can help document changes over time. Start where the singer is most comfortable, usually in the mid-range. Ask the singer to sing softly down the scale, pausing to breathe whenever needed. Notice any changes in quality as the lowest pitches are reached. Ask the singer to identify when it becomes more difficult to sing. Encourage the singer to stop singing if there is discomfort. Go back to mid-range and have the singer move up the scale, again singing softly and breathing freely. Document notes where there is a change in quality or anything that suggests greater strain. Ask the singer to stop if any note becomes uncomfortable. Remind the client to sing softly if loudness increases on the upper notes. Stop the singer if the production is noticeably strained. Ask how it felt to sing those high notes. Return to the mid-range and let the singer produce a few notes that are more comfortable, both for the brief physiological cool-down effect and for the psychological comfort to the singer.

It helps to use a notation system to write down the extent of the vocal range and to identify particular notes where the singer has difficulty or makes a transition in quality. One commonly used system references Middle C as C4, the first key of the fourth octave of the acoustic piano. Any note that falls within that octave has the number 4 after it. E4, two whole steps above Middle C (4) is often called the passaggio,[1] the passage between the chest voice (modal register) and the head voice (loft register) or falsetto (Colton & Hollien, 1973). A trained singer will work on technique that allows a smooth transition across the passaggio, balancing the work of the cricothyroid muscles that tilt the larynx and aid in higher pitch production with the work of the thyroartytenoid muscles within the vocal folds that shorten and relax the vocal folds. Observations will allow for development of therapeutic vocal exercises for specific notes or areas of the vocal range that the singer finds troublesome.

Documentation of the vocal range allows for demonstration of changes over time. Singers are appreciative of the information about the changes in their performance and will often request to check their range. Singers can use the information to help them when they are practicing vocalises or specific songs. The singer's range may vary somewhat from day to day, depending on factors including vocal and/or physical fatigue, hydration, failure to use warm-up exercises, illness, and hydration, as well as breath support and vocal technique.

[1] Richard Miller places this at D4 in *Training Tenor Voices*, p.3

A Transfeminine Singer's Fear

You aren't going to make me warm up my lower range, are you? My voice teacher kept insisting that I vocalize the entire extent of my range, and it really upset me to do that. I told her how I felt about it but she still made me do it.

– Transfeminine professional singer to Kozan during first therapy appointment

The transfeminine singer who has not used the falsetto range might not be able to vocalize in that range at all or might show a dramatic shift in quality. The highly trained transfeminine singer might have already been working on carefully developing her upper range. Some singers will want to demonstrate the entire range, including the male pitch range, while others will clearly avoid it. If the singer does not offer the information, ask how she feels about demonstrating her lower range. Be respectful of her wishes if she does not wish to sing any of her lower notes. Each singer brings her own special abilities and concerns. It is our responsibility to make sure that we know how to teach to each individual's needs.

A Transmasculine Singer's Fear

I was always known for my beautiful upper range. It's hard for me to think about never being able to perform those songs ever again like I did for so many years.

—Transmasculine professional singer to Kozan at the beginning of his transition

The transmasculine singer could show a wide variety of abilities, depending on how long hormones have been taken, how large a dosage has been used, and how the singer has responded to the medication. The desire for a lower-pitched voice sometimes creates a muscle tension dysphonia (MTD) that results in the singer reporting that very few of the pitches are comfortably sung (Adler,

Constansis, & Van Borsel, 2012; Constansis, 2008, 2009, 2013; Kozan, 2005, 2006, 2012). Some transmasculine singers do not want to have a high range anymore, wishing to concentrate only on their lower range, while other singers are sad to lose their upper range and wish to retain as many notes as possible (Adler et al., 2012; Constansis, 2008, 2009, 2013; Kozan, 2005, 2006, 2012).

All singers, no matter what their personal or vocal circumstances, deserve to be accepted where they are, and complimented on what they have achieved thus far. Whether they have just a few usable notes or more than three octaves worth, they are embarking on a journey of trust in placing their most precious instrument, the voice, in clinical care. It behooves every clinician to reach for the highest possible standard of care.

Videostroboscopic Evaluation

The intricate workings of the singer's voice are made visible through the use of videoendolaryngoscopy with stroboscopy. This evaluation is not required for the singer with a healthy voice, but is highly useful for understanding problems in the singing and the speaking voice, including vocal hyperfunction, vocal fold weakness, and changes in the surface epithelium of the folds. Even without stroboscopic light, the use of a flexible fiberscope, video camera, VCR, computer, light source, and monitor allows us to see the larynx and surrounding structures while voice is being produced. Examination using a flexible scope allows the singer to speak and sing in a fairly natural laryngeal posture. Comparisons of the laryngeal structures while the singer is speaking and while singing can provide important information that is useful in determining the best course of voice habilitation or rehabilitation. Evaluation using the flexible scope

with stroboscopic light allows for viewing of the vocal folds as if they were opening and closing in slow motion. The information about patterns of vocal fold vibration provides opportunities for important judgments that can help explain problems that the singer is experiencing.

Evaluation using the rigid endoscope provides a greatly enlarged view of the vocal folds and their patterns of movement. Judgments of singing voice are not possible because the tongue is extended during the examination and the pull on the vocal folds gives an inaccurate picture of vocal fold closure and ventricular (false) vocal fold positioning. However, the rigid scope is particularly useful for detecting lesions and injuries to the folds.

Both transmasculine and transfeminine singers can benefit greatly from this type of evaluation. The opportunity to view the vocal folds while the voice is being produced can be a powerful motivator as well as provide a picture to be visualized when rehearsing. The clinician should give the singer an opportunity to learn about the anatomy and physiology of the larynx before the examination is carried out, whenever possible. The singer can also choose certain songs or vocal tasks that are easy or challenging. Judgments of possible hyperfunction or other technical errors can be made.

Singing Voice Research

Transmasculine Singers

Prior to Alexandros N. Constansis' publications, no research on the transgender singing voice existed. A paper written by Max Gries, "Transgender Voices" (2004), surveyed the literature from medical, physiological, and therapeutic standpoints. His search revealed "a complete lack of useful data for transgender singers: when singing is mentioned, it is only cursorily" (p. 15). Adler and Van Borsel (2006) noted the need for research on the singing voice in transgender individuals. They cautioned transmasculine singers that taking hormones permanently alters the range of the voice and results in an overall reduction in pitch range (Van Borsel et al., 2000).

Alexandros N. Constansis, Ph.D., has made a major contribution to singing voice rehabilitation for transmasculine singers. A classically trained singer and teacher, Constansis was concerned about protecting his singing voice as he began his transition in 2003. The publication of his seminal dissertation research entitled *The Changing Female-to-Male (FTM) Voice* (2008, 2009) has resulted in Constansis' research being widely read and respected among the transmasculine and gender non-binary community, particularly by those who sing or aspire to do so. Constansis was one of three authors of Chapter 8 in the second edition of this book (2012) and presented his pioneering research findings in Amsterdam at the WPATH Conference (June 20, 2016) as well as at conferences in the UK, Europe, and Australia across the previous decade.

Constansis developed his vocal exercise regimen based on his own previous experiences and carefully nurtured his well-trained singing voice during use of gradual hormone replacement therapy (HRT), which began with much smaller dosages which were slowly titrated. After serving as his own pilot research subject for his Ph.D. dissertation research in Musicology (2008, 2009), he studied the changing transmasculine voice and systematically used diaphragmatic breathing and vocal exercises with his students as part of his research. His vocal exercises emphasized classic breathing and

speech warm-up techniques, based on the Accent Method of Svend Smith (1976) and on the work of Jo Estill, speech-language pathologist and teacher of singing, whose method was published posthumously by Steinhauser, McDonald Klimek, and Estill (2017).

Constansis' singing exercises included classic exercises from the *Bel Canto* method. The first major goal with each of the transmasculine subjects in his doctoral research was to retrain their diaphragmatic breathing in order to move away from a breathing style higher in the chest. He found it important to be in the room and supervise each subject while doing the work in order to facilitate learning the correct technique. He taught diaphragmatic breathing in the postures of lying down, standing against a wall, sitting, and then standing unsupported. He used a mirror for feedback for the research subjects (Constansis, Pedagogical Note 1, 2008, 2009). Constansis moved his research subjects to a set of exercises practiced daily, once diaphragmatic breath support had been established (Constansis, Pedagogical Note 2, 2008, 2009). Each subject began with 5 minutes of simple breathing exercises where he exhaled soundlessly through the mouth. He then performed 5 minutes of exhaling on /v/, slowly and then gradually accelerating his pace. This was followed by 10 minutes of rhythmic breathing exercises using /s/ and /z/, with variation in softness and rhythm. He then had the subjects produce 5 minutes of indefinite pitch exercises, such as "sirens" with the mouth shut or "ng" as in "sing" with the mouth open. Each subject was encouraged to explore his full range during this exercise. The fifth exercise was a more controlled pitch exercise using lip trills or rolled /r/ sounds on melody lines of easy to moderate difficulty. The next exercise was focused on carrying over the previously practiced principles and vocal placement to exercises with soft open and closed vowels. The subject was cautioned against using anything louder than a *mezzo piano* (medium soft) voice volume. The subject was also encouraged to use his falsetto when the notes became accessible, as this is a normal part of the male vocal ability. Finally, all of the previously practiced principles were carried over into parts of simple folk songs and ultimately to pieces from the Niccolo Vaccaj method (1999),[2] as referenced by Constansis (2008, 2009 Pedagogical Notes, footnote 3).

Constansis adjusted the key signature of the song to accommodate the available range of the singer. He took his subjects into more demanding sung literature only when they had reached the final stages of vocal transition. The singer subjects who had used an abrupt dosage of HRT, 250 mg bimonthly for 12 months, demonstrated moderate gains in pitches, with the subject in their 20s gaining an average of six pitches, and with the average gradually dropping across the age decades to a gain of four pitches for the subject in their 50s. Participants who used a gradual dosage of HRT, 100 mg bimonthly for 6 months, and then 200–250 mg for the remaining six months, showed improved results when compared with those who used an abrupt dosage. The subject in their 20s added nine pitches to their range and the subject in their 30s added seven pitches. The subject in their 40s added six pitches using gradual dosage, while the subject in their 50s added five pitches. Constansis concluded that using gradual HRT with soft vocal exercises can help the transmasculine singer not only to retain his singing voice quality but also to acquire a new, aesthetically pleasing quality, although there are challenges. His research documented the effects of the subjects' age

at transition as well as the value of using a gradual dosage of HRT along with a careful program of vocal exercises. Constansis reported that he considers his research paradigm to be outdated, and encourages transmasculine singers to seek information on the current best practices for hormone titration (2012). His research has also contributed to understanding the "entrapped" feeling some transmasculine singers and speakers experience after taking testosterone, caused by enlargement of their vocal folds within the fixed structure of the thyroid cartilage, which is not affected by taking testosterone.

Transfeminine Singers

Transfeminine singing voice development is also an important topic for research on the singing voice. There are no known studies reported at this time. However, Sandi Hammond, founder and former director of the Butterfly Transgender Chorus in Boston, MA, USA, will discuss the experiences of transmasculine, transfeminine, and gender non-binary choral singers in later sections of this chapter. The author also recommends the M.Phil. dissertation in Music entitled "The Very Model of a Modern, Major Gender Role: Toward a Transgender Voice in Musicology" (Univ. of Cambridge, 2014), Henry Stoll's tour de force examines the absence of focus on issues of transgenderism within musical studies, aspects of voice and trans identity, how trans singers on stage might affect the operatic institution, and what contributes to the erasure of trans identities. He describes how composers and performers such as Susie Self, a classically trained opera singer who has sung male opera roles, have shaken and stirred the establishment to see opera performance through a new lens, all of which will leave the reader breathless and delighted with Stoll's observations and challenges.

---

[2] Readers seeking books written by Niccolo Vaccai (Vaccaj) will also find them listed under Nicola Vaccai or Vaccaj.

Singing Voice Development and Rehabilitation

I know you said to sing softly and only for 15 minutes, but I was so excited to finally sing in my upper register as a woman that I sang for 45 minutes—loudly. Now I'm having problems and my voice hasn't come back.

—Transfeminine trained singer to Kozan when returning to therapy with a newly injured voice

The majority of transgender and gender non-conforming clients enter therapy with healthy voices and immediately focus on development of a new vocal range. Occasionally a client will demonstrate signs of a vocal injury at the beginning of therapy or rarely will injure their voice during the therapy process. Each singer will require the clinician's expertise in designing the safest recommendations for the individual's healthy voice rehabilitation and singing development.

The techniques used by Kozan with people who are transgender include ones used with cisgender singers, as well as techniques specifically adapted for trans singers. The "Singing Vocalises" section of this chapter also includes techniques used in Constansis' (2008, 2009) research with transmasculine singers. Those techniques are also based on techniques used by classically trained singers and were adapted specifically for the subjects in Constansis' study.

Warm-Up and Cool-Down Vocalises

The vocal development program for the singing voice begins with knowledge that the singer is also working on voice care of the speaking voice. If the clinician is satisfied that the speaking voice is being used in a healthy manner, work can focus on the singing voice. If there is concern about the speaking voice as well as the singing voice, rehabilitation of the speaking voice must come first or be done conjointly, particularly with the working professional singer. Simple singing voice exercises are often useful as an aspect of speaking voice rehabilitation that can segue into work on the singing voice. Vocal warm-ups can be demonstrated and written out for the client, demonstrated and imitated on a recording specifically made for the client such as on a smartphone, or carried out through use of a CD of recorded voice exercises such as *Healing Voices, Volume 1: Relax and Breathe* (Kozan, 2002). Vocal cool-down exercises are carried out after a person has used the voice in a demanding way, such as by prolonged or loud talking or singing. The same exercises as were used for the warm-up now act as a cool-down, flushing lactic acid from the laryngeal muscles, releasing heat from the muscles, and again acting as a massage. Kozan began recommending cool-down vocalises after hearing the concept presented by Alfred Lavorato (1984), speech and language pathologist, at the international Voice Symposium at the Julliard School of Music in New York. Although Lavorato brought the exercises to her attention, he noted that the concept of cooling down (or warming down) the voice was first presented in a column written by the editor of *Etude* magazine in the 1950s (A. Lavorato, personal communication, June 1984). Kozan used cool-down exercises only with singers at first. Now, all clients are encouraged to cool down the voice, both after prolonged speaking and after prolonged singing.

Warm-Up/Cool-Down Format for the Speaking Voice

Warming up the voice for speaking is part of every singer's voice care program. The vocal exercises begin with simple, descending glissandi (slides across pitches) proceeded by /h/, which helps the client learn to release air at the beginning of sound production and avoids a hard glottal attack. This exercise combines goals of good diaphragmatic breath support with a relaxed, soft, breathy production of sound. It also acts like a gentle massage of the vocal folds through use of soft voice and through lengthening and shortening the folds with increasing and decreasing pitches. Although some clinicians prefer to immediately focus on a technique with greater vocal fold adduction, the Kozan prefers the "massage" of this approach, which can be shaped toward a tone with greater adduction as the client progresses, if that appears to be helpful. Many singers prefer to continue with the more relaxed technique, especially for the first few exercises, because it is a less effortful and a safe technique.

The exercises continue with an increase in length of the utterance by going from consonant-vowel syllables, to initial /h/ words, to initial /hwh/ words, to imitated sentences with increased pitch inflection, and then to spontaneous sentence production. If the warm-up or cool-down vocal exercises are being used in conjunction with singing vocalises, the single syllables and sentence productions precede the warm-up vocalises. Cool-down exercises can consist of some vocalises alone, some of the speaking voice vocal exercises alone, or a combination of the two.

Speaking Voice Rehabilitation with Simple Singing Exercises

The simplest exercises can be carried out by singers and non-singers alike and are helpful for the speaking voice as well as for the singing voice. One of the goals for many individuals is to extend their vocal range, either to strengthen the upper notes for transfeminine speakers or to strengthen the lower notes for transmasculine speakers. The soft, slow movement of the voice from one note to a note just above it and then back down to the starting note is simple, does not depend on any knowledge of music, and is safe for the voice. It can be demonstrated by the clinician and imitated by the client. It is valuable even when the client does not produce the same pitch as the model, goes somewhat higher and/or lower than the model, and starts on a different note when repeating it. Untrained singers can use a soft voice and work independently on gradually training their vocal folds to produce pitches adjacent to their more secure pitches.

Transfeminine clients are usually able to judge when they are getting into the upper part of their range that needs strengthening. Working gently and softly on those notes helps to strengthen them. The same applies to the transmasculine client who can work softly and gently on those notes that are closer to the bottom of his range. These notes should be sung with caution. All trans and gender non-binary clients will benefit from use of an interval training schedule, which is discussed later in this chapter. Kozan acknowledges Jeannette LoVetri, founder of The Voice Workshop NYC, and creator and teacher of Somatic Voicework℠ The LoVetri Method (2006), for her decades of contributions to the international voice community, and for her valuable courses on how to use simple speaking and singing exercises to safely strengthen and increase vocal range and flexibility in the singing voice as well as the speaking voice. Her work on helping singers create a "mixed" voice quality by adding breath to their chest or modal register is comparable to classic voice therapy techniques used to help trans and gender non-binary speakers and singers achieve their voice goals.

Singing Vocalises

The vocalises discussed in this chapter were organized for dissertation research that investigated the perceptual effects of vocal warm-up on the singing voice (Kozan, 1995). Kozan's research results demonstrated that 20 experienced teachers of singing could consistently identify the warmed-up voices of 39 of 40 subjects, based on choosing the voice that had greater clarity and uniformity of voice quality. The judges correctly chose the warmed-up voice of 9 of 10 classically trained female singers, age range 20–29; 10 of 10 untrained singers who could carry a tune, age range 20–29; 10 of 10 classically trained singers, age range 50–69; and 10 of 10 untrained singers who could carry a tune, age range 50–69. Warm-up vocal exercises were beneficial regardless of the age and vocal training of the subjects. Transmasculine, transfeminine, and gender non-binary singers have successfully used Kozan's vocalises in their voice work since that time.

Most of the vocalises are familiar to trained singers. Singers who are untrained might need to have the vocalises written out or demonstrated on a recording. Some professional singers bring their guitars to the appointment to learn the vocalises, if they do not have a keyboard at home. The vocalises can also be sung a cappella (without accompaniment) if the singer has enough ability to do so. Regardless, the goal is focused on relaxed, soft singing. Although there is just one study of transmasculine singers and the effects of vocal exercises (Constansis, 2008, 2009) and there are no studies of transfeminine singers, a study of acoustic measures for cisgender singers, pre- and post-vocal warm-up, found that warm-up reduced frequency-perturbation and amplitude-perturbation values, increased the singer's formant amplitude, and improved the noise-to-harmonic ratio. Tone matching accuracy was not affected by vocal warm-up (Amir, Amir, & Michaeli, 2005).

Vocalises were compiled for use in research on perceptual judgments of the singing voice (Kozan, 1995). Musical charts were created by Rochelle Milbrath, trained singer and speech and language pathologist, using MuseScore (2011), free music composition and notation software (version 1.0). The first two vocal exercises noted in Figures 14-1 and 14-2 are self-explanatory, and may be done in the individual's comfortable range. Following are the vocalise exercises which are shown in Figures 14-3 to 14-7.

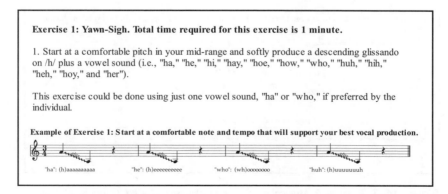

Exercise 1: Yawn-Sigh. Total time required for this exercise is 1 minute.

1. Start at a comfortable pitch in your mid-range and softly produce a descending glissando on /h/ plus a vowel sound (i.e., "ha," "he," "hi," "hay," "hoe," "how," "who," "huh," "hih," "heh," "hoy," and "her").

This exercise could be done using just one vowel sound, "ha" or "who," if preferred by the individual.

Example of Exercise 1: Start at a comfortable note and tempo that will support your best vocal production.

"ha": (h)aaaaaaaaaa   "he": (h)eeeeeeeeee   "who": (wh)ooooooooo   "huh": (h)uuuuuuuh

Figure 14–1. Exercise 1: Yawn-Sigh. Courtesy of Anita L. Kozan © 2011.

Exercise 2: Speaking sentences. Total time required for this exercise is 1 minute.
Read the following sentences, all beginning with initial /h/ (e.g., "hot" or "hike") or /hw/ (e.g., "what" or "whether") words, out loud. Say the sentences or phrases with a smooth, legato delivery, using a soft voice and a wide pitch range.

1. Hot weather comes in July.
2. Heat helps relax our muscles.
3. Hike up the trail to Lake Superior.
4. Haste makes waste.
5. Home is a great place to relax.
6. Help me to carry in the groceries.
7. Hoist up the sail.
8. When is your next client?
9. Why aren't you coming with us?
10. Which one do you like better?
11. How can I help you?
12. Whose pen is this?
13. Hug your family and friends.
14. Hawks soared lazily overhead.
15. Her voice sounds so beautiful.
16. Happy Birthday!
17. His voice is so soothing.
18. What time is it?
19. Where are my keys?
20. Whether we'll get to go is still unknown.

Figure 14–2. Exercise 2: Speaking sentences. Courtesy of Anita L. Kozan © 2011.

Exercise 3: Total time required for this exercise is 4 minutes.

1. Starting on a comfortable note in your lower mid-range, sing an ascending and descending glissando up and down an interval of a third (1-3-1), and then sing the notes one at a time (1-2-3-2-1), moving smoothly throughout all the notes.
2. Advance the starting note by a half-step and repeat.
3. Continue with this pattern until the top note sung approaches your higher range. Now repeat the entire exercise, beginning at your top starting note and descending the starting point of each repetition by a half-step. Proceed back to the initial starting note you used at the very beginning of this exercise.

Remember to sing all passages softly.

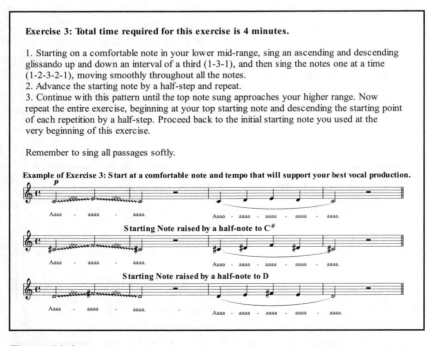

Figure 14–3. Exercise 3: Musical charts for vocalise exercise #3. Courtesy of Anita L. Kozan © 2011.

Exercise 4: Total time required for this exercise is 1 minute.

1. Starting on a comfortable note in your lower range, sing an ascending glissando up the octave (1-8), a descending glissando down the octave (8-1), followed by an ascending and descending glissando over the same octave (1-8-1), choosing from the sounds "nah," " næh" (as in "nap"),"no," "new," "mah," "mæh" (as in "map"), "mow," or "moo."
2. Advance the next starting note by a half-step and repeat.
3. Continue with this pattern until the top note sung approaches your higher range. Now repeat the entire exercise, beginning at your top starting note and descending the starting point of each repetition by a half-step. Proceed back to the initial starting note you used at the beginning of this exercise.

[Note: The starting and ending notes do not need to be precise, nor are you required to practice the exercise for every vowel sound listed. The goal is to freely slide across the pitches.]

Example of Exercise 4: Start at a comfortable note and tempo that will support your best vocal production.

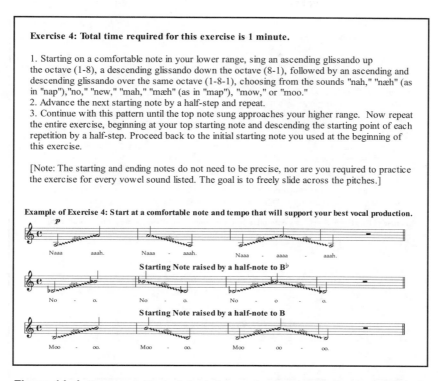

Figure 14–4. Exercise 4: Musical charts for vocalise exercise #4. Courtesy of Anita L. Kozan © 2011.

Vocalise #3 (see Figure 14–3) teaches an exercise that has proven to be of great value to many singers, regardless of their level of training or laryngeal status. It begins with an ascending glissando (smooth slide across pitches) across a musical third. The glissando slides steadily upward to the third and then just as smoothly slides back down. It sounds easy enough but many singers have to work to allow their larynx and vocal fold muscles to relax enough to make the slide. Some singers can produce it ascending the scale but not descending the scale. For others, ascending the scale is more difficult. If we remember that we are increasing longitudinal tension within the vocal folds as we ascend, and decreasing tension as we descend, this often will give us other clues on how to help the singer develop their voice, based on their strengths and difficulties with this vocalise. The versatility of Vocalise #3 was demonstrated by New York teacher of singing Jeannette LoVetri, faculty member of the Voice Foundation's Symposium on Care of the Professional Voice (1999). LoVetri taught a demonstration workshop for Broadway singers and was working with a singer with a huge, dramatic voice. The singer was able to sing loudly with great force. LoVetri asked the singer to imitate a soft production of LoVetri smoothly and gently sliding up a third and back down. The singer was unable to do it. LoVetri described the singer's difficulties as "muscling" the voice and using so much laryngeal tension that she was unable to relax enough to allow the laryngeal muscles to move freely. The other

Exercise 5: Total time required for this exercise is 4 minutes.

1. Start on a comfortable note in your lower mid-range (in the example, the starting note is Middle C). Sing an ascending and descending glissando up and down an interval of a fifth (1-5-1, where 1=C). Then sing the notes one at a time (1-2-3-4-5-4-3-2-1), moving smoothly through all the notes.
2. Advance the starting note by a half-step (i.e., 1 is now equal to C#) and repeat the steps.
3. Continue with this pattern until the top note sung approaches your higher range. Now repeat the entire exercise, beginning at your top starting note, and descending the starting point of each repetition by a half-step (i.e., if your top note was an A, where 1=D and 5=A, then lowering the starting point for the next repetition would make 1=C#). Proceed back to the initial starting note you used at the very beginning of this exercise. Remember to sing all passages softly (p).

Each individual should start at a note that is comfortable in his/her own range, and sing on one or more of the following sounds: "nah," "no," "new," "mah," "mow," or "moo."

Example of Exercise 5: Start at a comfortable note and tempo that will support your best vocal production.

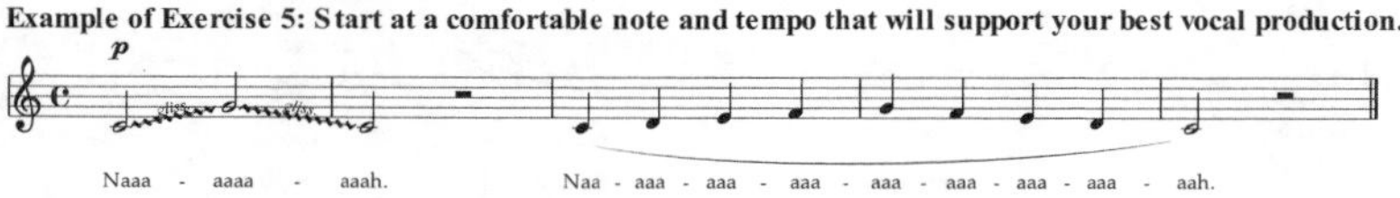

Naaa - aaaa - aaah.   Naa - aaa - aaa - aaa - aaa - aaa - aaa - aaa - aah.

Starting Note raised by a half-note to C#

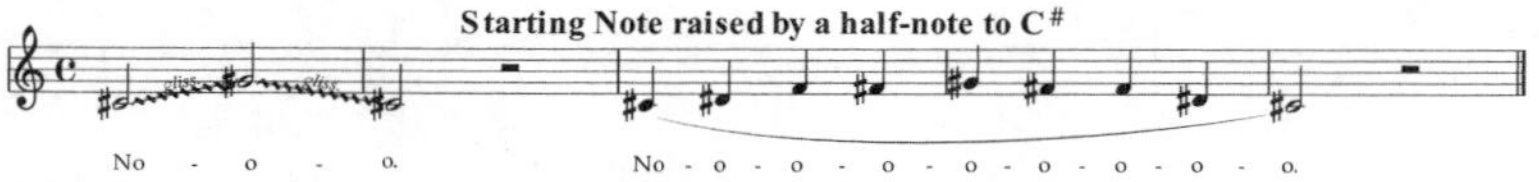

No - o - o.   No - o - o - o - o - o - o - o - o.

Starting Note raised by a half-note to D

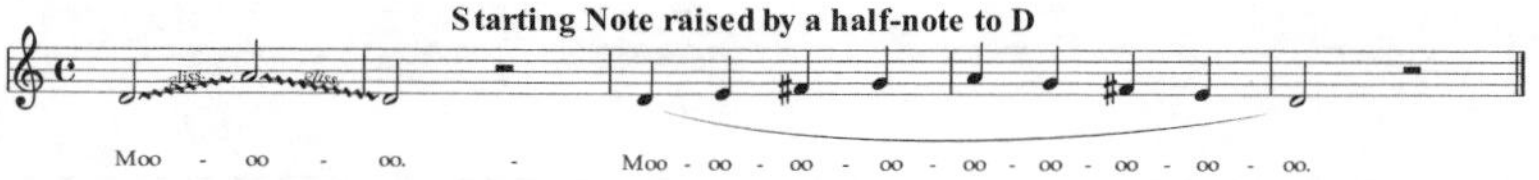

Moo - oo - oo.   Moo - oo - oo - oo - oo - oo - oo - oo - oo.

Figure 14–5. Exercise 5: Musical charts for vocalise exercise #5. Courtesy of Anita L. Kozan © 2011.

Exercise 6: Total time required for this exercise is 1 minute.

1. For this exercise, you will do an ascending and descending glissando across your whole range. You should make the total range of notes as short or wide as is individually comfortable. Using a soft voice, sing through your comfortable range of notes on "oo" (as in "boot") and then switch to an "ah" (as in "hot") as you reach your top notes. Continue to use an "ah" as you descend back down.

NOTE to MtF: You should not start on the absolutely lowest note in your range. It is strongly advised that your starting note be no lower than E below Middle C, but you should discuss this with your voice specialist before you begin.

Example of Exercise 6: Start at a comfortable note and tempo that will support your best vocal production.

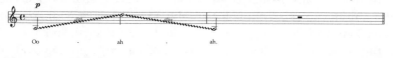

Oo   -   ah   -   ah.

Figure 14–6. Exercise 6: Musical charts for vocalise exercise #6. Courtesy of Anita L. Kozan © 2011.

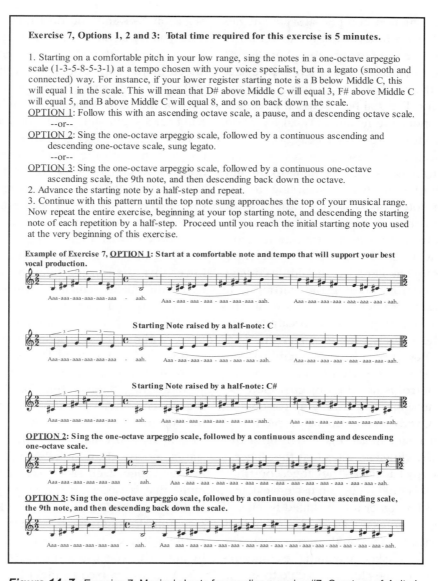

Exercise 7, Options 1, 2 and 3: Total time required for this exercise is 5 minutes.

1. Starting on a comfortable pitch in your low range, sing the notes in a one-octave arpeggio scale (1-3-5-8-5-3-1) at a tempo chosen with your voice specialist, but in a legato (smooth and connected) way. For instance, if your lower register starting note is a B below Middle C, this will equal 1 in the scale. This will mean that D# above Middle C will equal 3, F# above Middle C will equal 5, and B above Middle C will equal 8, and so on back down the scale.
OPTION 1: Follow this with an ascending octave scale, a pause, and a descending octave scale.
  --or--
OPTION 2: Sing the one-octave arpeggio scale, followed by a continuous ascending and descending one-octave scale, sung legato.
  --or--
OPTION 3: Sing the one-octave arpeggio scale, followed by a continuous one-octave ascending scale, the 9th note, and then descending back down the octave.
2. Advance the starting note by a half-step and repeat.
3. Continue with this pattern until the top note sung approaches the top of your musical range. Now repeat the entire exercise, beginning at your top starting note, and descending the starting note of each repetition by a half-step. Proceed until you reach the initial starting note you used at the very beginning of this exercise.

Figure 14–7. Exercise 7: Musical charts for vocalise exercise #7. Courtesy of Anita L. Kozan © 2011.

difficulty the singer had was fulfilling Lo-Vetri's request to sing softly. The singer always sang loudly and did not have the control to decrease the amount of pressure she used and still be able to control her pitch. LoVetri recommended that the singer improve her technique by working on simple glissandi sung softly which would require her to release the tension that she habitually created. Kozan began using this vocalise successfully with a variety of singers, including transfeminine, transmasculine, and gender non-binary singers. Transmasculine singers often develop hyperfunctional voice production compensatory strategies when they try to force out the lower notes in their emerging lower range. Vocalise #3 has been helpful to many singers, regardless of their specific vocal needs. The use of this vocalise will be discussed in greater length under the heading "Vocal Exercises for Transition across the Passaggio."

Vocalise #3 also includes a legato (smooth) major scale ascending to the musical third and then descending to the starting note. This is usually easier for the singer than is production of the glissando. The focus is on a legato transition across notes without "bouncing" or accenting each note. The clinician should discourage the singer from holding the starting note too long before beginning the ascent. This will allow the singer enough breath to complete the exercise. If the singer does not have sufficient breath, recommend pausing at the top of the scale before descending. Pitch control is not the objective here because the singer is warming up (or cooling down). Overly zealous focus on pitch control can result in laryngeal tension. However, if the clinician notes that the singer is consistently flat across the range, contributing factors could include muscle weakness, de-conditioning, or a less skilled listener. If the singer's notes are sharp, this often indicates a lack of focus on the target pitch. The singer may be asked to match the clinician's own voice (if the clinician is able to sing in that range) to see if this improves the pitch control compared with when a keyboard is used. Including the singer in the diagnostic process will help with analysis as well as treatment design. Asking the singer to make observations will often provide another avenue for investigation or rehabilitation.

The singer continues with Vocalise #3 by going up the scale one step at a time for the starting note. If C4 was the beginning and E4 the top note, the next repetition will begin on C#4 and end on F4. The starting note will be advanced for each repetition, staying well within the easiest range produced by the singer. Sometimes the singer will note a slight strain in producing the top note of the third. More likely, the clinician will hear a slight shift or loss of quality and decide that the singer is now ready to start the descent with the vocalise. The starting note is now going to be lowered down one step at a time. If the singer had vocalized up to a third beginning at F4 and ending at A4, the descent would start at E4 to G#4 and back down to E4, then D#4 to G4, and so on. The clinician can take the singer slightly lower than the starting point by a note or two, if the quality remains consistent.

Vocalise #4 (see Figure 14–4) gives the singer a chance to increase the vocal range without the restriction of a specific starting and ending note. The octave range is given as a reference point but is not an absolute. In demonstrating for the singer, the clinician should mention that matching the starting pitch is not necessary. Trained singers are more likely to match pitch, or start an octave above or below the clinician in their range. Each singer can choose the range that is easiest. If the range goes too high or too low, specific feedback can be given on altering the range. The goal is vocal flexibility without precise control, note by note. This vocalise is sung softly.

Vocalise #5 (see Figure 14–5) is a variation of Vocalise #3. The singer is now challenged to produce an ascending and descending glissando across a fifth on the musical scale. For singers with injured voices, this vocalise might take them across their entire accessible range, within just a few repetitions. The singer must understand that this is not a contest to see how high or low a note can be reached. Testing the singer's range when teaching this exercise will help to set parameters for the extent of the range that is safe for exercise. The decision-making process should be explained to the singer. The clinician should write down the range that is safe for exercises, and the client cautioned against pushing too far beyond it or singing louder. The more the singer understands about the larynx and vocal conditioning, the better the singer's decision making when the clinician is not around to provide feedback.

Vocalise #6 (see Figure 14–6) is an extension of Vocalise #4. This vocalise can be added to the singer's warm-up when it is certain that the singer can perform it safely without pushing for volume at either end of the range. The transmasculine singer is free to vocalize across the entire range, maintaining a soft voice volume throughout. The transfeminine singer might wish to vocalize no lower than E below Middle C (approximately 165 Hz) because research by Spencer (1988) revealed that 160 Hz was the threshold for perception of male voice. Gelfer and Schofield (2000) reported that a pitch of at least 170 Hz was needed for perception of a gender-ambiguous speaker. The experience of vocalizing in or near an appropriate gender pitch range gives the transfeminine client the opportunity to experience the lowest range that could be considered for gender appropriate speech production, as well as for singing.

If the singer needs to push with volume or with significant tension to reach either end of the range, those notes should be omitted from this vocalise. If the singer wishes to "test" the higher notes, advise the singer to lightly slide up to the notes but to avoid sustaining them. Some singers, even with good training, are prone to sustaining a note with increased tension, as if creating a crescendo (increase in loudness). The clinician can advise some singers of a safe technique to check their highest notes by recommending that they "think" coming in

on a high note or imagine the high pitch before they come in, and then slide down. The visual imagery of descending gently onto a soft cloud has been helpful to some singers wanting to test their high notes. When the singer alights on the top note and slides down, the longitudinal tension is gradually decreased, whereas ascending the scale results in a lengthening of the vocal folds. The increase in tension could result in overdriving the voice where it is most vulnerable for some singers with injured or de-conditioned voices. Once again, this vocalise is always performed softly.

Vocalise #7 (see Figure 14–7) is a one-octave arpeggio, a chord separated into its individual notes, followed by a one-octave scale. The scale can be performed with the ninth note added for variety, if the singer wishes. The singer with less training or one who has traditionally performed this vocalise across an exact octave will do better if the ninth note (the tone a whole step above the octave) is left out. Some trained singers have learned this vocalise as the first one in a warm-up routine performed while singing in a choir or while studying privately. The singer is encouraged to refrain from using this vocalise until all previous vocalises in this warm-up routine have been mastered. Interestingly, a previously learned exercise will likely elicit old habits of performance, some of which could be antagonistic to the goals of the singer's current program. Vocalise #7 is written here in the key of C. The arpeggio is sung legato: C4-E4-G4-C5-G4-E4-C4. The legato scale is a traditional eight-note major scale, sung legato, with the ninth added for variety. In the key of C4, the ninth would be D5, sung at the top of the scale before descending back to C4. If the singer has progressed satisfactorily, voice volume can be increased to a moderate level. The challenge to the singer is to keep the volume as consistent as possible while ascending to the higher notes. Pushing more volume is not an appropriate goal until the singer can sing every note in the vocalise at a soft level. If the higher notes can only be sung with greater volume, they are not ready to be sung at all.

As was discussed earlier in this chapter, Constansis (2008, 2009, 2013) studied the changing transmasculine voice and systematically used diaphragmatic breathing and vocal exercises with his students as part of his research. The reader is referred back to the section titled Singing Voice Research to review his vocal warm-up regimen. Kozan's vocalises are compatible with Constansis' exercises and have been used successfully with transmasculine singers who sought voice therapy after having completed their transition. Constansis' work is particularly relevant for trained transmasculine singers who want to preserve and protect their singing voices as they approach their transition.

Soft Singing

Soft singing is harder to accomplish than loud singing. Singing softly requires more control of vocal technique. The clinician needs to explain to the singer how the vocal folds work for speaking and singing softly. The increasing duration of the closed phase of the cycle as voice volume increases should be demonstrated and explained. The clinician should suggest a pitch that is within the singer's range and give the number of Hz (cycles per second) for that pitch. The hands may be used to represent the inside edges of the vocal folds, or a video or DVD may be shown of vocal folds in motion, contrasting soft, moderate, and loud singing.

The technique of singing softly is used with all singers, whether gender binary or non-binary. Singers with a healthy voice might progress much more rapidly toward singing with a moderate or loud voice volume. Some clinicians might prefer to teach

a healthy technique with tighter adduction as a first step. Kozan views soft singing as the first step in successive approximations toward the goal of firmer vocal fold adduction. Occasionally trans singers, including well-trained singers, must sing softly for a number of months because of the demands of the conditioning process for the new range of the voice. Constansis (2008, 2009) emphasized the importance of singing softly with his transmasculine singers. Every singer, whether gender binary or non-binary, is cared for as an individual. If it takes more time for the vocal conditioning, the singer has enough information to understand the importance of the conditioning process. Every singer wants success "right now," but the rewards experienced along the way are usually sufficient to keep the singer motivated and moving forward. The singer's language should be used whenever possible, except when a term is used incorrectly, such as the use of "flat" to mean "straight tone" and "without vibrato." The singer's attempts to use musical terms should always be acknowledged even while the clinician is correcting any errors. Most singers do not use the technical words for loudness and pitch (i.e., intensity and frequency), so Kozan uses these words only with singers with a background in physics or acoustics.

Easy Onset of Vowels

The technique of eliminating a hard glottal attack from words that begin with a vowel is a respected technique among classically trained singers and voice clinicians. Kozan teaches this to all transgender and gender non-conforming singers to use both for speaking and for singing. It is described by Richard Adler and Christella Antoni in Chapter 8 and can be found in most texts on voice rehabilitation. It is easily adapted for the singing voice, once the technique is mastered.

Indeed, it is actually easier to sing than to speak with an easy onset on the vowel because the singer uses a smooth release of breath when beginning to sing. The legato line of many singing styles helps the singer to flow into the next phrase after the breath pause. Easy onset on vowels is rehearsed specifically on songs and literature sung by each individual singer. The music text or lyric sheet is marked, when available, to aid the singer in anticipating the easy onset.

Cooling Down the Voice After Singing

Use simple vocalises to cool down the voice after rehearsing or performing. The goal is to reduce any swelling that has occurred in the vocal folds by using soft, gentle vocalises to help to dissipate the heat generated by the more demanding singing, flush the lactic acid from the muscles, and decrease the demands on the vocal folds made by loud voice production, prolonged singing, and/or singing at the extremes of the vocal range. Rock and roll singers who are transitioning have been particularly thrilled with their experiences using some of the easier vocalises (#3 and #5 are favorites) as their cool down. Simple descending "yawn-sigh" glissandi and soft production of sentences with moderate inflection patterns, such as tracks 4 and 6 on *Healing Voices, Vol. I Relax and Breathe* (Kozan, 2002), are also helpful in cooling down the voice. There is no magic combination of exercises. The focus needs to be on soft vocalization across the mid-range of the singer's voice for at least 5 minutes. The sooner the cool down is accomplished after the singer has finished rehearsing or performing, the better. Singers routinely report that their voices sound clearer and their throats feel better, both after the cool-down is completed and the following morning.

Transition Across the Passaggio

The classic passaggio is E4 (see also footnote 1) in the octave of Middle C. This is the primo (first) passaggio for the soprano, while pitches in the range of B4 to D5 comprise the secondo passaggio for the soprano. The passaggio is the point at which a singer transitions from using pure chest voice (below E4) to using a blended voice created by a balanced use of the thyroarytenoid muscles within the vocal folds and the cricothyroid muscles, which help to elongate the vocal folds (Colton & Hollien, 1973). Kozan's experience is that many altos tend to push their chest voice quality up to A4 and then make a noticeable breathy transition into their head voice. Many male singers show a noticeable transition into falsetto or head voice at E4 or an octave below, at E3. However, these data are based on cisgender men and women. Work with the transgender singer offers multiple opportunities for voice exploration before, during, and after transition. Hammond's section on the Butterfly Transgender Chorus later in the chapter will include her observations on the vocal ranges of transmasculine, transfeminine, and gender non-conforming singers.

Simple Vocal Exercises for the Development of the Singing Voice

---

Descending Glissandi

Descending glissandi are useful and versatile simple vocalises. The singer can be taught the basic exercise, starting on a note that is fairly secure in the singer's range. The goals stay consistent: soft voice, relaxed easy onset on /ɑ/ or /u/. Avoid /i/ because of the tension created by the tongue posture.

It can give a false sense of security to the singer, whose success is based solely on sound quality. The glissando must be sloppy so that it does not create a legato scale in which the singer smoothly descends from one discrete note to the next. The legato scale is a worthwhile exercise in itself, but it is easier than a glissando for singers who cannot quite let go of muscle tension. A legato scale is harder than a glissando for singers who have a sudden loss of quality or range. Experimentation will help determine how to best organize the exercises for the individual.

Ascending Glissandi

Ascending glissandi (slides from a target pitch going up the scale to another target pitch) are occasionally easier for a specific singer than are descending glissandi. An ascending glissando requires that the singer increase vocal fold longitudinal tension as the pitch is increased. This exercise is most helpful with a singer who has some vocal fold weakness, in that it takes advantage of the increase in tension created by the rising pitch as a compensation for the loss of muscle stamina created by the demands of sustained phonation. However, some transfeminine singers without any vocal fold weakness have also found it easier to use the ascending glissandi. Ultimately, the clinician will recommend the exercises in order of difficulty, having the client go first in whichever direction is easier for the client.

Combinations of Ascending and Descending Glissandi

Combinations of ascending and descending glissandi can be used as a next step when the singer has mastered production of a glissando in one direction. Adding on a return to the starting pitch, whether ascending and then descending or descending and then ascending, gives the singer an opportunity to increase the difficulty of the exercise while staying within the guidelines set by the clinician. Breath support is a problem for some singers who are exploring a new range. The singer should be encouraged to stop at the top of the ascent or at the bottom of the descent before reversing direction, if there is not sufficient breath to complete the exercise.

Speed of Ascent and Descent

Experiment with the singer and find the speed of ascent/descent that is most successful. Some singers are more relaxed when the glissando is produced very slowly, while others are more successful in moving uniformly across the notes when producing a faster slide. Variations of speed can be used to increase the difficulty of the exercise, once the easiest speed is mastered.

"Holes" in the Passaggio

The term "hole" or "holes" in the passaggio refers to a note or notes that are missing when the singer glides or sings a scale across a vulnerable part of the range that requires a transition or blending of tone quality to successfully transition across the "break" or passage. A "hole" might be as great as the loss of a grouping of notes up to an octave, particularly in the adolescent voice. It might take the form of a single note that drops out. It can refer to a fluctuation in voice quality shifting between "chest" and "head" or falsetto on the same note or on adjacent notes. Some singers will describe this as a "flutter," where the quality truly does rhythmically or inconsistently flutter between chest and head voice quality.

The most familiar passaggio is at E4, sometimes called the first or primo passaggio for sopranos. Some sopranos might have trouble anywhere from B4 to D5, sometimes referred to as the second or secundo passaggio. Altos and mezzo sopranos who push their chest voice quality across E4 usually will be forced to transition into head voice at A4. Baritones who have always pushed their chest voice and never sung in their falsetto will approach unknown territory when they consider learning how to make that transition. Tenors might have the range but not the resonance they desire. Basses top out at E4 (Vennard, 1967). The transgender singer might have specific limits of vocal range physiologically or psychologically. However, working on expansion of vocal range and strengthening of singing ability can be addressed through adaptation of the vocal exercises described above, regardless of the singer's previous range.

The transfeminine singer will have the opportunity to make any number of decisions about how she wishes to develop her voice for singing. The larynx has some limitations of range, but development of the head voice and/or a head voice quality is an option, if she has not already had some development while singing in falsetto. The glissandi described above, whether practiced across a small number of notes such as a third, or whether practiced across a fifth, an octave, or more, can be useful in helping extend the singer's range, or to mend troublesome areas of the vocal range. A discussion of the long-term goal or goals of voice training will help to determine the first exercises undertaken.

The transmasculine singer often "pushes" the voice to lower pitches or through vulnerable places in his range. He is not alone in this behavior. Pushing the voice or the desire to "push on the cords" is a familiar description of a dangerous technique used by both men and women, including some trained singers as well as some untrained singers. Somehow the act of pushing or creating pressure and tension in the larynx has become synonymous with being strong and creating a powerful voice. One untrained but widely acclaimed cisgender singer even reported that her church choir director had used her faith as a lever to get her to work and push her voice harder! The muscle tension created by pushing can be a devastating act to any singer's voice, regardless of the motivation. The transmasculine singer often has used the same misguided technique to develop the speaking voice as well as the singing voice, usually with a generalized muscle tension dysphonia resulting. The focus on the desire to lower the vocal range must be tempered with the knowledge that the larynx is adjusting to the increased testosterone in the body and that the lowest (and highest) notes of everyone's vocal range are always more vulnerable. The singer is particularly vulnerable with his emerging lower notes. Again, the glissandi vocalises are invaluable in helping the singer gradually deepen and strengthen his range. Constansis (2008, 2009) has used slides across pitches as part of the research protocol with transmasculine singers.

Adjustments in Resonance

Work on resonance can be undertaken by the clinician as part of development of the singing voice. Variations in tension at the level of the glottis can affect the listener's perception of breathiness and nasality. Tighter vocal fold adduction will create a tense tone and will mask the listener's perception of breathiness, while a more relaxed laryngeal posture will result in a breathier tone which will mask nasality, assuming breath is being taken in and released. These differences will be most audible if the singer's mouth is open and the tongue relaxed. Palatal posture of greater height allows for more resonance in the oral cavity and can enhance the tone. Acoustic analysis of "forward" placement of the singing voice revealed that voice quality correlates with higher frequencies of the second (F2) and third (F3) formants, as well as with a more salient "singer's formant" in the voice (Vurma & Ross, 2002). Constansis reported that several transmasculine singers have achieved a singer's formant in their new vocal range (A. Constansis, personal communication, January 2, 2017). Untrained singers will likely need more guidance and will progress more easily if they are given just one behavioral change at a time. Trained singers might be able to handle several changes added quickly in succession. The resonance and tone focus are shaped in step by step approximations, always protecting the singer from any task that is too demanding for the mechanism's stability.

Imitation of a model is useful in helping the singer understand what is being requested. Exaggerated models of breathiness (Sade or Marilyn Monroe's voice) and nasality (a country-western twang) often help the singer to change more easily than would a lengthy description of what is desired. Models of accents such as speaking and singing with a Southern drawl or British accent, where the vowels are prolonged, can also help develop resonance. Again, one example presented for imitation can open up a whole new area for exploration. The untrained singer might also benefit from using recorded songs of favorite singers. The clinician will need to work with the singer to make sure that the songs are vocally appropriate. A transfeminine singer can also work with a recording of her sister or another female family member as a model for the singing and speaking voice. The trained singers and performers will benefit from

professional observations. The speech and language pathologist or singing voice specialist should give the clients opportunities to be observed in their preferred performance venue. The singer can receive positive feedback on what was correct, as well as a constructive critique of errors, preferably at the next private session with the client. Guiding the singer toward increased accuracy in self-monitoring will heighten the potential for safe and insightful practices at home.

Interval Training Schedule

Interval training is one of the most useful exercise physiology models that can be applied to teaching singing to individuals who are working to begin singing in an untrained vocal range. The basic concept is that periods of training (singing) are alternated with periods of rest (being quiet). The schedule of regular intervals of rest keeps the vocal fold muscles and surrounding laryngeal musculature from becoming fatigued from the effort of attempting new vocal tasks. Intervals of singing can be as brief as five seconds, with a five-second rest before singing again for five seconds. The cycle of sing–rest–sing–rest continues on for a given number of minutes or repetitions. The avoidance of vocal fatigue is paramount. If the singer feels fatigue, a longer rest period and/or a shorter period of singing is initiated before singing is continued. If the fatigue returns, the singer observes the conditions that led to the fatigue, such as number of minutes sung, specific range used, breath support, loudness, tension, and any other observation that might be relevant, including interrupted sleep, esophageal reflux, stress, or other demanding voice use. Although there is no research on transgender or gender non-conforming singers with regard to the effects of using an interval schedule, Yiu and Chan (2003) reported that hydration and vocal rests were useful strategies to preserve voice function and quality during karaoke singing. Singers who engaged in long periods of singing without hydration and rest experienced a loss of voice quality, as shown by greater jitter measures, and a loss of the notes on the top end of their range. This example uses an interval training schedule with a transfeminine singer who wanted to work on improving her upper range. She started with descending glissandi beginning on notes easily accessed within her upper chest voice range. She sang softly with a relaxed breathy voice, never pushing, and rested after every minute of singing. Her rest periods were one minute long. Her starting pitches ascended after several repetitions on each starting note. When she felt that she needed to push harder in order to get the pitch, she refrained from doing so, and began the process of gradually taking her starting note back down the scale, step by step. Each day of rehearsal, she would "test" herself by seeing if she could go a little higher, but then always came back down, knowing that she was not using her voice optimally by pushing too hard or ascending the scale too fast.

> *It's been so difficult to wait for my voice to develop. I want to have a strong voice right now! But I can tell that my voice is gradually getting stronger by practicing very carefully and keeping my voice volume at a consistently soft level. I'm happy that I'm making progress.*
> —Transfeminine singer of classical literature and folk songs to Kozan

The men want to push, too, but their vocal fatigue reminds them that pushing for loudness or low pitch is not worth it. Most transmasculine speakers are so grateful that their throat stops hurting after they start using a relaxed voice production technique for speaking that they readily embrace the same guidelines when they work on development of their singing voice. Working with descending glissandi, always staying soft, and pausing to rest, sometimes even after every single descending glissando, has helped some singers be able to vocalize to the bottom of their range with minimal, if any, discomfort. All singers, trans or cis, come to face the fact that no one's vocal folds can close tightly at their lowest pitches and thus are incapable of producing a loud and clear sound, no matter how strong the breath support (Kozan, 2005). Each singer must also learn that today's voice might not be the same as yesterday's voice. Variations in pitch range and stamina are familiar to all singers, but most of all for the transitioning transmasculine singer. The singer should be encouraged to do his vocal exercises carefully every day, and to avoid competing with his performance from the day before. Staying in the present and respecting and caring for the voice will ultimately result in the healthiest development, especially since Constansis' (2008, 2009, 2013) work has brought us a better understanding of the effects of the "entrapped" transmasculine larynx.

> *Some T-men really want to have a beard. Others want the change in the shape of their body. Some men really want a deep voice. You take testosterone and then see what happens. Sometimes you get what you want but sometimes you don't.*
> —Participant in the Transgender Voices Festival, St. Paul, MN, April 24, 2004

Voices change and develop over time. Testosterone will continue to affect the voice as the transmasculine individual continues to take it. The transfeminine singer will not experience any changes in her voice secondary to increased estrogen in her body. However, both individuals have the potential to improve their vocal quality in their desired pitch range through continued, careful use of vocal exercises.

Mouth Opening and Jaw Movement

Singers who have excellent diaphragmatic breath support, an open laryngeal posture, effortless technique, and a well-blended pitch range are still not going to achieve their full potential if they do not open their mouth with a relaxed jaw posture. Exercises that release jaw and tongue tension are valuable to singers as well, and can be pivotal in helping the singers improve their technique and find a more beautiful sound. The tongue is the most powerful muscle in the body for its size. Reduction of tongue tension can be achieved by trying the exercises that are described here.

The "tongue buckle" exercise begins by placing your tongue tip behind your lower teeth. Buckle your tongue outward so that it forms a big curve out from just beneath your top teeth and then back in behind your bottom teeth. Watching yourself and your client in a mirror while you demonstrate the exercise will provide a model and give you an opportunity to watch for tongue fatigue. Demonstrate the exercise while you face the mirror and then let the singer see your tongue posture from the side. Your goal is to round your tongue outward as much as possible. Try to hold the tongue posture while doing a "yawn-sigh" or descending glissando on /a/, as in "hot" and on /æ/ as in "hat." Stay in the easiest range of the singer's vocal range. Tongues

that are tense will tend to flatten, shake, or pull back into the mouth while the exercise is carried out. Stop and take a rest if you or your client shows fatigue. Many singers can do only one repetition each of the vowels /ɑ/ and /æ/. You can make the exercise increasingly difficult by encouraging the singer to imagine pushing from the rear superior surface of the tongue. Ask the singer to do four repetitions of each vowel, with rest periods as needed, before going on to the next exercise.

The second part of the "tongue buckle" exercise is carried out with the tongue tip placed between the lower teeth and the lower lip. The exercise is more difficult because the tongue is farther out of the mouth in the starting posture. Again, if you notice that the tongue is starting to flatten downward in the mouth or retract back into the mouth, let the singer rest. Once a muscle is fatigued, it needs to rest at least a few seconds before the exercise is attempted again. Try to do four repetitions, using an interval training schedule of 10–30 seconds rest in between each production of /hɑ/ and /hæ/.

The next tongue tension release exercise is a bit of work and a lot of fun. The goal is to talk with your tongue extended all the way out of your mouth, using jaw opening and partial closing to "articulate" your speech. Before you begin, ask your client to curl the tongue back in the mouth so that you can see the lingual frenulum, in order to judge what is a reasonable expectation for tongue protrusion. Demonstrate the exercise in front of a mirror, if possible. Call attention to your jaw movement as you speak. If the client is unable to move the jaw up and down, you know that the tension is so great that you will need to start at a simpler level. One sequence that has been successful with some singers starts with simply opening and closing the mouth, using the "duh" posture. No sound is produced. Some singers will need to practice this until the next appointment. Gradually go from simple jaw opening and closing to adding sound on /ma/ along with the jaw movement. Next, guide the singer through gradual increases in tongue protrusion, starting with the tongue just touching the inside of the lower teeth, then extended slightly over the lower teeth. Again, add sound after the singer can move the jaw up and down freely. The tongue is gradually protruded a little farther after each successful production with sound.

Eventually, the singer will be ready to imitate your production of words and simple sentences. Encourage the client to let the speech be sloppy, to have fun and to laugh! Try again when the tongue starts gradually being retracted or suddenly darts back into the mouth. Explain that if the lingual frenulum is quite short, it might be sore from being stretched across the teeth, even if the tongue is not tense. If the singer does tend to carry tension in the back of the tongue, the tongue and/or the muscles in the neck might feel sore. However, after the exercises are completed, the singer might have a wonderful sensation of the tongue floating in the mouth, or feeling loose and free. Singers with hyperfunctional voice production might experience a clearer voice. There are a number of singers who have made steady progress in improving their singing voice by doing a series of tongue tension release exercises before they warmed up with their singing vocalises.

My girlfriend noticed the change in my voice as soon as I got home. It made me happy that she could hear it.
—Transfeminine speaker, after previous therapy session with Kozan that included tongue tension release exercises, glissandi, and upper body posture changes

Mirror Work

A wall or two of mirrors in your voice rehabilitation area can be an exceptionally strong feedback mechanism. First of all, if the singer's eyes tend to close when singing, they will have to be open in order for the singer to look in the mirror. Observations can be made on head and neck posture as well as overall body alignment. "Entanglement" is a term used by Wesley Balk (1977), teacher of singing and acting, to describe the unnecessary involvement of muscles in a particular motor act. Singers are most likely to show entanglement of the eyes and eyebrows when singing. Lifting the eyebrows or furrowing the forehead for higher pitches is not necessary to produce a higher pitch. Some singers are well aware that they have extraneous movement, while others have no idea. The mirror helps them concentrate on staying relaxed while working on the vocalise or song. Occasionally a singer will have some other idiosyncratic entanglement of a limb gesture, shoulder movement, or head tilt associated with breath inhalation. Working at home in front of a mirror has helped many singers improve more quickly.

A mirror can be a drawback if singers like to watch the keyboard while you are leading them through vocalises. Instruct the singers to position themselves so that they cannot see the keyboard directly or reflected in a mirror. This will free them up to concentrate on their technique and not attend to how close you are to their difficult note or notes. Singers who tend to tense up on certain notes will have more trouble with their technique if they know those notes are part of the vocalises they are singing.

Making the Transition from Vocalises to Sung Literature

Singing literature, whether it be classical or contemporary, is usually a joyful step, only occasionally fraught with fear. Most singers, especially those with injured voices, have trained so carefully using vocalises that they are thrilled to get to sing an actual song and know that they can do it safely. It is easier to work with a singer who is a little shy about doing something wrong than it is to work with an established singer who cannot wait to get back to the old playlist or repertoire on stage.

Start with a new song or one that is familiar but previously unrehearsed. If you work on a song that the singer already knows, any bad habits will likely still be present, even if you have shifted the key in order to accommodate the singer's new range. Save the familiar songs until you have helped the singer establish healthy habits and solid technique on new material. At this point, the singer might also ask about studying with a teacher of singing. If the singer has an injured voice in addition to making a transitional voice change, the recommendation is to hold off on private lessons until the voice is nearly or totally healed, unless the teacher of singing has experience with helping transgender singers and is knowledgeable about care of the injured voice. As a general guideline, working on sung literature is not recommended until the singer is well on the way to a healed voice. It helps that sometimes the vocal range is so narrow that very few songs can be sung until the range develops and the vocal hyperfunction decreases. Constansis (2008, 2009) suggests that a transmasculine singer limit his singing to just the part of a song containing accessible notes while he is developing his male voice.

Songs are easiest when the vocal range is within the singer's reach and when the tempo is slow. The singer has more time to make adjustments in technique and can stay relaxed. Any song can be sung more slowly, whether or not it is a ballad. Nor are there any rules about phrasing within the song. The singer is encouraged to breathe whenever air is needed and to not push to the end of the breath, causing more tension. "Air is free" becomes the phrase of encouragement. Clients should be encouraged to work on prolonging the breath as they become more confident, especially after the chosen vocal range is more secure.

Work on familiar songs can proceed when the singer is more consistent in following through on warm-up and cooldown, as well as on carryover of technique into new literature. If the singer is working with a teacher of singing, regular communication will help the singer to maximize improvement. When working on a familiar song, the singer may be asked to perform the song, preferably using live or recorded accompaniment, so that the singer does not have to think about playing an instrument as well. Observe for carryover of technique and reinforce the singer for all the successes. In seasoned pop music performers, a sloppiness of articulation might be noticed, to the point that some words are unintelligible. This then becomes an additional goal of work with the singer.

Solo singers and band members who accompany themselves should bring their instruments to their appointments so that observations can be made about posture and habits that need altering. The singer's technique should first be secure without the instrument being used, before work begins with the singer playing the instrument.

Whenever possible, the singer should be observed in performance, wherever that might be. Observations can be reviewed at the next appointment, so that the performance is not affected by remarks. If DVDs, CDs, videotapes or recorded performances on the internet are available, these can also be helpful in giving constructive feedback to the singer who performs.

Performing on Stage

The singer who does a solo act or sings and plays in a band has unlimited opportunities for vocal strain. There are many topics that can be reviewed as part of the ongoing discussion with the singer. Some of these might come up in the initial evaluation, but more likely they will be revealed as discussion unfolds across the weeks of voice rehabilitation.

Vocal monitors are absolutely critical for the singer whose music is amplified. The singer needs to be able to hear the vocal line without it being overshadowed by the instruments. If there is more than one singer and separate monitors are not available, the mix in the monitor should be balanced so that the singers are equal in loudness. The transgender singer might still be using a soft to moderate voice volume, in which case the singer's microphone will have to be turned up, both on stage and in the monitor. Instruments should be run through separate monitors so that their volume does not overpower the vocals.

Set lists or play lists are constructed keeping the strengths and difficulties of the singer(s) in mind. Transgender and gender non-binary singers will want to choose songs that stay within their vocal range. Learning the song in a new key is an option. Singing some lines higher and other lines lower can also be a way to use songs from the existing repertoire. Although some songs might have to be dropped from the play list because they are too high or too low, new songs can be added.

Many singers have to make decisions about exposure to smoke when performing in clubs. Helping singers to cut down on or avoid tobacco usage can enhance their voice and their vocal control. The effects of alcohol usage on the voice must be addressed. The transfeminine singer is especially vulnerable to the negative effects of smoke and alcohol, which can make her voice sound hoarse, husky, and dry. The transmasculine singer usually complains of tightness and fatigue when exposed to smoke. Helping singers reduce or eliminate tobacco usage and refrain from using alcohol when performing have been worthy goals frequently pursued, regardless of whether the singers are transgender or not. All singers, without fail, are so buoyed up by the improvement in their voices that they continue to succeed in reducing or eliminating tobacco and alcohol from their performances. They conduct themselves as professional singers, warming up, cooling down, and being proud of their accomplishments.

Singing in a Choir or Chorus

This section begins with information about the first transgender choirs that had an internet presence between 2005 and 2011. The San Francisco Transcendence Gospel Choir was formed in 2001, the first transgender choir in the United States, and by 2006 had become the subject of a documentary movie, *The Believers*. The Trans Voices Chorus was formed at the Transgender Voices Festival in 2004 in St. Paul, Minnesota and was only the second chorus of transgender people in the United States. A transgender choir was formed in Kathmandu, Nepal in 2009 and has since released a CD. There are many transgender singers who perform in choruses or choirs that include gay, lesbian, bisexual, and transgender singers in various cities. The discussion presented here is intended to help voice specialists best serve their transgender and gender non-binary clients who sing or want to sing in a choir.

A discussion group met in 2005 to discuss what had transpired during the first year of the Trans Voices Chorus in St. Paul, Minnesota. Each member of the group provided important observations on the experiences of the trans choral singers. Jane Ramseyer Miller, director of One Voice Mixed Chorus and original director of Trans Voices, and Kevin Wojahn, interim director of the chorus at the time of the discussion, agreed that the most important skill that the singers developed was pitch matching. This became particularly important for those members who were new to taking testosterone and who were still developing their pitch range, let alone their ability to match pitch. Wojahn noted that listening skills, breath support, and learning to blend the voices together were the same goals that any church choir would have. J. Michele Edwards, then Music Director of Calliope Women's Chorus and Music Director/Conductor of the Minnesota Center Chorale, discussed the voice as an important part of a person's identity. She noted that grieving the loss of the voice is part of the process for a person who is transitioning. Max Gries, founding member of Trans Voices, noted the empowerment that comes from singing once the transgender person breaks a self-imposed or society-imposed silence and allows the voice to come out and be heard. Dorothy Williams, at that time the accompanist for Trans Voices and for One Voice Mixed Chorus, an LGBT chorus, observed a huge difference

in the members of the chorus. Some did not care what part they sang, while others would only softly sing low notes. Still others sang only in their chosen range. Gries observed that feeling free to sing the part as it was written but then dropping down an octave when it got too high might work fine when an individual was singing alone, but it could throw off the other singers in a choral setting.

Ramseyer Miller set a good example for all choir directors as well as for speech-language clinicians when she said that she always demonstrated sectional parts within her range. The singers then had to imitate the part within their own range. Wojahn added that if the director modeled a sectional part with a gravelly voice because the part was too low, the singers would imitate the gravelly quality as well as the pitch. His directions for vowel placement/neutralization on high pitches described the preferred sound as gender neutral, as open and relaxed and as beautiful as possible. Ramseyer Miller spoke to the singers by calling attention to the part that they were singing, such as tenor or alto, rather than using any gender-specific noun or pronoun. She also stressed the importance of warm-up, observing that 50–80% of the benefit was in the focus that was achieved by the singers. CD recordings were used for the singers to work on their individual parts at home, since many of the singers did not read music and learned their part from the CD.

The transgender singer can be aided by the speech and language clinician, who helps the singer find the range that is comfortable, both physically and psychologically, and then helps the singer develop the voice. The gifts that we can give to the singer are the encouragement to sing and the acceptance of the singer's choices regarding vocal range and sectional part. As Wojahn so aptly described it, the chorus members develop an intuitive solidarity that bonds them, no matter if they are transfeminine or transmasculine, or whether they are transitioning or not. The empowerment comes from finding the voice and using it. The joy comes from singing with others and, according to Gries, knowing that others want to hear you sing.

Butterfly Music Transgender Chorus, Boston, MA

Sandi Hammond, Founder and Director, 2014–2016

Formation of the Butterfly Music Transgender Chorus

The idea of the Butterfly Music Transgender Chorus was born on the Facebook Transgender Alliance, when chorus founder, Sandi Hammond, posted the idea on September 1, 2014. In fewer than two hours, 123 comments followed on the thread from all over the world, including Sydney, Australia; Leipzig, Germany; and Houston, Texas and Boston, Massachusetts, USA. That day, two Boston-area singers signed up and the founder began a mailing list, announcing that as soon as she had six or more members, they would find a free rehearsal space and schedule an initial rehearsal and community meeting. One of these singers, a trans activist and speaker in her 60s, began listing the new choir in various LGBT listservs and mailing lists serving the greater Boston area. The sign-up list grew to almost 12 and an initial gathering was held in November of 2014 with 35 people attending. Hammond was able to secure free rehearsal space at a Unitarian Church via a clergy person who was transgender.

After Butterfly began in the fall of 2014, a wave swept across the country over the next 12 months, with all-transgender choirs forming in Chicago, Atlanta, Los Angeles, Kansas City, Missouri, and Manchester, New Hampshire. Although San Francisco and Minneapolis–St. Paul, Minnesota had successfully started choirs in 2001 and 2004, respectively, they were no longer active in 2014. Boston Butterfly Music Transgender Chorus got up and running with an all-volunteer staff during that first year. The first fundraising effort was conducted in June of 2015 via Kickstarter and raised $12,500. By September of 2016 Butterfly had 31 members in its Repertory Chorus, which rehearsed weekly and had an 80% attendance policy (singers needed to attend four out of every five rehearsals). The chorus gave concerts and made educational presentations that were a combination of singing and speaking. As an alternative for those who could not be fully out or wished to not appear in public (risk of photography outing them, exposure on social media), Butterfly created an adjunct program called "Trans Song Time," which was a closed, confidential drop-in singing class with a more flexible format, no performances or public events of any kind and no attendance policy. After year one, the chorus gave a public debut concert in April of 2016 in downtown Boston to a sold-out crowd of over 300 people. A second date was added a week later at a nearby venue for overflow sales, which sold out at 200 seats.

Purpose/Rationale and Inspiration

The Butterfly Music Transgender Chorus was created to provide a safe space for trans and gender non-conforming singers to reclaim their voices and find community. The group was non-auditioned and explicitly recognized that many trans singers were coming back to singing after a long break. The format of the chorus was designed to include extra warm-ups and vocal function exercises to accommodate changing voices and/or those who had not sung in a long time. The following comments were made by new chorus members upon enrollment:

"I stopped singing when I transitioned. I couldn't find a safe space that really included me so I just gave up—until now."

"My voice changed so much with testosterone that I found singing difficult and my voice tired easily."

"I tried to find a voice teacher who could help me after transition and one teacher I met said, 'I don't work with people like you.' This was so discouraging that I gave up for several years, until I found the chorus."

"I never knew if I could achieve a strong upper singing register, after going through male puberty, but I really want to achieve a feminine sound. I didn't know where to go for help with that. Technically would this be called developing falsetto? I didn't know. And, as a trans woman I wasn't sure I would fit into a 'regular' women's choir."

"I joined a women's choir but I couldn't sing in alto or soprano range. I was more like a baritone and they didn't know where to put me. They just said 'sing higher!' Well HOW is the question! I felt like the Director didn't really know how to accommodate me."

"I was very involved in choral singing growing up—all-state, auditioned groups, all through college. Then at 27, I went on testosterone and my voice became raspy and weak. I was so frustrated. I didn't sing for 10 years—not even happy birthday at an office party. This chorus has given me a safe space to explore my voice again, to get feedback and to reclaim my singing."

"Traditional choirs—most of them as far as I can tell anyway—have highly gendered concert attire requirements and that will just never work for me."

The repertory chorus "incubated" its own development in year one by committing to no public or ticketed concerts. A very few select engagements were taken in private settings (for example, a Unitarian worship service where not even the congregation knew in advance that the chorus would appear, in order to avoid possible mention on social media). This strategy was designed to maximize a sense of safety, allow the chorus to build its own internal culture, and allow the chorus time to develop musically without the pressure of outside factors. The founder and chorus members based many decisions on the results of the landmark publication "Injustice at Every Turn" (National Gay and Lesbian Task Force and the National Center for Transgender Equality, 2011). The report contained devastating statistics regarding the status of transgender and gender non-conforming people in the United States. This laid a clear rationale for the creation of a positive, safe, social, and musical all-transgender space in the form of a singing chorus. Hammond also observed what she believed to be "highly gendered" choral spaces that used a soprano-alto-tenor-bass format which did not adequately include or accommodate the transgender singers. This provided additional rationale for the formation of an all-trans chorus. The chorus was structured using its own vocal paradigm, identifying unique "Trans Vocal Ranges" 1, 2, and 3 (Upper, Middle, Lower), based on range assessments of all participants. Singers were allowed to switch sections at any time during rehearsal, sing in different sections depending on the repertoire (for example, singing Upper on one song and Lower on another) and adapt written musical parts by switching octaves at any time.

Demographics

The Butterfly Music Transgender Chorus was made up of a diverse range of gender identities and included people across ages 17–65. Self-reported gender identities included the following: "f2m" and/or "transmasculine," "m2f" and/or "transfeminine," "non-binary," "gender queer," "gender fluid," "agender," "3rd gender," "intersex," and "bi-gender." The chorus consisted largely of Caucasian members but at times had three to five people of color (Korean-American, African-American, Latinx). The goal was to continue to develop a more racially diverse roster.

Program Characteristics

The chorus structure included the following guidelines:

- The group was non-auditioned and has an explicit "musical safety policy." More experienced singers did not "eye-roll" or criticize beginners or those who might be struggling to learn. All levels and abilities were truly welcome.
- Upon enrolling in the chorus, each individual singer received an "Individual Vocal Evaluation," which focused on range assessment and desired vocal goals of the singer.
- Enrollment was open for only two weeks at a time, three times a year for three different seasons beginning in September, January, and June.
- Warm-ups were longer than for most choirs and included:
  - □ Techniques based on the research of the other author of this chapter, Anita Kozan, particularly the use of glissandi
  - □ Exercises using mindfulness and mind-body relaxation techniques and beginning every rehearsal with a guided relaxation
- Weekly rehearsals had an attendance policy requiring singers to attend 80% of rehearsals, which enhanced musical learning and helped build community.

- Weekly rehearsals always included warm-ups, repertoire rehearsal, and time for community.

Vocal Range

General Observations

It must be noted that some trans singers had very binary goals and some did not. Some trans men in the chorus elected to go on testosterone or already had; others did not and preferred to experiment with range without the effects of testosterone. For trans men not on testosterone, many wanted to explore a lower register, and yet achieving any pitch below E3 proved difficult. One masculine-identified individual who elected not to go on testosterone wanted to use their high register because: (a) they liked it and didn't want to give it up, and (b) they wanted to find a way to use it without it feeling like "the stereotype of a soprano."

All transgender women in the chorus had no choice but to go through male puberty. None had the benefit of a childhood in which a physician and/or the family repressed testosterone and put the singer on estrogen at a young age. Therefore, all trans women in the chorus essentially had a "male" vocal mechanism altered by testosterone during male puberty. Not all trans women had the goal of achieving an upper register akin to that of a cisgender female. A few trans women, particularly younger ones, were very comfortable singing in their lower register and had no desire to alter their singing voice or speaking voice in terms of pitch. The chorus retained a significant population of singers who identified as non-binary and/or gender fluid. It must be observed that non-binary singers had their own goals and needs that required more nuance and flexibility in addressing, and therefore the chorus allowed singers to change sections at any time except in the six weeks leading up to a performance.

Trans Male/Transmasculine Singers

For trans men/transmasculine individuals who elected to take testosterone, the most common goal observed by Hammond was to achieve a lower register with resonance. It was observed that for most trans male singers on testosterone, the lowest achievable pitch was usually A2. Of approximately 25 trans male singers evaluated, only 2 were able to sing below A2, one by an entire 4th, which was highly unusual. This range limitation appeared significant and indicates the need for further research. Quantifying range for trans male singers also deserves further study. In addition, for the same population, techniques for achieving resonance need to be incorporated. Most trans men on testosterone reported that while they were pleased with the pitch drop, they felt they "couldn't sing loud enough" in the lower register. Also, trans male singers reported a loss of range in their upper register of at least a 4th to a 6th. In the words of one singer, "I knew it was going to happen, but still, it was a shock when it finally did." One singer reported that the loss in upper register "happened really fast, like in three weeks. It was just gone."

Most transmasculine individuals who went on testosterone as adults reported that sight-singing and pitch-matching had to be learned all over again. It felt as if "my brain and voice connection disappeared." In the words of one singer, "I was an excellent sight-reader as a soprano and had years of experience. After going on T [testosterone], I could not match pitch. I couldn't believe it. I would think one pitch and a different one would come out of my mouth. I had to learn to match pitch and sight-read all over again." Many trans men found it helpful during rehearsal to use an app on their smartphone

called "Tunable" or another app originally designed for tuning instruments. Singing into the phone, holding the phone up to their mouths, and observing the screen during rehearsal gave them immediate feedback about whether or not they were on the correct pitch and if that note was in tune.

Trans Female/Transfeminine Singers

For trans women/transfeminine individuals who had to unfortunately go through male puberty earlier in life and essentially had a male vocal mechanism, achieving falsetto was not easy. In Hammond's experience, only a handful out of several dozen trans women were able to achieve a legitimate falsetto voice with any significant volume and power. Most trans women had a range limited to A4, just a 6th above middle C, before the voice began to fatigue and strain significantly. Not all trans women in the chorus had the goal of achieving an upper register, but most did. One trans woman in the chorus quit, saying, "for a while the chorus helped my dysphoria, but now it's just getting worse. I can hear what the other women are able to do. They have such strong voices and I am comparing myself and feeling worse and worse. I have to take a break." It is Hammond's opinion that a trans chorus is best served with an adjunct private voice teacher who can "pull singers out" of rehearsal intermittently for private lessons in an adjoining room.

Range Implications for the Choral Setting and Repertoire

If in fact it is true that most trans men on testosterone cannot achieve a pitch below A2, and most trans women cannot achieve a pitch above A4, then this has implications for any chorus that wants to accommodate the trans singer, especially an all-trans chorus. Choral arrangements for trans singers should generally remain within these two octaves. All of the Butterfly repertoire was arranged or composed to accommodate trans ranges and generally stayed between A2 and A4. In fact, the Butterfly chorus commissioned the first known choral compositions in the world that rejected the soprano-alto-tenor-bass paradigm, and used language on the written score "Trans Upper, Trans Middle, and Trans Lower" or "T1,T2,T3."

Future Considerations

Choral directors and voice teachers interested in helping trans singers would do well to consider ways to help trans men acquire resonance and help trans women with range extension. Study of countertenor technique may become especially relevant for trans women who did not have the benefit of repressing testosterone during male puberty. Warm-ups specific to each section could be further developed in collaboration with a speech-language pathologist who specializes in transgender singing voice development. It is also Hammond's belief that using singing warm-ups can enhance learning and mastery for the gender transition of the speaking voice; in other words, working on the singing voice can enhance work on the speaking voice.

Unanticipated Outcomes

Hammond observed a number of unanticipated outcomes during her tenure as founder and director of the Butterfly Music Transgender Chorus of Boston.

- Chorus became a hub for conversations around voice (speech-language pathology referrals, singing teacher referrals, even trans support group information exchange), which was a very positive outcome.

- Intense media interest at the local, national, and international levels was a surprise. Coping with intense interest from the media was a double-edged sword. While at times this was exciting for some members, for others it was threatening. Many conversations were had about how to proceed, and special community meetings were sometimes held to debrief on a media response.

- Tension between those who were not out and wanted more discretion (no photos at concerts, for example) and those who wanted to be fully out and "loud" and "visible" as activists emerged in the culture. Some members of the group wanted the repertory chorus to scale back and be less public and other members of the group wanted to push forward and be on the "edge" of leading a movement for social change and public education. At times this felt like a very negative outcome.

- While not entirely surprising, the founder was surprised by the number of inquiries received from organizations that wanted the group to come and do a "Trans 101" presentation, while incorporating music and storytelling into the format.

- Tension evolved around not having a director who was transgender. This escalated to the point where Hammond, the cisgender director, felt she had to step down.

- Fundraising and organizational development required an Executive Director but this chorus did not have one and the work fell to Hammond, the artistic director and founder. The sheer volume of work was overwhelming and unsustainable.

- A cultural schism developed between the vision of a performing chorus that was fully out versus a closed music program that was more therapeutic and had no outreach or performing objectives. This became a great source of tension within the community, particularly in the context of interest from the media (*Oprah* magazine, Associated Press, Boston Globe, NPR, ABC News, Refinery29, *New York Times, Washington Post*).

Recommendations for Future Research and Program Development

Hammond recommends that individuals and groups interested in forming a transgender chorus consider the following structural elements and procedures in order to increase the efficacy and potential for success of their endeavors. The concepts listed below might also provide opportunities for research investigation of their application to chorus creation and development.

- A trans artistic director and a trans pianist are recommended.
- An adjunct voice teacher, adjunct music therapist, and adjunct gender psychologist to advise cisgender staff are all recommended.
- The board of directors must have an appropriate mix of cis and trans members.
- Longer warm-ups are recommended for a trans chorus.
- Singers need to take "vocal breaks" intermittently throughout rehearsal.
- Warm-up routines should be refined in conjunction with a speech pathologist to customize the goals for different trans populations.
- Fundraising is crucial to the success of an organization such as this. A particularly strong source may be surgeons and clinicians from the medical community who see the value of a trans chorus (i.e., hospital executives,

physicians, surgeons, speech-language pathologists, and mental health providers).

- The chorus could partner with a speech pathology lab to conduct research and to support development of therapeutic vocal exercises for trans singers.
- Chorus leadership should decide if the chorus is fully out and performing or is more of an insular community-based closed group that does not seek an audience and/or publicity of any kind.

While Hammond attempted to offer two separate programs (Trans Song Time was a drop-in class offered at no cost and with no attendance policy), somehow the class seemed overlooked by the community and tension developed about what Repertory Chorus should actually look like. Should it be public and performing? Should it allow media interviews with some if not all individuals? These questions were flashpoints for strong feelings within the community and resentment was sometimes directed at the founder.

Conclusion

The community would benefit greatly from further research and program development. Doctoral candidates in vocal pedagogy, speech-language pathology, or choral conducting would do well to take on specific populations such as: (a) trans men with binary goals who are on testosterone, (b) trans women with binary goals who are on estrogen and had to endure male puberty, (c) trans women who have had the benefit of the suppression of testosterone prepuberty and have been on estrogen as young adults, and (d) non-binary singers with a wide range of goals and needs. Choral directors, music teachers, speech pathologists, and others working with trans singers who are cisgender themselves would do well to meet with activists in the community to learn the basics of "Trans 101" and beyond. The language and culture of the transgender community are always evolving, and connecting with activists prior to engaging in services is critical. Having ongoing "advisors" who are embedded in the trans community will help to keep the program current and relevant.

There is a great need and interest in such a chorus. Singers from all over the world contacted Hammond and made comments like "I wish we had something like that here" (Leipzig, Germany). The challenge to sustaining such a group is fundraising. While Boston has a strong LGBT community and a strong individual private donor track record in supporting the arts, it has one of the worst scorecards for funding for the arts when evaluated nationally in comparison to nine other major metropolitan areas in the United States. "Boston has relatively few foundations and government organizations making grants to the arts, and what funding is available is skewed toward the larger organizations. Relative to other cities, Boston's small and mid-sized arts organizations do not receive significant foundation support. Boston receives the lowest amount of government funding per capita among the comparison cities" (The Boston Foundation, January 2016). While great strides were made in developing a donor list in less than 18 months, making the program fiscally sustainable became an enormous challenge.

Addendum

It should be noted that as of this writing, Sandi Hammond, founder and director of the Butterfly Music Transgender Chorus, has stepped down as Artistic Director and is no longer directly involved. The chorus has been much less active since October 2016. While a small group of volunteers has continued to facilitate weekly rehearsals in a donated space, the organizational development has paused and no concerts have been scheduled as of this writing. A member of the transgender community has stepped forward to facilitate a search for hiring a new Artistic Director. At the time of the founder's stepping down, the Butterfly Music Transgender Chorus had $21,000 for future program development. In good faith, Hammond turned all funds over to the core group of transgender volunteer musicians in the hope that a new program would be developed.

Gender Non-Binary Singers

There are singers who identify as transgender or gender non-binary who choose to avoid all hormones that might have any effect on the singing voice. Kozan has consulted with a number of trained and untrained singers, transmasculine, transfeminine, and gender non-binary, who chose to maintain their singing voice in a healthy manner and wanted to consider ways in which they might change their singing voice without vocal injury. Again, the client is the ultimate decision maker and is cautioned only if a particular behavior might irritate or injure the voice.

Erik Peregrine, a classically trained singer who holds a Master of Music degree in Conducting, shared his experience coming to recognize his non-binary gender identity during his undergraduate vocal performance work and his conducting work while in graduate school (E. Peregrine, personal communication, February 16, 2017). He started singing Baroque opera "trouser roles" while an undergrad, male roles originally written for castrati and in the last century sung by females. Peregrine noted that when singing those roles, his voice was where he most felt at home and he was able to explore his gender identity through music performance. He describes himself as a transmasculine non-binary person and uses the pronouns they/them and he/him interchangeably. He did not start at a reduced dosage of testosterone, as some transmasculine binary and gender non-binary people do. He began HRT between his first and second years of graduate school after he realized that being perceived as male reduced his own gender dysphoria and allowed him to be present in his body. Peregrine moved to Minneapolis after finishing graduate school and was hired as the part-time Youth Outreach Coordinator for One Voice Mixed Chorus (OVMC) by Jane Ramseyer Miller, Artistic Director of OVMC, Minnesota's LGBTA Mixed Chorus. Ramseyer Miller, a cisgender female who has conducted OVMC for over 22 years, has worked for inclusion of minority performers, composers, and conductors with the chorus and has contributed to earlier discussions presented in this chapter.

Ramseyer Miller and Peregrine discussed the experiences of Sandi Hammond, contributing author to this chapter, and Founder and Artistic Director of the Butterfly Music Transgender Chorus until mid-2016, when some members of the chorus decided that the directorship should be held only by a transgender or gender non-binary conductor. Ramseyer Miller and Peregrine understood the dilemma that faces transgender choruses that want a transgender conductor, but agreed with Kozan that a chorus needs to have the best possible conductor to work with them, whatever the gender identity of the director. Hiring a cisgender conductor and a transgender assistant conductor would seem to be the most workable solution when a well-qualified

transgender candidate is not available. It was hoped that eventually a strong candidate would be available or that the assistant conductor would continue to develop their skills with the help of the cisgender conductor, and eventually take over the directorship of the chorus (J. Ramseyer Miller and E. Peregrine, personal communication, February 16, 2017). Kozan recognizes the challenges faced by Hammond and by the former Butterfly Music Transgender Chorus members and thanks them all for their significant contributions to educating people around the world about their work and their quest to sing again, a legacy that will endure.

Mind-Body-Spirit Connections within the Transgender Singer

Role of Self-Talk

Transgender and gender non-binary singers will reach their greatest potential if their vocal development is complemented with goals that take the whole person into consideration. An important part of singing voice development is attending to the content of the singer's self-talk, that is, what the singer is thinking and saying internally while singing, as well as when they are discussing the development of their singing voice. This focus often begins when Kozan observes the singer while working on learning the vocalises. If the singer tenses up, grimaces, or makes an audible negative comment, more than likely there is negative internal self-talk. Ask the singer what they are thinking or saying internally. That will be the starting point for any recommendations on changing self-talk. What we as clinicians say to ourselves is incredibly powerful and can influence the outcome of our work. If we believe that our work with a particular singer is going to go well, it will go well. If we doubt our abilities or believe that a given singer is not going to benefit from voice rehabilitation, the singer will likely not benefit. We must have a positive intent when we do therapy. We must coach ourselves to be positive in our thinking, just as we coach our singers to do so. If we ask singers to change to a more positive message of self-talk, they might get mad at themselves when they forget. Part of the challenge here is to help them to stop from getting angry when the old behavior crops up, otherwise they are still engaging in negative behavior. One helpful strategy is to encourage clients to acknowledge whatever comes into their minds and then to say some variation of this: "I notice that I just thought _____, and that is no longer helpful to me. I release that thought and accept that I will be making mistakes while I learn. That's normal. I want to think of something positive right now. I'm happy to be having the opportunity to work on my singing voice and to hear the changes in my voice." Whatever the goal might be, decreasing smoking, drinking more water, or being more consistent in doing vocal exercises, singers are encouraged to focus on the positive changes in their voices that have resulted from what improvements they have made thus far. The positive reinforcement of the clinician can play a huge role in helping singers change their self-talk and ultimately improve their self-image and confidence.

It is also important for both the client and the clinician to be emotionally present during the therapy session, as discussed with Christine Wing (C. Wing, personal communication, February 27, 2017). Wing is a speech and language pathologist whose doctoral research, clinical work, and teaching focus are on the relationship between early communication skills and social-emotional development. Discussion of Kozan's work with transfeminine, transmasculine, and gender non-binary clients elicited Wing's observation that the amygdala is activated during emotional presence and increases the activation of the hippocampus, which is the first level of memory (Phelps, 2004). She noted that we need to bring our emotional selves to that learning. As clinicians, our clinical knowledge and experience form the basis from which therapy techniques are remembered, applied, and created. We bring our empathy and draw from the art and the science of our work. In Wing's observation regarding therapy with transgender individuals, clients who are grounded in their purpose and are focused and open to their feelings will have greater success in attempting the therapy tasks while exploring and naming their feelings and progressing through the session than will the client who is controlled in seeking perfection in production of the very first sound they make. Thus, Kozan often brings up the importance of self-talk in the first therapy session. Clients begin their work learning to listen to their quiet thoughts as well as to their first attempts at seeking their own voice, and come to accept their inner and outer voices in that moment, no matter what is revealed. When both the clinician and the client work within this model of self-acceptance, the outcomes can be achieved in genuine harmony of spirit.

Role of Spirituality in Singing Voice Development

The spiritual nature of each person can be a source of healing and motivation for that person as the voice rehabilitation program continues. It does not matter whether the person participates in a faith community or not (Kozan, 2001). What can be of value is the individual singer's sense of spirituality, in that it can be a source of support and security for the singer who is embarking on the journey of voice development. Encouraging individuals to accept themselves where they are, to believe that they have a purpose, and to ask for help when they need it can be an affirming start. Prayer or meditation helps some individuals feel relaxed and connected to their spiritual selves. Others want to commune with nature or to follow a wiccan or a pagan philosophy, while still others are atheists. Whether the individuals have a sense of working for the common good, a feeling of simple faith, a specific belief system, or a belief in the Divine Voice, we have the wonderful possibility of getting to know our clients better and using their beliefs to help them to heal and develop their voices. We can speak about our own belief systems if it is helpful to the singers in finding the words to express their feelings. However, we have no need to encourage them to adopt our beliefs. Rather, this is an opportunity to look for language that can be used to support each singer individually. If there is a relationship that the singer finds particularly healing, perhaps that can be a source of comfort to the singer who struggles with goals.

At its best, the therapeutic relationship between the singer and the clinician is a powerful, healing one. Each of us feels called to do the amazing work of helping to heal the planet by touching the lives of the singers who come to us for voice therapy. Keeping our minds filled with good intent and our hearts open to healing, we will continue to help the singers who come to us. They, in turn, will offer us opportunities equally blessed, to grow and learn and heal.

Remember to Listen, to Speak, and to Sing

Kozan concludes this chapter with a story about the experiences of a gifted artist whose life journey began before birth with congenital dysplasia of hips, feet, and the right knee, a condition in which the major joints are dislocated. Catherine Louise Johnson was born in the 1950s, when the best treatment available was to place the infant in a splint in hopes that the dislocated and not fully formed joints were malleable enough to develop and reshape. Her reconstructive surgeries began at age 6 months, in a full body cast that restricted all movement from below her knees up to her clavicle. She lived in a hospital for "crippled children" where cribs were lined up close together, row after row. Johnson was bound face down in her crib, her movement and vision were limited, yet she could hear those around her. Only one parent was allowed to visit, once a week for two hours, but there could be no physical contact with the child. Parents were not allowed to be with their children before or after any surgical procedures. The yearning for touch was demonstrated by the wild groping of tiny hands and arms through the slats of their cribs when a parent would visit. Johnson's mother recalled this as a heartbreaking time (C. Johnson, personal communication, November 13, 2017). The infants and children in the ward were alone most of the time and if they cried or became upset, they were given Demerol, a powerful synthetic opioid pain medication with a long half-life. Johnson recalled the terror experienced once sedated because she felt disconnected from her surroundings. She learned not to cry because when she would receive the drug, her body cast was so tight that it was hard to breathe if she cried. She began making hushed, rhythmic humming sounds and over time gradually offered her self-soothing song to the other children who were inconsolable. At night, her keening would begin at the first sound of a whimper, a lullaby for their pain which helped them stop moaning and crying, until all Johnson could hear was the beautiful hushed sound of the children's calmed breathing as they finally fell to sleep (C. Johnson, personal communication, November 12, 2017).

Johnson left the hospital only once, for two months when she was 18 months old, because her father demanded and fought with the physicians and authorities until they allowed her to come home. She had never seen blue sky or green grass or colored flowers. Her mother saw her daughter's senses bang open when her father laid her down on the grass by his parents' garden. Johnson heard a bird's song and felt the wind across her face, astounded in wonder at the sensations she experienced. Then she reached for the red, purple, and yellow flowers—and ate them! Eight weeks later she was back in the hospital continuously until age 3, and then thanks to the demands of her father, her care was transferred to another hospital, where she began a series of stays and would have a surgery and recover, go home for two months, and then go back for another surgery. Johnson's head was shaved so the nursing staff could observe for the onset of bedsores, a common occurrence with hospitalized bodies whose movement is restricted. When she went to visit a nearby men's surgical ward, all the patients called her "Lad" because she looked like a boy. In the hospital, a girl child with a shaven head did not receive the conventional gender training. Instead, she learned humanity.

Johnson never went to a full year of school until fifth grade. She was very shy and hardly spoke except when asked questions. She was frozen in reticence as she entered a foreign land and culture of vertical moving and noisy children. The children would ask, "What is wrong with you?" Johnson made a lifelong friend when a girl asked, "What happened to you?" Johnson knows that she had been seen for who she was by that little girl.

The unspoken rule at home was that her story was not welcomed; she was expected to bury what she knew. No one talked of her terrible ordeal. Johnson learned shame and embarrassment, a new phenomenon. She was a visitor to what was normal. She used crutches in order to walk, bearing not only the weight of her body but also the heavy weight of plaster casts. Johnson adapted to her crutches and they became her wings, the determined vehicles of mighty locomotion to move fast. Her prolonged use of crutches required more surgeries on both her hands and arms to rehabilitate nerve damage. As of this publication, she has endured and accomplished 47 surgeries. She has used her fortitude, perseverance, grace, and resilience throughout her life to propel her to literally stand up and become more alive with each breath. Johnson chose to work with gifted trauma psychologists in order to remember and come to terms with what had happened to her. This reclamation demanded courage and yielded freedom (C. Johnson, personal communication, November 13, 2017).

When we are bound and cannot breathe, even when the binding is released, we still are frozen in that posture. The body holds the truth of one's life: the prison of fear and despair and others' limited perceptions, the freedom fighters' songs of I Shall Overcome and Amazing Grace, and the sacred release of being seen for all the things you are. One chooses which ship to live in.
—C. L. Johnson, personal communication, February 25, 2017

Johnson's art continues to be a sacred vehicle for her to express what had been repressed, unknown, hidden, and kept quiet for all of those years. Long before she could shape the words of her narrative, her art was a loving oracle that told the truth. Her writings, readings, and exhibitions share the soul's grace of song and the freedom of living with integrity. Johnson has received prestigious national and international merit awards for and because of her art, including a MoMA P.S.1 International Studio Residency and a Bush Artist Fellowship. Her art is in corporate and private collections nationwide. Johnson noted that she has never been asked to disclose any information about the circumstances of her birth and life when applying for awards and grants. Her art is what draws the recognition. Viewers experience a dynamic and quiet, electric power in the presence of her art. Johnson lives her belief: that her life purpose is to tell the truth, live her True North with integrity, and rise and choose joy (C. Johnson, personal communication, November 13, 2017).

Kozan is struck by the similarities of some of Johnson's experiences and those of the transfeminine, transmasculine, and gender non-conforming people with whom she has worked over the past decades. Transgender clients have spent their lives trying to be who they are not, trying to act and talk like their gender assigned at birth. Trans women are often still stiff, not easily moving their face or body, not opening their mouths and not showing emotion. They have often shared that they were worried while growing up that they would be perceived as being effeminate or gay and would be bullied, so they refrained from any movements or gestures that they thought would make them suspect. Trans men talked of literally living in bodies bound with binders and bandages to keep their upper chests from moving, experiencing physical as well as psychological pain, with some experiencing physical injury, being unable to breathe diaphragmatically because of the ribs being so tightly bound, forcing themselves to use clavicular breathing, with shoulders elevated and tense, and with neck tension and laryngeal strain. Being forced by society to

live your life by being who you are not is a terrible burden. It includes excruciating repetition of so many behaviors and habits that have been learned in order to survive because the person's life did depend on it. Our work with our clients, whether transfeminine, transmasculine, or gender non-binary, is work that helps our clients learn new behaviors and gently release the behaviors that protected them but are no longer needed.

Listen. Listen. *I HEAR THE BLOOM WITHIN THE SEED.*
—Catherine L. Johnson, Interdisciplinary Artist, LIBRETTO, 1994

There is little that is intuitively obvious in becoming who we truly are, especially when we have worked so hard to be who we were not. If you are reading this chapter because of your own personal journey, be gentle with yourself and respectful of all the work involved in the many changes that you are undertaking. You are stronger now than you've ever been and will become even stronger in the months and years ahead. If you are reading this chapter for professional knowledge, know how important your work is in helping people find their true voice. We are helping to give voice to some tender and incredibly strong, courageous individuals whose voices have been silenced far too long. Whatever has motivated you to read to the end of this chapter, may you approach your work believing, as Catherine L. Johnson has written above, that you can hear the bloom within the seed. Remember to listen, to speak, and to sing. May the black and white photograph of Johnson's work of art, HER-HYMNS: BE BRAVE (2013), created after remembering how she sang to soothe herself and the children around her in the hospital ward, inspire you to continue to heal

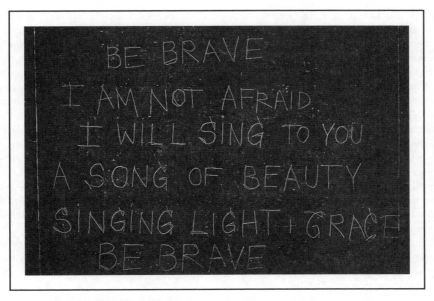

Figure 14–8. HERHYMNS: BE BRAVE Photo. Courtesy of Catherine L. Johnson.

yourself and to help heal those around you (Figure 14–8).

References

Adler, R. K., Constansis, A. N., & Van Borsel, J. (2012). Female-to-male considerations. In R. Adler, S. Hirsch, & M. Mordaunt (Eds.), *Voice and communication therapy for the transgender/transsexual client* (pp. 153–185). San Diego, CA: Plural Publishing, Inc.

Adler, R. K., Hirsch, S., & Mordant, M. (2006). *Voice and communication therapy for the transgender/transsexual client.* San Diego, CA: Plural Publishing, Inc.

Adler, R. K., Hirsch, S., & Mordant, M., (2012). *Voice and communication therapy for the transgender/transsexual client* (2nd ed.). San Diego, CA: Plural Publishing, Inc.

Adler, R. K., & Van Borsel, J. (2006). Female-to-male considerations. In R. Adler, S. Hirsch, & M. Mordaunt (Eds.), *Voice and communication therapy for the transgender/transsexual client* (pp. 139–167). San Diego, CA: Plural Publishing, Inc.

American Speech-Language-Hearing Association (2005). *The role of the speech-language pathologist, the teacher of singing, and the speaking voice trainer in voice rehabilitation* [Technical Report]. Retrieved from www.asha.org/policy.

Amir, O., Amir, N., & Michaeli, O. (2005). Evaluating the influence of warmup on singing voice quality using acoustic measures. *Journal of Voice, 19*(2), 252–260.

Balk, W. (1977). *The complete singer actor.* Minneapolis: University of Minnesota Press.

Colton, R. H., & Hollien, H. (1973). Perceptual differentiation of the modal and falsetto registers. *Folia Phoniat, 25,* 270–280.

Constansis, A. N. (2008). The changing female-to-male (FTM) voice, *Radical Musicology, 3.* Retrieved May 17, 2009 from http://www.radical-musicology.org.uk

Constansis, A. N. (2009). *Hybrid vocal personae.* Doctoral dissertation. University of York, UK.

Constansis, A. N. (2013). The Female-to-male singing voice and its interaction with queer theory-roles and interdependency. *Transposition: Journal of Music and Social Sciences, 3.* http://transposition-revue.org/The-Female-to-Male-FTM-Singing.http://transposition-revue.org/The-Female-to-Male-FTM-Singing

Constansis, A. N., Kozan, A. L., & Hammond, S. (2016a). Development of the transgender singing voice: clinical implications for voice, speech and beyond. Paper presented at the American Speech-Language-Hearing Association Conference, Philadelphia, PA.

Constansis, A. N., Kozan, A. L., & Hammond, S. (2016b). *Trans vocality: Succeeding against all odds!* Paper presented at the WPATH Biennial Symposium, Amsterdam, Holland.

Davies, S., & Goldberg, J. (2006). *Changing speech: Guidelines for people in gender transition.* Vancouver Coastal Health, Transcend Transgender Support and Education Society and Canadian Rainbow Health Coalition. Free download from http://www.vch.ca/transhealth/resources.

Gelfer, M. P., & Schofield, K. J. (2000). Comparison of acoustic and perceptual measures of voice in male-to-female transsexuals perceived as female versus those perceived as male. *Journal of Voice, 14*(1), 22–33.

Gries, M. (2004). Transgender voices. *IDIM Final paper.* U. of MN GLBT 3993.

Johnson, C. L. (2013). Artist. HERHYMNS: BE BRAVE. https://catherineljohnson.wordpress.com/about/

Jourdain, R. (1997). *Music, the brain, and ecstasy.* New York, NY: William Morrow Press, Harper Collins Publishers.

Kozan, A. L. (1995). *Perceptual judgments of the effects of vocal warm-up on the singing voice.* Doctoral dissertation, University of Minnesota, 1995. UMI Dissertation Services, No. 9537878.

Kozan, A. L. (2001). *The role of spirituality as a clinical tool in the rehabilitation of adults with voice, speech and language disorders.* Paper presented at the Minnesota Speech-Language-Hearing Association Convention, Duluth, MN.

Kozan, A. L. (2002). *Healing voices, vol. I, relax and breathe* [CD]. Crow White Records.

Kozan, A. L. (2005). *Rehabilitation of the speaking and singing voice for female-to-male transsexuals.* Poster presented at the Harry Benjamin International Gender Dysphoria Association Conference, Bologna, Italy.

Kozan, A. L. (2006). The singing voice. In R. Adler, S. Hirsch, & M. Mordaunt (Eds.), *Voice and communication therapy for the transgender/transsexual client.* San Diego, CA: Plural Publishing, Inc.

Kozan, A. L. (2012). The singing voice. In R. Adler, S. Hirsch, & M. Mordaunt (Eds.), *Voice and communication therapy for the transgender/transsexual client* (2nd ed., pp. 413–458). San Diego, CA: Plural Publishing, Inc.

Kozan, A. L., Constansis, A. N., & Hammond, S. (2016a). *Development of the transgender singing voice: Clinical implications for voice, speech and beyond.* Paper presented at the American Speech-Language-Hearing Association Conference, Philadelphia, PA.

Kozan, A. L., Constansis, A. N., & Hammond, S. (2016b). *Trans vocality: Succeeding against all odds!* Paper presented at the WPATH Conference, Amsterdam, Holland.

Kozan, A. L., (2017). *Singing exercises—a clinical tool for trans* voice development.* Paper presented at the USPATH Inaugural Conference, Los Angeles, California.

Lavorato, A. (1984). *International voice symposium.* New York, NY: Julliard School of Music.

LoVetri, J. (1999). Workshop Session. The Singing Voice. 28th Annual Symposium: Care of the Professional Voice. Philadelphia. Curtis Institute of Music.

LoVetri, J. (2006). Somatic Voicework: (SM) The LoVetri Method. lovetri@thevoiceworkshop.com

Miller, R. (1993). *Training the tenor voice.* New York, NY: Schirmer Books.

MuseScore: Free music composition & notation software (version 1.0, release date February 7, 2011) [Software]. Available from http://musecore.org.

Phelps, E. (2004). Human emotion and memory: Interactions of the amygdala and hippocampal complex. *Current Opinion in Neurobiology, 14*(2), 198–202.

Sataloff, R. T. (1997). *Professional voice—the science and art of clinical care.* (2nd ed.). San Diego, CA: Singular Publishing Group.

Smith, S., & Thyme, K. (1976). Statistic research on changes in speech due to pedagogic treatment (the accent method). *Folia Phoniatr (Basel) 28*(2), 98–103.

Spencer, L. E. (1988). Speech characteristics of male-to-female transsexuals: A perceptual and acoustic study. *Folia Phoniatrica, 40*(1), 31–42.

Steinhauer, K., McDonald Klimek, M. & Estill, J. (2017). *Estill voice model: Theory & translation.* Pittsburg, PA: Estill Voice International.

Stoll, H. (2014). *The very model of a modern, major gender role: toward a transgender voice in musicology.* MPhil Disertation, Music: University of Cambridge, UK).

The Boston Foundation (January, 2016). *Understanding Boston. How Boston and other Amer-*

ican cities support and sustain the arts. Funding for cultural non-profits in Boston and 10 other metropolitan centers. A report issued by The Boston Foundation, copyright 2015.

Vaccaj, Nicola (1999), *Metodo Practico di Canto*, (Italian and English) Ed. Elio Bataglia. Milano: Casa Ricordi.

Van Borsel, J., De Cuypere, G., Rubens, R., & Destaerke, B. (2000). Voice problems in female-to-male transsexuals. *International Journal of Language and Communication Disorders, 35*(3), 427–442.

Vennard, W. (1967). *Singing: the mechanism and the technic.* (rev. ed.). New York, NY: Carl Fischer.

Vurma, A., & Ross, J. (2002). Where is a singer's voice if it is placed "forward"? *Journal of Voice, 16*(3), 383–391.

World Professional Association for Transgender Health, Standards of Care 7th Version (2015). Available from www.wpath.org.

Yiu, E. M. L., & Chan, R. M. M. (2003). Effect of hydration and vocal rest on the vocal fatigue in amateur karaoke singers. *Journal of Voice, 17*(2), 216–227.

15

Meeting the Needs of Gender Diverse Actors: Personal, Clinical, and Artistic Perspectives

*Christine Adaire, Delia Kropp,
Sandy Hirsch, and Rebecca Root*

Every actor has a very possessive feeling toward their voice. Far more than non-performers, even. Why? Because their voice is what they use to tell the truth. In real life we lie all the time, with our bodies and voices and minds. Hundreds of times a day, we mask the truth, misrepresent, warp it into something else for our benefit or protection. Actors, if they're any good, instinctively see through all that deception. And their voice is the instrument to reflect the truth inherent in their character. Their age. Their social background, geographical location. Emotions and thoughts. Their character's complexities and contradictions and those dark nuggets of truth most people hide from themselves and seldom confront in other people.

—Delia Kropp, Transgender Actress

The Dual Perspective of a Transgender Actress and Voice Coach: Rebecca Root

The craft of acting necessitates not only a keen perception of the human condition, but also the ability to translate that observation into representation. In other words: how to present human life on stage or film and make it look as if it were *real*.

Professional actors tend to rely less on personal experience than *imagination*. This informs the creative journey undertaken during rehearsal and performance. The audience accepts that what they see on screen or stage is no more "real life" than is playing "shop" with their 5-year-old child—no one would suggest that an actor have experience with killing somebody in order to realistically portray a Bond villain.

When the gender diverse person transitions to their gender identity, they may well feel like they are absorbing a character in this way. But this is no temporary transformation—accepting one's gender and fulfilling that identity requires lifelong commitment. The unique needs and goals of the transgender actor deserve and require a different training focus than that of the transgender person learning a permanent life skill. By definition, when an actor prepares a role, he or she knows that the role will end: when the curtain falls each night, and ultimately when the show is "broken down" for good. Actors know that they are developing an overlay to everyday communication, and the contract requires that they maintain this overlay for the length of each performance. They can then go out for a beer and revert back to who they are in real life. Gender diverse lay people learn a life skill that becomes them, every minute, every day for the rest of their life, and they therefore have to maintain a cognitive, emotional, and vocal consistency that an *actor* is able to mete out over the life of a play, versus the play of life. "This ain't no show, it's the real thing," you might say. For this reason, the processes of coaching a gender diverse client, versus a gender diverse actor playing an opposite gender role, are indeed closely related, and yet ultimately there are a number of distinctions requiring illumination.

While both training approaches draw on the same vocal skill set and must be approached with the same level of vocal intelligence and care, the actor has to apply those skills differently for every role. This is dependent upon the particulars of character requirements and directorial goals and expectations. Preparing for a theatrical role, or "building a character" requires a unique blend of psychological insight coupled with an innate understanding of the text and character as presented by the writer.

As a performer and voice coach who is also transgender, Rebecca Root has experienced for herself the vocal re-gendering that both actors and gender diverse clients may seek when addressing these demands.

A Trans Actress's Personal Perspective and Advice: Delia Kropp

Part 1: The Danger of the Single Story

When speaking about the diversity of trans people, I like to reference the TED Talk by Nigerian author Chimamanda Ngozi Adichie, here speaking eloquently and passionately about race:

> *the single story creates stereotypes, and the problem with stereotypes is not that they are untrue, but that they are incomplete. They make the one story become the only story.*
>
> —Adichie, 2009

Later in this section, I share a great deal of my personal transition and voice story to graphically demonstrate how even we trans feminine trans persons bring very different skills, histories, and needs to their instructor. Equally important, we need to acknowledge that trans masculine and non-binary actors also exist in the entertainment profession, with their own specific needs as both groups and individuals. Failure to recognize these performers is not just unfair, but unrealistic, as an ever-growing number of projects and audition calls focus on these performers.

Indeed, when given this opportunity to represent trans actors, my first concern was that once again a trans woman would be hogging the mic. I wondered if my concerns are even the same as masculine and non-binary performers?

An Informal Survey of America's Trans Actors

I am an administrator of America's largest Facebook group for transgender actors. As such, I had the opportunity to post a survey, open to all members, to talk about voice. While the responses do not represent a rigorous cross-sampling, they do suggest that voice is a special issue for most trans performers.

A Profile of Respondents

The majority of this sampling was actually trans men or non-binary individuals. Eighty percent of all respondents were actively auditioning for stage parts. Thirty percent had received some stage training and sought some professional voice help. Only 50% of the respondents had attempted to modify their regular voice. Indeed, there was a higher level of satisfaction with everyday voice (60%) versus 40% being "mostly satisfied" with their stage voice. Asked to elaborate about how voice factors into their career, comments indicated far more concern about external pressures, such as the perceptions of casting directors, agents, etc. than their own personal expectations related to self-image.

Voice instructors need to be aware of this trend. No matter how happy one may personally be with one's voice, it's a highly gendered world out there, so if a client seeks help to feminize or masculinize a voice in order to be cast in more parts, then varying strategies may be necessary.

Avoiding the Pitfalls of That Single Story

Some of my suggestions may seem obvious, but with the multiplicity of trans identities and varying voice needs today, they are worth a review.

1. *Acknowledge Your Personal Perceptions and Assumptions.*
   Where primal things like gender identity are concerned, we're wired to make snap decisions about others. When you first hear or see a trans person, it may be natural to jump to conclusions or make certain value judgments. Don't deny these reactions, but listen carefully to them. Let your own little internal voice say what it wants, even if it's rather harsh or judgmental, such as:
   "Oh, he looks rather butch. Must want to sound that way too."
   Or, "What a lovely delicate voice they have, it's a shame that testosterone is affecting it."
   Or, "She has such a deep voice, is she really serious about playing female parts?"
   This is not unlike what therapists do with their clients. With the help of their own therapists, they work hard to identify their personal prejudices, in order to set them aside when helping their clients.

2. *Listen to Your Client.*
   Even if it eats up class/session time, encourage your client to speak. Use open-ended questions. Learn how they feel about their voice in real life, and on the stage. How have people reacted to it? What opportunities have been created by their voice, or perhaps eliminated?
   You are already an accomplished listener—but we trans actors may be your biggest challenge yet. We have built high walls, fashioned elaborate personas to protect our vulnerability. Once you establish trust, however, and have an open dialogue, your clients' answers will surprise you, and probably up-end many of those initial gut reactions and assumptions. By establishing trust and an open dialogue, you have also

signaled to the client that they have an active role in their voice development.

3. *When You Do Speak, Be Non-Judgmental.* Steer clear of any value-oriented language—even if you're inclined to say something positive. For example, telling us how feminine or masculine or gender neutral we sound just minutes after some salesperson misgendered us on the phone just undermines your credibility.

This may also already be part of your toolset, but remember, trans people are generally skeptical about cisgender attempts to figure us out, or to make our voices "better." Your expert, professional, and well-meaning critiques might feel a lot like the body of those other reactions, large and small, positive and negative, that have become a part of our self-image, and have influenced the sound and speech we use. So go especially easy with the "good and bad," or any language suggesting judgment tied to an external standard or model. Rather, tie all feedback directly to the client's vocal goals, and the voice narrative they have shared with you.

Part 2: Further Debunking the Single Story

Sharing details from my own journey seems to be one way to demonstrate the uniqueness and unstereotypical nature of trans actors. Let me start by offering a personal profile, contrasting myself with some commonly accepted narratives about trans actors.

We Don't All Know from Birth

Beware the wildly popular "I've always known I was a (man/woman)" narrative. I did not experience substantial gender dysphoria until the age of 47, and did not begin my transition in earnest until 50. For five decades I had lived as a cisgender, heterosexual man. Did I have some general confusion, and unhappiness with myself? Certainly. Did I think I was a woman? It wasn't even on my radar. It was unthinkable.

The "always known" narrative is concise, emotionally compelling, and for some trans individuals it's certainly true—but not for everyone. Like much of our reality, this narrative is crafted as much for your benefit, so as to be easy to digest, as for ours.

As yet, there are no hard data on this, but from hundreds of conversations with other male or female identified trans people, I can vouch that for many others, our gender identity evolved over time. It was not an immediate slam dunk.

Other Challenges for the Late Transitioner

For my generation, transitioning can be burdened with shame; lots of it. Growing up male we learned our feminine traits are disgusting, laughable, and worthless. My childhood was a minefield of confrontations with bullies, or being labeled "sensitive," and a host of other cues that meant "less manly," and by inference, less of a human being. Decades of such conditioning almost requires a "de-transitioning" prior to transitioning. This takes time and some hard work. I needed three years just to accept that I might be trans, and another five to complete my counseling and physical changes prior to "coming out."

One reason some older trans persons may be more prone to "gendering"—seeking "passability"—is to protect ourselves, to feel more safe in public. And the voice, both personal and professional, can be part of that armor.

We Aren't All Laverne Cox— Or Want to Be

TV and films (and also the stage, though perhaps less so) are historically biased toward young, attractive, and very binary "passable" actors. You've probably noticed a slew of female trans actors and models who are exceptionally beautiful even by cis female standards. Well, I'm not. I am not passable, and I'm no great beauty.

Beauty, of course, is linked directly to "passability." Why? Besides the safety factor noted above, cisgender people basically want performers to look like them—decidedly male or very female. Ambivalence about a performer's gender—their face, body, voice, or clothing—can form an unconscious negative impression when looking to cast most roles. Too often, "passability" for trans people isn't just about being extraordinarily pretty or handsome, it is about being accepted as "normal" too.

Again, talk about this with your client. Discuss casting challenges and other external, social realities, but also what's going on inside of them. Because some of us have internalized the beauty/"passability" thing— and some have not. From my experience, I again find we older trans are more likely to subscribe to that notion; and it's no wonder. We grew up with attractive, passable trans celebrities like Caroline Cossey (Tula), tennis player Renee Richards, and Christine Jorgensen. There were literally no other models. This was not least of all because doctors made that impossible. Until the past 15–20 years, if diagnosed with gender dysphoria, you got your counseling and were routinely scheduled for a sex change—end of story.

Not "Fully" Transitioned

So far my transition has entailed no surgeries of any kind. Yes, I have undertaken certain other physical modifications. My beard has been permanently removed through electrolysis. And hormone therapy has changed a number of secondary sex characteristics: obvious things like substantial breast growth (without implants) and more subtle characteristics like softer skin, hair, and a redistribution of body fat which softens male musculature and partially emulates ladylike curves.

My reasons for these specific choices are complex, and might not be the reasons of other trans persons. Some facial surgeries are too expensive for me, and must wait until money is available. Other procedures (breast and "butt" implants) will never align with my self-image, and so will never be considered. Right now, on the whole I'm pleased with what I see in the mirror, and feel it expresses my internal gender perception pretty well.

As a result of these choices, I am keenly aware that when stepping on stage or before a camera I am not what most people expect, or perhaps even what they want to see. Considering that my instrument is my voice and body, that's a lot to work through. But with my patchwork of feminine and male characteristics, it's inevitable that I don't read as female to all people. I accept this, as I must accept that it is harder to get certain female-identified roles.

I Didn't Transition "On the Job"

Currently, I know of several young trans persons who continue to audition and work in the midst of their transitions, while still "a work in progress," as it were. This requires courage and is not easy by any means. I chose to leave theatre altogether to transition not because I lacked such courage but because my situation was quite different. In 2006, trans acceptance was even more hit and miss than it is now, virtually nonexistent both socially and within the theatre community. The term "transgender" hadn't even entered into common usage yet. And also, being an older trans person who had lived as their assigned gender for many decades, I first needed to transition out of that former identity before exploring my truer gender expression.

I had been acting professionally since 1976. I loved theater, loved acting and directing, and I knew it was my calling. But for 40 years my male-ness had become thoroughly embedded in my career. So I just knew I'd not feel able to grow; to shed the old facade, while working in the profession. So I consciously decided to cease all acting and directing until completely comfortable and confident in my female identity.

But when that finally happened in 2011, and I legally changed my name and gender marker and formally came out, I then had another obstacle. Until January 2015, I was convinced there was no place for me in the theatre profession. Who would want a woman that looked and sounded like me? I couldn't bear the prospect of re-entering the profession only to be negatively judged and rejected just for who I am. Indeed, if I hadn't been offered a few opportunities "out of the blue" to prove myself, I might still be enjoying theater only from the audience seats.

Whose Voice Does a 50-Year-Old Use as Model?

In part, most young trans people just absorb their idea of gendered (or non-gendered) voice from the world around them—famous singers, actors, announcers, and of course their family members and peers. This is unconscious, and that's a good thing.

My process, however, turned out to be a little different.

I knew about the popular "voice feminization" programs on the market from my trans girlfriends. I tried some of them, for a time, but found them tedious. They seemed geared to "civilians," people afraid to journey outside the box with their voice. Heck, I not only ventured outside the box of my old male voice . . . I frolicked there.

During my 10 years offstage, I experimented with voices that echoed what I saw in the mirror. For the most part, they grew from models of extreme femininity, and perhaps because I intuitively sought softer tones and a broader pitch range. I even modeled other dialects like British or American Southern. With my actor's temperament, I had no problem sounding silly and ridiculous on the way to finding something true. Within a relatively short time I established a baseline sound, my "Female Voice," and even employed it with little self-consciousness in small, public social gatherings.

However, I soon learned that "my voice" struck other people as eccentric—different—somehow out of step with how women talk *today*.

From Life, or Imagination?

As an actor, I draw largely from my life, and embellish only where I need. Earlier in this chapter, Rebecca Root, in the first of four perspectives on acting, stated that actors tend to rely less on personal experience than imagination. My perspective is that an actor's truth—all the demands of their character, the period, and other details—comes foremost from their own personal experience.

But what about my process? Was my new voice, and indeed my entire female persona, just a complete fiction, having nothing to do with my true, innate identity? It honestly didn't feel so, but I worried about that for a long time.

Working with What You've Got

It eventually dawned on me that, in my own strange way, I was doing what all women—cisgender or transgender—intuitively do: I was referencing norms from my childhood. For me, that meant female role models going back to the late 50s and early 60s. My mother, grandmothers, neighbor ladies, and of course media personalities from those impressionable early years, all these had created a "composite female" voice in my head. You might say my voice came out of a mid-century time capsule, with additional qualities of gentility and feminine self-possession few women reference today, regardless of age. And yet even if it sounded like a relic to others, this voice was born of my own experiences. It felt real, reinforced my sense of femaleness, and even gave me confidence when socializing.

So my challenge became this: to let my voice "grow up"; to progress through the 70s, 80s, 90s, and into the 21st century. Or otherwise stated, to let it evolve out of adolescence and into adulthood; to embrace a woman's need to convey authority and gender equality with her voice; to include more contemporary word choices and expressions, each with their particular musicality; and finally, to let the progress of my voice reflect the gravity and maturity commensurate with an intelligent woman nearing her 60s. This was an entirely personal, intuitive process: totally my own.

Back in the Spotlight

After three and half years living as Delia, performance opportunities suddenly came my way. I auditioned for a role that brought me into final call-backs, but where I was ultimately deemed "too feminine" for the part. I participated in staged readings, seated behind a music stand to read trans and cis female parts. Then came the chance to understudy cis female roles. Then, in less than a year, I was offered a leading role. A trans character, yes, but one who had lived "stealth" (as a cis woman) for over 30 years, and whose voice would therefore be 100% passable.

That vocal challenge finally prompted me to seek professional voice instruction. For the first time since my year at the Drama Studio of London in 1979, I was open to letting someone else tinker with my vocal identity.

New Doubts

Luckily I had a few months to prepare prior to rehearsals. I met about 10 times, one session per week, with a top actor's voice coach, here in Chicago.

These were the goals we agreed upon: first, after 10 years off, to find a viable stage voice again, fully audible, flexible, and at my command even when gripped with stage fright. Already I'd accepted that "My Voice" wouldn't cut it professionally. What worked in intimate conversation would feel too soft, too lacking in color and power to hold an audience's attention for two hours at a certain distance. Secondly, we'd seek to identify places in my newly restored instrument that might strike the audience's ear as less masculine—or even, possibly, as feminine. Total "passability" was never a real goal because I knew that would just make me anxious and distract me from other aspects of my demanding role.

First Responses

As an actor, my reviews were uniformly positive; commending my ability to tell the story, command attention, create empathy, and generally engage the audience. I was thrilled to get notices one would give an actress, not a trans actress. None of the reviews specifically mentioned the "passability" of my voice or appearance.

Still, part of me was unsure if I'd earned that acclaim, wondering if journalists were afraid to broach such delicate matters as my female presentation. Fellow actors were supportive, too, but that's their job, and they too might be reluctant to pierce that membrane surrounding trans-ness. Certainly no artist wants to tell another "you sounded like a guy," even when asked directly. I learned that it's not always easy to find reliable feedback as a transgender performer.

To my own ear, I was unsure. I had sufficient volume, dynamic range, and colors. But I also leaned a bit on "female impression," occasional breathiness and certain pitch choices that might have served more as a crutch, devices to anchor my personal femininity; not necessarily the best choices for this specific character.

Due to financial constraints, I could not continue formal lessons through the entire rehearsal process and into the run. My voice teacher graciously offered some general observations anyway, all very supportive, but from here on I felt rather on my own.

A Turning Point

My next lead role was, again, a transgender woman, but with a twist. It had never before been acted by a transgender actress. It was Charlotte Von Mahlsdorf, in "I Am My Own Wife."

Written as a one-person show, it's usually performed by a single cisgender man—partly because the other 30-some parts are male, and partly because the actor who cre-

ated the role—winning a Tony Award for his superb work—was a cis man. Doing all 30-some parts was a problem for me, because I'd resolved never to perform male roles, for a variety of personal and aesthetic reasons.

But there was Charlotte, this beautiful trans part embedded in a matrix of cis maleness. I decided to approach a prominent LGBT theatre with an unusual concept—to involve multiple actors: myself embodying only Charlotte through the entire play, and three more actors to cover the rest. After mounting a test read, and obtaining permission from the author, I went on to play Charlotte Von Mahlsdorf, and create a little theatre history.

My work was well reviewed in the media, and praised by theatre people whom I knew and trusted. Along with other aspects of my instrument, my thinking about stage voice also moved forward.

Turning the Page

Pre-transition, my greatest acting challenge was vulnerability. Like many men, I had that quality pretty much beat out of me by social conditioning. I could approximate emotions, yes, but not so faithfully as to create a solid truth for myself or audience. The exceptions, of course, were anger and humor—the feelings most accessible to cisgender men.

Post-transition, after years of real-life weeping, feelings of suicide, worthlessness, and delving into childhood memories too dark to share here, I had developed a pipeline to feelings never before accessible, on stage or off. Acting has become a whole new experience, and I am a more powerful performer.

My voice requires very specific techniques to serve those emotions. I'm now extremely aware of how powerful emotions cause physical changes that sabotage my voice: they tense my jaw, constrict my throat, and freeze my diaphragm. As a result, I now warm up a LOT, employing whatever exercises feel necessary to bring my voice forward and get the chords flexible. On stage, I consciously keep my jaw relaxed, and use plenty of breath support. If successful, my voice can handle almost any feelings I throw at it.

Do I sound more passable now? Objectively, probably not. But I do connect with my female-ness through emotions seldom accessible as a man, a different but equally important kind of gender connection and authenticity.

Part 3: What I Most Seek in Voice Coaching

I look for humility, because none of us has all the answers. Our Western conception of gender has evolved more in the last decade than in the previous millennium. We are all figuring this out as we go along. We are feeling our way toward a truth and a language able to describe it, without decades of scientific research or precedence. Gender identity is a new land, and the landscape can be pretty scary at times. I know this, and want you to appreciate that empathy.

I respond to compassion, because we trans people get so many negative messages, and internalize too many of them, often becoming our own harshest critics. Sometimes we need support more than professional judgment. If we come with specific goals, we ask for compassionate support of those choices, no matter how lame they seem.

I appreciate respect for how we trans people see ourselves. The idea of masculine, feminine, or gender neutral still held by a majority might not be ours. Expertise is

appreciated, but should also include room for us and our ideas.

I appreciate respect for our creative needs, and the strange wiring that comes with being an artist. We're kind of the opposite of other people, in real life: our job is to tell the truth with our voice, not to lie or mislead. Regardless of how gender factors into things, our instrument has a very intimate connection with our feelings, our sensations, and our very soul. Just like all other actors.

Most of all, I admire and need your patient persistence. There will be frustrations, resistance; dead ends. Please don't give up on your trans clients. Even when we fight you every step of the way.

The Voice of the Clinician: Sandy Hirsch

Paramount to the role of the clinician with any actor is to ensure that the voice is being trained with a view to health and sustainability (see Chapter 8), and that training includes an interdisciplinary approach.

If all goes well, the role of the voice clinician with actors, indeed all performers, should be less prominent than that of the voice coach. In the hands of a skilled voice coach, an actor will learn what they need regarding the best approach to the voice, given the character assigned and studied.

As regards trans actors and their specific needs vis-à-vis gender specificity (or not) and voice modification, multiple chapters in this text (8, 9, 10, 11, and 12, in particular) address those approaches and the tools needed to nuance using the voice across the gender spectrum.

The balance of roles between coach and clinician is vital. Clinicians must have the understanding and humility to refer to a theater voice coach when their knowledge of the arts side of voice comes up short. By the same token, it is critical that the voice coach and trans actor understand that if the voice is consistently not performing as expected and hoped, there may be a need for medical and clinical approaches: a referral to an ENT and ultimately a voice clinician may be what is required. Coaches and clinicians alike must understand the boundaries of their role, and use interdisciplinary tools available to best serve the actor, regardless of gender identity.

A Voice Coach's Personal Experience and Viewpoint: Christine Adaire

I have worked in the professional theatre for over 30 years as an actor, director, and voice coach. In the past few years my experience as a voice coach has included work with transgender and gender non-conforming actors. Many more plays, television shows, web series, and films are including transgender and gender non-conforming characters. I am certain that future actor training programs will increasingly encounter more young artists who choose to transition to another gender or who are gender non-conforming. As a teacher, I want my transgender students to have the skills to be able to play whatever role they want; whether it is a transgender role or a cisgender role. I want the professional trans actors with whom I work to feel confident and successful in meeting the demands of the production.

Following I will share some of my expertise and experience as a voice coach. I am aware that the gender spectrum is very diverse. For the purpose of simplicity, however, whenever I refer to "transgender actors," I am referring to gender non-conforming actors as well as transgender actors.

The Linklater Voice Method

There are many different voice methodologies that are used in the world of the theatre. Kristin Linklater, Cecily Berry, Patsy Rodenburg, Roy Hart, and Arthur Lessac are the creators of the methods that are most widely used. In my 35 years in the theatre, I have been introduced to all of these methods and have used exercises from them at different times. However, my major point of reference is with the Linklater method.

I am a Designated Teacher of Linklater Voice, trained by Kristin Linklater, who created her method in the 1960s for the actor's speaking voice. Ms. Linklater is originally from Scotland and trained as an actor at the London Academy of Music and Dramatic Arts (LAMDA). She trained with Iris Warren, an innovative voice teacher at LAMDA. When Iris died, Kristin herself taught voice at LAMDA. In the early 1960s she came to the United States and was based in New York City. I was lucky enough to meet her in the early 1980s when I was an actress with Shakespeare & Company. Kristin was the Director of Training as well as an actress in the company. She published *Freeing the Natural Voice* in 1976. A second edition of this book with the revised title *Freeing the Natural Voice: Imagery and Art in the Practice of Voice and Language* was published in 2006. In addition, Kristin wrote a book about Shakespeare in 1992, *Freeing Shakespeare's Voice*. Ms. Linklater has continued to research the voice and develop her method for over 50 years. She is now based in Orkney, Scotland, and has established The Kristin Linklater Voice Centre.

Linklater Voice: What Is It?

Linklater Voice, known as "Freeing the Natural Voice," is a comprehensive progression of exercises by which the actor can explore and develop the voice for authenticity and the full range of expression. Its fundamental goal is to hear the individual *through* the voice.

"The natural voice is transparent. It reveals, not describes, inner impulses of emotion and thought, directly and spontaneously. The person is heard, not the person's voice" (Linklater, 2006, p. 8). This approach is psycho-physical, not merely technical. The voice is our "acoustic mirror," it expresses who we are.

"To free the voice is to free the person, and each person is indivisibly mind and body. Since physical processes generate the sound of the voice, the inner muscles of the body must be free to receive the sensitive impulses from the brain that create speech" (Linklater, 2006, p. 8). Ms. Linklater's assumption is that everyone was born with a "free voice" that is capable of expressing all of an individual's feelings and needs. The infant's voice has stamina, strength, and a huge range to express its many needs. Parents or caregivers can attest to the duration and range of expression in an infant. However, as each of us is "socialized," we adapt our behavior to meet the constructs and constraints of society. We learn to use our "indoor voices." That primary impulse for vocal expression is supplanted by a secondary "learned" impulse. That learned impulse might help us to get what we want. Unfortunately, the cost of suppressing the primary impulse is often a reduction of spontaneity and a narrower range of expression. The repression of the primary impulse is very often achieved by muscular tension. That tension might reside in the breathing muscles, the tongue, the jaw muscles, or many different places in the body. Certainly, this learned behavior is important for the civil functioning of society. However, an actor needs to tap into that primary

impulse. Stanley Kowalski isn't concerned about waking up his neighbors when he's calling for Stella in *A Street Car Named Desire*. Since the Linklater method is about expressing who you are through your voice, it is a very useful technique for working with transgender performers. As an individual is transitioning, finding one's new voice is a crucial step in establishing their gender identity. Through their voice the transgender individual can actualize who they are.

The Role of the Voice Coach

Being a voice coach in the theatre requires sensitivity, whether one is working with cisgender or transgender actors. When working on productions, the goal of the voice coach is to serve the vision of the play as it is defined by the director. The voice coach's specific task is to help the actor realize this vision. The approach to the work has to be tailored to the needs of the individual actor. One of the most challenging parts of the process is to determine HOW to work with an individual. What is their learning style? What do they feel are their strengths as actors? In what areas do they feel less secure? Each actor is different. Frequently, the voice coach is regarded with suspicion or fear. I've sometimes heard coaches referred to as the "Voice and Speech Police." The main job of the voice coach is to support the actor so that they can perform to the best of their ability and be successful. A big part of this process is accomplished by helping the actor feel confident, supporting them and giving them the space to explore. One of my students recently wrote to me: "Every time I left your class, I felt more confident and comfortable as myself and as an artist. You always made me feel like I was enough as a person and didn't have to sacrifice who I was to make art." Being an actor takes a lot of courage and the desire to reveal the self. The transgender actor has had to access a tremendous amount of courage in their own life. I don't ever want any actor to feel they had to compromise who they are in the rehearsal process. Transgender performers need even more support and affirmation.

Use of Language

The language we use has a major impact on the quality of our experience. You might even say that language *determines* our experience. Eve Ensler, who wrote *The Vagina Monologues*, said: "I believe in the power and mystery of naming things. Language has the capacity to transform our cells, rearrange our learned patterns of behavior and redirect our thinking" (Ensler, 2006).

It is crucial that the language the voice coach uses with actors is accurate and respectful. The goal of that language is to encourage exploration, not to shut the actor down. The specificity of language is even more important with transgender actors. Liz Jackson Hearns, a voice coach and singing teacher in Chicago, refers to language which is "trans affirming or trans harming." One of the first things the coach needs to do is to ask the actor what pronoun they use. It's also helpful to use language that doesn't reference gender, especially when describing different vocal qualities. Ms. Jackson Hearns goes on to say: "Because as soon as you say 'Can you make that sound more masculine? 'More feminine?' the singer's vocal quality and timbre become tied to their gender identity/expression. If you, as the teacher, are looking for a sound that's fuller, deeper, rounder, then use adjectives! Describe what you're looking for instead of taking a shortcut by using gender-assumptive language!" (Jackson Hearns in Castanho, 2017).

Some time ago, I was working with a trans woman on a scene which was very emotional and difficult. The character had to confront her father about an abusive situation. The actor was struggling to find more power and size in her voice. Without thinking, I asked her if she could tap into her "masculine voice." As soon as I said that, I knew those words were harmful. That comment profoundly hurt that actor. I apologized to her, but it took a long time for her to trust me again. As has been mentioned on numerous occasions in this text, the language for transgender/gender nonconforming individuals is constantly evolving. The voice coach needs to stay up to date with the most current terminology.

Most importantly, I like to think of the role of the voice coach as a *collaboration* with the actor. The coach is the "expert" in the field of voice and has trained for many years to gain that expertise. However, the needs of the actor vary tremendously from production to production and actor to actor. There is rarely one answer or definitive solution to a problem. Instead of being prescriptive, it is helpful for the coach to make suggestions. As Delia Kropp states above, listen to the actor. I prefer to ask open-ended questions. For example, questions that start with "What do you think about . . . ?" and "How would you . . . ?" or "What is your experience with . . . ?" As coaches listen to actors' answers, they will get a deeper understanding of the actor's process. Listening also provides the opportunity to cultivate empathy and build a relationship. My experience of working with transgender actors is a much more recent development in my career. I need to learn from my transgender actors; perhaps even more than they need to learn from me. Finally, the most important piece of this collaboration is a sense of fun and exploration. Once the coach and the actor have defined the problem, they can play with a solution. If that doesn't work, explore the next possibility. They can try something else, and perhaps that will open the door to another acting/vocal choice.

The Thought/Breath Connection

If an actor doesn't have enough breath to speak a thought, then different muscles engage to "help" the speaker. The most common "helping muscles" that tighten are: the abdominals, the throat, the back of the tongue, the soft palate and the jaw. Actors each have their own way of compensating for this scarcity of breath. The result is a voice that is "pushed" or strained. In addition to this pushed quality, the range of expression is usually diminished. The inflection gets flattened out.

"The role played by breathing in the art of acting has occupied me professionally for fifty years and, in the art of acting, the goals are believability and a sense of limitlessness. We search for truth in the language of extremity and in the most intimate emotional expression. The alchemy of inspired communication is a mix of emotion, intellect and voice. The 'prima materia' is breath. This fundamental element of truthful speaking is accessible for anyone involved in speaking publicly—or indeed privately" (Linklater, 2009; https://www.linklatervoice .com/resources/articles-essays/39-the%20 alchemy-of-breathing).

Linklater explains the mechanics of speaking in the following simplified way (Linklater, 2006, p. 13).

1. "There is an impulse in the motor cortex of the brain.
2. The impulse stimulates breath to enter and leave the body.
3. The outgoing breath makes contact with the vocal folds creating oscillations.

4. The oscillations create frequencies (vibrations).
5. The frequencies (vibrations) are amplified by resonators.
6. The resultant sound is articulated by the lips and tongue to form words."

Perhaps the most important part of this sequence for the actor is the very beginning. The connection between thought and breath. A crucial part of this connection is the need to communicate. It is that need (or in acting terms, the motivation or intention) that stimulates the breathing muscles. Each new thought initiates a new breath. The word is the last part of the whole sequence. However, in the theatre, we START with the word. The actor needs to track back to the beginning of the sequence to find the thought/breath connection. In Hamlet, Claudius says: "My words fly up, my thoughts remain below: Words without thoughts never to heaven go" (Shakespeare, *Hamlet*, Act III, Scene 3, p. 1095). Claudius is praying and saying the words, but he cannot repent his sin. Therefore, the words are meaningless. The words always need to have that thought/breath connection, otherwise it sounds like actors are saying "lines." When working with actors, it is extremely useful to slow down. There is so much pressure in the rehearsal room to produce that often actors push forward, without really connecting to what or why they are saying something. In a voice session, the actor can take the time to slow down and connect to each thought. I like to use Cecily Berry's exercise of "Walking the Text" (Berry, 2000, p. 179). Berry has the actor walk in a straight line and change direction with each punctuation mark. I like to have the actor change direction with each new thought. Sometimes punctuation will signal the new thoughts, but not always. When a new thought comes, the actor will let the breath come in and change direction. It is crucial that the abdominal muscles are relaxed, so that each thought can drop down to the belly. This will allow the actor to "embody" the thought.

Open Mouth versus Closed Mouth Breathing

"For actors, nasal breathing is utterly counterproductive to truthful speaking" (Linklater, 2006, p. 48). The Linklater Method places a big emphasis on breathing with an open mouth. The jaw is released and the lips are slightly parted. There are several reasons why open mouth breathing is helpful for acting.

1. It provides a direct connection to the emotions. The actor is more emotionally available.
2. It helps release the jaw. Many times when people close their mouths, they clench the jaw muscles. Tense jaw muscles can inhibit expression and affect the voice.
3. It encourages spontaneous speech. In speaking, if you close your mouth to take in your breath, the breath goes in much more slowly. Because of this slower intake of breath, there is a delay in the speaking. It produces a measured or stilted quality. However, that stilted breathing pattern might be an interesting character choice. Lady Bracknell in *The Importance of Being Earnest* comes to mind!
4. It is much easier to receive from your partner when listening with an open mouth. The impulse to speak happens *while* the other person is speaking. If the actor waits to find that impulse until the partner is finished speaking, it will sound like the actor is saying "lines."
5. The facial muscles are much more responsive and expressive with an open mouth.

Those "micro expressions" are especially important on camera.

Releasing Muscle Tension: Jaw and Tongue

As discussed earlier, if there isn't enough breath, the muscles will push to compensate for the inadequate breath. The muscles of the jaw and tongue are the main offenders. Also, both of these muscles are experts at repressing emotion.

"One of the strongest and universal muscular defense systems is in the jaw hinges. Clenching the teeth is a sure way to avoid opening the throat wide enough for a scream of fear to escape, so a bulging jaw muscle comes to represent bravery and strength. Rage is nailed down in the muscles of the jaw" (Linklater, 2006, p. 131).

Relaxing the jaw will not only help free the voice, it will also allow the actor to connect more fully with their emotions. Massaging around the jaw hinge and up along the temporal bone is helpful. The Linklater Jaw shake is really useful (Linklater, 2006, p. 135). Take a hold of the lower jaw with both hands. Swing the jaw down and back and then up to meet the teeth. Repeat this action multiple times. Be careful to not have the teeth hit each other. This swinging action lengthens the jaw muscles. Like any muscle that is habitually tense, the jaw muscles will shorten. This action will create more space in the mouth, especially in the back of the mouth. Make sure the actor is breathing and not holding their breath. It's useful to do this first sighing out with breath, then you can add a sigh with vibrations. The jaw shake is especially useful for trans men who need to create more space to access fuller resonance. Many times, trans men will open the jaw wider to access more space within the mouth cavity. The space that's crucial is the space in the BACK of the mouth, between the upper and lower molars. Opening the mouth wider actually adds to the tension. It pushes the larynx down, and makes it more difficult to breathe. If the jaw is pushed down, it obstructs the trachea.

Tension at the back of the tongue is one of the major contributors to strained voices and a diminution of range. The tongue is an excellent "helper" muscle to compensate for a lack of freedom in the breath. Also, the tongue is a great repressor of emotion, especially sadness. If you've ever gotten "choked up" or had a "lump in your throat," that's the back of the tongue tensing to repress the feeling. Trans men will depress the back of the tongue to create more space in the back of the mouth. They also may use tongue tension in an attempt to find more power or to deepen the voice. The problem with these strategies is that the base of the tongue is attached to the hyoid bone, which is attached to the larynx by a membrane. When the back of the tongue is tense, the tongue pulls back and down. Therefore, the larynx is depressed. This is one of the reasons trans men's voices are often pressed and lack variety in range. Releasing the back of the tongue is essential to open up the voice. For trans women, often the back of the tongue takes over to push the voice higher.

The Linklater tongue stretch (Linklater, 2006, p. 142) is an excellent way to release the back of the tongue. It's helpful to do this initially with a mirror. Anchor the tip of the tongue on the bottom gum ridge, right below the back of the bottom front teeth. Think into the middle of the tongue and stretch it out of the mouth. Make sure that the tongue is wide and flat as it stretches out. Then let the tongue release back into the mouth, keeping the tongue tip anchored. Repeat this action multiple times—stretch and release. Make sure the actor is

breathing and not holding their breath. Like the jaw shake, it's helpful to do this first sighing out with breath. After a sigh with no sound, add a sigh with vibrations. Start at a comfortable pitch and go up by half steps.

Toning the Soft Palate

Unlike the tongue and jaw muscles that are overachievers (they work too hard), the soft palate is usually lazy. The idea behind the Linklater approach is not to hold up the soft palate but rather to exercise it so that it is more responsive to thought. Also, if the soft palate is toned, in its resting position it will be higher in the mouth. This is helpful for both trans women and trans men. For trans men, a more responsive soft palate will create more room in the back of the mouth, which will help them find a fuller resonance. The soft palate is also the trapdoor to the upper resonators. Trans women need to access their upper resonators. If the soft palate is stiff, it won't lift to let the vibrations resonate off the bony hollows of the sinus area. A responsive soft palate can help trans women find those higher tones, without pushing. Yawning is an excellent way to stretch and activate the soft palate. The Linklater voice work suggests a "horizontal yawn." Keep the tip of the tongue in contact with the back of the bottom front teeth and direct your yawn sideways. This sideways stretch keeps the jaw in its hinge, and keeps the throat open. Another Linklater exercise for the soft palate is the "whispered KAH" /kɑ/. Whisper a KAH /kɑ/ on an incoming breath, and then whisper the KAH /kɑ/ as the breath goes out. Swallow and repeat. Don't allow the tongue to pull back. Keep the tip of the tongue anchored to the back of the bottom front teeth. This is another exercise in which it is helpful to use a mirror. As you look in the mirror, make sure the soft palate is lifting as high as it can go with each KAH /kɑ/.

Unique Challenges

Managing Emotional Lability and Acting Challenges

An actor's job is to *express* rather than to *repress,* therefore open mouth breathing will facilitate that emotional connection. However, sometimes actors might be in an emotional state which is not useful for the work at hand. Several times I've worked with trans actors who have become very emotional. Sometimes that emotional rollercoaster has been influenced by a shift in the balance of hormones. One actor in particular was so emotional that she felt out of control and wasn't sure she could continue to work. I suggested that she close her mouth and breathe through her nose. Breathing through the nose calms the nervous system. After a few minutes of breathing through her nose, she felt calmer and more in control and was able to continue with the rehearsal. I don't mean to imply that emotional states are counterproductive to the acting process. Not at all! Emotion is certainly a huge part of the tapestry of acting. However, in a professional situation it's helpful to know a way to disconnect with the emotion, if that gets in the way of a rehearsal or performance.

Binders for Trans Men

Working with trans men who are wearing binders is very similar to working with actresses in period plays who are wearing corsets. The ribcage is immobilized, it is therefore vital that the belly be free and expansive. Open mouth breathing will help.

There is a connection between the intercostal muscles and nasal breathing. Nasal breathing stimulates the intercostal muscles; therefore, open mouth breathing will be beneficial when the rib cage is immobilized. Trans women (as well as cis women) need to be encouraged to let go of vanity and let their bellies expand.

Sometimes costumes will be too tight around the waist to allow that expansion. The voice coach can be an advocate for the actor to talk with the director or costume designer to help make the costume as comfortable as possible. If the character is wearing heels, it's helpful to do some sessions without shoes so that the lower back can open up. Working on the floor with the knees up is another way to free up the abdominals and lower back (refer also to Chapter 9).

Finding Tone

The Resonating Ladder

Resonance (refer also to Chapter 11) is a key factor in working with trans performers, in helping them develop the voice that is congruent with their gender identity. Kristin Linklater has a unique system for working with resonance. She talks about the "resonating ladder."

"We will be looking at the resonating system as if it were a kind of ladder. The resonators are a series of cavities going from big and broad at the base and gradually getting smaller and narrower toward the top—like a type of ladder. They have many different shapes as well as sizes, built in as they are to the skeleton" (Linklater, 2006, p. 187). She defines the different rungs of the ladder as: chest, mouth, teeth, sinuses, nose, and skull. She has exercises that strengthen and develop each of these areas of resonance. There are several of these Linklater exercises that are particularly useful for the transgender performer.

Chest Resonance

The trans man usually needs to develop and strengthen his chest resonance. The following Linklater exercise develops chest resonance (Linklater, 2006, p. 188). Lengthen the front of the neck so that the head can drop back. Be careful to not collapse the neck or the shoulders. Picture the channel for sound that widens into your rib cage and descends into a great hollow cave of your belly. Sigh warm breath on a HAAAH from the depths of your belly. Make sure the abdominal and throat muscles are free and not engaged. When the head is back, it is almost impossible to use the throat to support the sound; the breath must take over (Linklater, 2006, p. 183). Now sigh deep, lazy, warm vibrations from that cave of your belly on a HAAAH /hɑ/. Three times. Put your hand on your chest and feel the vibrations. Let your hand become a fist as you thump your chest. Bring the back of the neck up, head floats on top. Relax. Chest thumping helps when an actor is working on text and the voice seems high in the body. Jumping up and down while speaking a text is another way to ground a voice. Accessing this lower part of the voice is particularly challenging in highly emotional material or if great volume is required. If you use too much force, the voice will usually jump in pitch. If the voice is pressed down in pitch using tongue tension, the result will be an unpleasant sound and possible vocal strain.

Teeth Resonator

Linklater divides up the resonators into six different areas: chest, mouth, teeth, sinus, nasal, and skull. The teeth resonator is unique to the Linklater method (Linklater, 2006). It's extremely useful for both trans men and trans women. It has clarity and a great deal of volume; however, it is in the mid-range, not in the upper part. It is on the third rung of the resonating ladder. It still has a quality that feels grounded; however, it's a few steps higher than the chest or the mouth. It is also very forward focused. It's helpful for trans men because they will be able to access some power without pressing down at the back of the throat. For trans women, the teeth resonator will help them move their sound forward. They can find a higher pitch, but without becoming breathy. I think this resonator is kind of "sassy." To explore the teeth resonator, let your head drop slightly forward. With the tip of your tongue feel the back of your front upper teeth and the upper gum ridge. Put a hand on your diaphragm and send a powerful whispered "KEE" /ki/ to the back of the upper teeth. Feel that explosion of breath, powered by the action of the diaphragm. Now change to a "HEE" /hi/ on vibrations. Imagine the vibrations were a laser beam cascading off the back of your teeth. Explore pitches until you feel the maximum resonating feedback in your front top teeth. Make sure you are using 100% vibrations and not a mix of breath and vibration. Repeat. HEE-HEE-HEE /hi hi hi/.

Sinus Resonator

This resonator too is unique to the Linklater method. It is above the teeth resonator, but still in the middle register. This is a really useful resonator to develop and strengthen for the trans woman. It is a very transparent part of the voice. It is powerful but can also be very vulnerable. "It is the voice's most revealing area, and perhaps for that reason it is often the least freely used. The resonating corridors here are labyrinthine compared with the simple chest and mouth chambers. . . . Easily triggered defense mechanisms develop early in life to make the most revealing part of the voice the best guarded" (Linklater, 2006, pp. 245–246).

The muscles of the face can sometimes be held and become "a mask." This "mask" is an excellent way to hide this part of the voice and the thoughts/feelings that might live there. Some actors I've worked with have had cosmetic surgery or injected "fillers" in their faces. As a result, their facial muscles are less responsive and can "muffle" their voices. It is necessary to free any tension that might be held in the facial muscles. This can be accomplished by using the fingers to massage the face. It's also useful to wake up the responsiveness of the facial muscles by doing facial isolations while looking in a mirror (Linklater, 2006, p. 247). The following exercise will help to identify and strengthen the sinus resonator (Linklater, 2006, p. 250): Take your two middle fingers and massage the area along the nasal labial folds and under the cheekbones. Let your head fall slightly forward so that your fingers feel some of the weight of your head. "Let the tip of your tongue fall loosely forward onto your lower lip. The tongue should slide, thick and relaxed, forward and out of the mouth. . . . Now with the tip of your tongue still out on your lower lip, sigh a whispered "heee" through the narrow space between the front of the tongue and the top teeth" (Linklater, 2006, pp. 250–251).

Now, sigh a "heee" /hi/ with vibrations as you move the sinus muscles up and down with your fingers. Use a pitch near the bottom of the feminine range, say E3. Sigh out easily on that pitch and go up by half steps. It is important to keep the tongue out and wide. As the pitches get more demanding, the back of the tongue will want to engage and the tongue will slide into the mouth.

Go up only as high as is comfortable, without any pushing or going into falsetto. When you've finished, intone a sentence or two on a comfortable pitch in the range you just explored. After the intoning, speak it. A helpful instruction is: "Speak through your eyes."

The Vowel Scale

All vowels have an intrinsic pitch. This is a result of the different spaces that the vowels create in the mouth. The tongue and the lips determine the shape of the mouth cavity for each vowel. The tongue is in its highest position for the vowel [i], which means that the vibrations move through the smallest amount of space. Therefore, [i] has the highest pitch of all the vowels. Hirsch refers to this in the *Acoustic Assumptions* discussed in Chapter 11. Linklater terms this "the Vowel Scale" or "the Vowel Tree."

The mouth and throat are like a wind instrument that changes musical pitch by making the aperture through which the breath escapes larger or smaller. Each vowel has a different set of frequencies and its own intrinsic musical pitch. When the musculature of the mouth and throat is free of habitual tensions that distort organ vowel formation, music is a natural component of speech, with the Vowel Scale covering at least two octaves. When there is tension in the back of the tongue or throat, the music flattens and the range diminishes to a monotonous two or three notes (Linklater, 1992, p. 19).

Of all of my Linklater training, the Vowel Scale has been the most useful for me as a performer and as a voice coach. Whenever I explored a text through the intrinsic pitch, there was an opening up of the language for me. Of course, I would marry meaning and sense with the pitch of the word. But there was usually something interesting that would emerge. As a voice coach, I've noticed that whenever actors are straining in a section of the text, almost always they've made vocal choices that go counter to the Vowel Scale. This shows up in a major way if the text is highly emotional or the actor has to fill a large space. When I was acting, I performed mostly outdoor Shakespeare, so I had the opportunity to explore emotionally charged texts in a large venue. I've also had the opportunity to coach at several outdoor venues: the Oregon Shakespeare Festival, the Old Globe in San Diego, and Shakespeare & Company in Lenox, Massachusetts. Linklater also attached these different vowels to different parts of the body: the lower vowels in the lower part and the higher vowels in the upper part of the body. As I explored, I could FEEL the words in different places in my body. Embodied language!

Years ago I had an experience, coaching an actor in the role of Hamlet. He was a conservatory trained actor with an expressive, mercurial voice. I had coached him the year before as Troilus in Shakespeare's *Troilus and Cressida*, and he was crystal clear even in the most demanding parts of the play. Suddenly, as Hamlet he was experiencing vocal strain. Curious! I was in rehearsal one day, listening to him do the soliloquy, "Oh what a rogue and peasant slave am I!" He got to the climax of the speech:

"bloody, bawdy villain!
Remorseless, treacherous, lecherous, kind-
less villain!
O, vengeance!"
　　　　　—Shakespeare, *Hamlet*, Act II,
　　　　　　　　　　Scene 2, p. 1086

As he said "vengeance" I could hear his voice break. When he spoke the "O," he was in the bottom of his range, but he also spoke "vengeance" using the same register. "O" is a low-pitched vowel. However, "vengeance" has two high vowels. Once he found the resonance of those vowels, the word powerfully soared out! Plus, he discovered by saying the word in that higher part of his range that his acting choices were more supported. Vengeance isn't something that sucks you down, but it propels you forward. The intrinsic pitch helped the actor connect to Hamlet's action in that moment, and preserved the actor's voice.

The Vowel Scale and Gender Diverse Actors

The Vowel Scale has a direct application to working with trans actors. For trans men, the coach can help the actor identify the lower vowels and use those as "anchors." Words that contain an [u] [ʊ] [oʊ] [ɔ] or the diphthongs [aʊ] [ɔɪ] [ju] are examples. Those are sounds that can drop down. In addition to feeling the lower resonance of those words, it is also important to connect image. For instance, an actor who has the word "woe" can feel the vowel low in their body. The actor also needs to connect to the meaning and image of "woe." For trans women, the coach can help the actor identify the higher vowels and those can be "handles." They can be words that can soar. Words that contain [i] [ɪ] [eɪ] [ɛ] [æ] [aɪ] [ɪɚ] [ɛɚ]. Again, it's important to connect sound to image. The word "grief" is a synonym of "woe," but the places of resonance for the vowels are completely different in the body. The consonants are also vastly different. In "woe" there is the /w/, which is a glide and classified as a semi-vowel. There is no consonant at the end of that word to stop /oʊ/. The vowel continues until the breath stops. "Grief" begins with the stop plosive /g/ and follows with the very tense /r/. The /i/ explodes from that abrupt beginning and then is silenced by the unvoiced fricative /f/, which is essentially just breath. Even though both words are synonyms, the experience of speaking the words is very different. Actors need to sensitize themselves to the difference of feeling for the sounds of words, so that the language is more specific. If the actor is experiencing the language, the audience will HEAR that experience and they will then experience it.

"When today's actor starts to *experience* Shakespeare's language as a whole-body process, s/he is led to a larger and deeper experience of thought and emotion, and from there to a more fundamental, more individual and enlarged experience of 'truth.' Understanding the text is immediately illuminated" (Linklater, 1992, pp. 6–7).

A Whole Body/Voice Warm-Up Using the Vowel Scale in Practice

This is a warm-up that organizes the intrinsic music of the vowels with the resonating ladder. It also attaches each of the vowels to a body part. A consonant has been added before each vowel, to avoid onset with a glottal attack. Also, the vowels are experienced as either long or short (Linklater, 2006, p. 337). I have adapted Linklater's sequence to include an additional vowel and slightly different positioning. In this exercise, actors should begin at the bottom of their pitch range with /zu/ and move up their range to /ri/ (coaches should be sensitive to ranges that might trigger dysphoria, as mentioned earlier).

/ri/ TOP OF SKULL—Spirals upward
/kɪ/ MIDDLE OF THE FOREHEAD—Pops out suddenly
/peɪ/ EYEBROWS—Allow to widen

/dɛ/ EYES—Pops out suddenly
/bæ/ CHEEKBONES—Pops out suddenly
/hɜ/ (i.e., British er) UPPER LIP—Allow it to widen
/fə/ BOTTOM LIP—Pops out suddenly
/ma/ HEART—Allow it to widen
/gʊ/ BREAST BONE—Pops out suddenly
/ʃɔ/ SOLAR PLEXUS—Allow it to widen
/woʊ/ BELLY—Swirl it around
/sʊ/ THIGHS—Pops out suddenly

START HERE AND GO UP /zu/ KNEES DOWNWARD. Swirl around the sound. Feel it from the knees as it bores down into the floor.

Having gone all the way up the ladder, go all the way down. Let each sound arouse its different energy and mood. Make sure to allow each sound its true pitch frequency. This scale should warm you up through a wide spectrum of sounds and pitches, but if that is all that happens you have missed the point. The sounds are intrinsically connected to energies and moods as nuanced and diverse as the spectrum of the rainbow and the gamut of human nature. This scale provides an aerobics of the inner self and it is your inner self that desires communication and needs a language sufficient for its most complex expression" (Linklater, 1992, pp. 24–26).

The voice coach can help trans actors as they explore and widen their range of expression in their gender identity. Through using the Vowel Scale and other exercises, the coach can help awaken the actor's sensitivity to the particular sounds in a language and strengthen those parts of the actor's range that are less familiar. The goal is to have a voice that will express the full range of the human experience. As Linklater states above, an actor needs a voice that is as "diverse as the spectrum of the rainbow and the gamut of human nature." With the guidance and collaboration of the voice coach, hopefully the actor will be more confident and successful in performance.

Conclusion and Summary

All actors are challenged with the Herculean task of using the voice in a healthy, functional manner that allows for the full expression of self and character. The challenges of gender diverse actors are greater: they must learn to coax vocal ranges and a spectrum of sounds from their instrument, using the voice in a healthy, sustainable manner, while staying true to their identity and embodying multiple roles. Voice coaches and clinicians must perfectly blend their artistic creativity with scientific knowledge and expertise, in order to not just adequately train gender-diverse actors, but to prepare them for the task of auditioning for and being cast in a wide range of roles; roles that heretofore have largely been conferred upon cis actors. Alexandra Billings, a trans actress in *Transparent*, made this point herself in an interview with Michelle Ruiz in *Cosmopolitan* (Ruiz, 2015) when she said, "I'm an acting teacher myself, and I'm tired of trans actors coming up to me and asking me how they can get in a reality show. I turn to them and say, 'Look, let's study. Let's work on your skills before you become famous, shall we? Let's take ourselves a little bit more seriously.'" Coaches, trainers and clinicians must take their actors seriously. We must be of service, and always begin with "I am here to serve you. What do you need?"

References

Adichie, C. N. (2009). *The danger of the single story*. TEDGlobal, July 2009. https://www.ted.com/talks/chimamanda_adichie_the_danger_of_a_single_story?language=en (Retrieved January 16, 2018)

Berry, C. (2000) *The actor and the text*. New York, NY: Applause Theatre and Cinema Books.

Castanho, C. (2017). Gender diversity and education in musical theatre. *Huffington Post*, March 7.

Ensler, E. (2006, March 20). The power and mystery of naming things. *NPR: All Things Considered*. Retrieved from https://www.npr.org/templates/story/story.php?storyId=5285531

Linklater, K. (1992). *Freeing Shakespeare's voice*. New York, NY: Theatre Communication Group, Inc.

Linklater, K. (2006). *Freeing the natural voice*. Hollywood, CA: Drama Publishers.

Linklater, K. (2009). The Alchemy of Breathing. In J. Boston & R. Cook (Eds.), *Breath in action*. Retrieved November 14, 2017 from https://www.linklatervoice.com/resources/articles-essays/39-the alchemy-of-breathing.

Rodenburg, P. (1992). *The right to speak*. London, UK: Routledge.

Rodenburg, P. (2000). *The actor speaks: Voice and the performer*. New York, NY: St. Martin's Press.

Root, R. (2009). There and back again? Or, adventures in genderland: An investigation into the nature of transsexual voice, its presentation in performance, and the perception of gender. In Rena Cook (Ed.), *The moving voice: The integration of voice and movement studies. The Voice and Speech Review* (pp. 144–155). Cincinnati, OH: Voice and Speech Trainers Assoc., Inc.

Root, R. (2011). Stepping off the stone: Transsexual and transgender voice modification and presentation. A practical resource from a personal perspective. In Knight (Ed.), *A world of voice: voice and speech across culture. the voice and speech review* (pp. 254–261). Cincinnati, OH: Voice and Speech Trainers Assoc., Inc.

Ruiz, M. (2015, October 19). Trans actors and Hollywood insiders discuss the complicated reality of trans casting: Should trans roles always go to trans actors? And are trans actors still being pigeonholed as damaged characters? A conversation. *Cosmopolitan Magazine*, Retrieved November 14, 2017 from http://www.cosmopolitan.com/entertainment/celebs/a47797/trans-actors-casting-roundtable-interview/

Shakespeare, W. (1603/1992). *Hamlet*. In Bevington (Ed.), *The complete works of Shakespeare*, (4th ed.), New York, NY: Harper Collins.

16

Considerations for Discharge and Maintenance

Leah B. Helou and Sandy Hirsch

Discharge: How Do We Know "When" with a Gender Diverse Client?

General Considerations

For "traditional" voice therapy populations, a survey of voice-specialized speech-language pathologists (SLPs) revealed 85% agreement that the single most important factor in determining discharge readiness is the patient's ability to independently transfer voice techniques to conversational speech (Gillespie & Gartner-Schmidt, 2017). Four other factors were also shown to be of high relevance to discharge readiness: the patient's ability to function with the new voice production in activities of daily living, skillfully differentiate between the good and the bad voice, take responsibility for voice, and use a voice that sounds better compared with baseline. We have every reason to believe that these same factors are critical in discharge readiness for transgender clients, even in the absence of vocal pathology or impairment, and many of the recommendations in this chapter will underscore the importance of these factors

in discharge. Indeed, the report by Gillespie and Gartner-Schmidt recapitulates the findings of Ziegler et al. (2014), who examined perceptions of voice therapy from patients who underwent voice therapy either for muscle tension dysphonia or benign mid-membranous vocal fold lesions. Their participants, all of whom had undergone direct and indirect voice therapy, reported that transfer of techniques to conversation was one of the most useful aspects of treatment. Further, the findings of this study point to the value of incorporating carry-over/maintenance activities early on in the therapy process for optimal satisfaction and success in treatment.

Particularly in the context of transgender voice training, one consideration is that clients' long-term goals need not be the same as their discharge goals. For instance, if a client's stated long-term functional goal is to be appropriately gendered by others when they speak, then the measurable long-term goals for that client might involve achieving and maintaining a target average pitch during speech, using a particular resonance pattern, and so on. However, these same goals needn't necessarily be the discharge goals. Rather, at a broad level, a set of appropriate goals for discharge should be that clients (a) know what they are trying to achieve, (b) have acquired ample tools and techniques to achieve their aims *in due time* and troubleshoot any challenges *in the meantime*, and (c) know how and when to access resources (e.g., the clinician) if their skill set becomes overburdened. Stated differently, clients can be discharged from training when they are capable of functioning as their own clinicians, even if their long-term functional goal (e.g., being appropriately gendered by others) has not yet been fully realized. Thus, as in the context of the above example, clients might be discharged before they can independently maintain their target voice at a high level of accuracy. However, if the client and clinician agree that the client has the tools to eventually meet that goal given what has been learned, then discharge can be deemed fully appropriate.

If, as described above, clients are showing their ability to function as their own clinician, then they can reasonably begin to move away from SLP/voice trainer support. Note that this factor has also been shown to influence adherence to therapy overall (van Leer & Connor, 2010), thus the sooner the client feels ownership and agency in the voice change process, the better. This shift toward independence is typically accomplished by moving from weekly sessions to twice-weekly or monthly sessions. Indeed, titration is optimal for many clients, as an abrupt end to regular weekly sessions can sometimes backfire.

Of course, clients should *feel prepared* for discharge, and it should not be a surprise to them that they are being discharged from training. Preparation for discharge from training is best achieved if its foundation is laid from the outset of training. Such a foundation can be established in a number of ways, some of which are

bulleted below. This list is not exhaustive, and likely recapitulates principles of training discussed elsewhere in this text.

■ At the beginning of training, the clinician should **indicate a rough time line for when it might be appropriate to consider moving to twice-weekly or monthly sessions** (e.g., after two months of weekly sessions). Actual discharge dates can be completely flexible based on clients' individual needs and progress, but giving clients a mid-horizon goal for assessing discharge readiness helps them to expect and prepare for a foreseeable end point.

■ **Clients should be guided to take ownership of their voice change process**. For instance, if clinicians open each session with questioning along the lines of "How did you use the information presented in our last session?" and "What would you like for us to work on today?," they send an implicit message that they expect the client to take ownership of the session and, in fact, the entire process of communication change. Indeed, it has been shown that a sense of agency governs adherence to voice therapy (van Leer & Connor, 2010), and it is reasonable to expect that this finding extends to the context of transgender voice and communication training even when clients exhibit no medical voice impairment.

■ **Clients should learn how to pin tasks and techniques onto a conceptual framework** so that they have clarity about the process of communication behavior change. This building of a conceptual framework generally emerges by way of the discourse that occurs in training sessions. Helou (2017) refers to this process as "meta-therapy," and posits that how clinicians talk about *what we are doing here* will dictate how clients perceive the nature of training and their role in it, and thus how clients choose to practice and apply new tasks and techniques.

- **Clients should understand that discharge may come not when their voice is perfect**, but rather when they know how to work toward their ideal voice with minimal to no regular support. This can be simultaneously intimidating and empowering, but once clients realize that progress, not perfection, is the immediate goal for training, the path toward their ideal voice often feels less bumpy.

Readiness for Discharge

If expectations for discharge have been well defined at the outset of therapy, the decision to end training or change its timing will ideally be anticipated by both the client and clinician simultaneously. Various situations might arise that impact the discharge timeline and clients' readiness for discharge. Some such situations are described below.

Fine-Tuning

Some clients are tempted to "fine-tune" their voice *ad nauseum*, which can lead to frustration and boredom on both sides of the desk. Fine-tuning can turn into a trap for the clinician, who feels obligated to deliver the final product within the course of direct training. Rather, in the fine-tuning stage, the clinician is often most helpful in identifying what portion of the communicative signal is sounding "off." Clients often have a hard time identifying what it is they don't like about a recording of their voice when they talk. In that event, clients can provide an example (e.g., speech recording) that highlights or at least includes the

undesirable qualities, and clinicians can be valuable in helping parse out the root issue. It is uncommon that voice- and speech-related behaviors that clients wish to fine-tune require a vastly different set of skills and techniques, compared with those that were employed for the bulk of training (i.e., prior to the fine-tuning stage). Thus, if clients are capable of troubleshooting problems and employing their skills independently at a broader level, they can be guided to apply the same skills to independently fine-tune once they can grasp the source of their dissatisfaction. The final ~15–25% of communication development often comes just from living with that voice for a while, and exhaustive fine-tuning efforts in the training setting are no replacement for real life experience.

Difficulty Accepting Success

Some clients may have difficulty accepting success, and this often occurs for reasons that might best be explored most deeply by a counselor. Common comments and themes that have emerged in the course of our training experience are as follows:

- Clients subconsciously feel they don't deserve to achieve their goals.
- Internalized transphobia.
- Clients worry that others will feel they are trying to trick them or be dishonest about who they are.
- Clients do not feel they have permission, from society and/or themselves, to emerge in a gender identity–congruent way.
- Clients are somehow not able to embrace certain facets of the target voice, perhaps because they feel it conveys an identity or trait that they are not willing to adopt.

Clinicians should each decide whether they have the appropriate skills for exploring why clients might have difficulty accepting their own success in communication training. Social and emotional issues might not need to be unpacked, or they might be critical to address, but the clinician is not the person to take on that task. Regardless of whether and how clinicians choose to address social and emotional issues in the course of their training, they should bear in mind that such barriers might be at play, particularly when a client is able to readily achieve the target voice within the session but cannot generalize it despite weeks of continued practice. For example, sometimes clients will use a voice they think pleases the clinician, but because it does not please *them* personally or they do not feel worthy of it, they are challenged to implement it outside the training environment. Social, emotional, and psychological barriers to success can present themselves in myriad ways, and can also be easily overlooked by both client and clinician. It is hoped that open and explorative discussion will reveal core factors in due time, particularly when the dynamic between client and clinician is healthy. Clinicians should also maintain regular and open communication with counselors and therapists, to sharpen their skills and better recognize the boundaries of their professional scope and skills (see Chapters 2 and 3).

"Premature" Discharge from Training

At times, clients will withdraw from training early for logistical or financial reasons. Other clients will self-discharge if they feel their needs are not being met. Such instances are fairly straightforward. If a clinician has a high proportion of clients who self-discharge before their goals are met, they might consider reflecting on their own practice, asking themselves questions such as "Is my approach effective?," "Do my clients feel safe in my practice?," "Have I successfully created an atmosphere of dignity and respect for my clients?," and so on. It is well documented that transgender individuals have experienced discrimination, prejudice, bias, and micro-aggressive behavior by health care providers (e.g., Safer et al., 2016), and even well-intended clinicians might struggle to create a space and experience that feels comfortable for their clients. Clinicians might also consider ways to solicit feedback, ideally anonymous, from all outgoing clients.

In addition, therapists should be aware that clients might also discontinue training because they feel that they sound "good enough," even though they have not yet achieved their stated goals. In this situation, some clinicians might feel that their clients are "giving up," "being lazy," "lowering their standards," "suffering from low self-esteem," and any number of other such judgments. However, this situation might very well be more a cause for celebration and pride than for disappointment. Clinicians working with transgender individuals will hopefully make it clear to their clients from the first session that in their eyes, clients are each good enough just as they are, without ever changing the way they communicate. When clients cease training because they also have come to share this perspective, it is a moment to celebrate, even if the clinician thinks "they could have had such a good voice." Truly, if clinicians have succeeded in making clients their own clinician, then change will be ongoing over time if the client desires it.

Finally, some people find that the mental effort required to maintain their target voice for extended periods of time is simply not worthwhile. These clients might spend a good deal of time trying to learn how to maintain their target voice, but then decide that they are okay functioning primarily in a "default voice" that is closer to their baseline or somehow "short of" their target voice. Such clients are often satisfied with knowing that they can achieve their target voice when it is needed, but accept that they won't live with it 100% of the time. Not only is this a perfectly acceptable outcome, it is also one that clinicians can present as an option to clients early on, and particularly when maintenance of the target voice is evasive over time.

Duration of Therapy

Training duration is quite dependent on the person and their particular skills and situation, the clinician's level of expertise, and the unique interaction between client and clinician. However, the majority of clinicians working with gender diverse populations on voice and communication report that treatment may take anywhere from two to nine months to achieve desired results. This time line is usually based on a weekly session, allowing for obvious breaks such as holidays, vacations, illness, and other unforeseen interruptions. As stated above, there is value in expecting to assess discharge readiness at a set point in the future (e.g., after the first two months of training) rather than allowing the process to be fully open-ended. Of course, more sessions can be scheduled as needed, but clients should be working toward their goals with the knowledge that an assessment point is on the near horizon. This creates the expectation that active engagement and change need to happen *right now*, not just at some point in the future when the client is somehow more advanced.

Clients who pursue biweekly or irregularly scheduled sessions from the outset, whether for scheduling or budgetary reasons, should know that this schedule might prolong the total training duration. If a client requests an even less frequent schedule, the clinician should caution the client about the possibility that progress may be delayed and perhaps in some cases not achievable. Due to a lower chance for success, the ethics of agreeing to a very irregular schedule of therapy should be in the forefront of any clinician's mind. If requests for infrequent meetings are based on financial considerations, clinicians might suggest that clients consider waiting to initiate training until they have the resources to commit to two months of weekly sessions, with the aim of transitioning as soon as possible to a less frequent schedule. In sum, it is essential that the client and clinician have a clear understanding as to the seriousness of commitment to a schedule.

Defining Successful Therapy and Criteria for Discharge

Defining success of therapy should be an integral part of the assessment, but the definition of success for a given client might also be a shifting target. As such, discharge goals can be reassessed at any point in training, and should be revisited at least once between intake and discharge. It is most important that therapy outcomes meet the daily needs of the client, in terms of both satisfaction and communication ability. For example, if the client has stated during the intake process that being properly gendered on the telephone 100% of the time is the primary consideration, then regardless of acoustic metrics pertaining to vocal pitch and inflectional measures, this must be the driving criterion used to measure success. That said, clients should also be counseled to understand that 80% is a more realistic measure of competence in any therapy process, given the number of possible impeding variables at any moment and in any context.

If therapy objectives are written well and the client has met them, there can usually be little argument as to whether therapy has been successful. However, as therapy draws to a close, it is not unusual for a client to recognize the need for adjusting or adding higher-level goals, just as is the case with other types of communication therapy. Sometimes clients will be reluctant to "graduate" from training because their voice is not "perfect" yet (see previous subsection, "Fine-Tuning"). The client's definition of success is going to be based on a more subjective everyday level of satisfaction and expectation, whereas the clinician needs to have established objectives and measurable outcomes with the client. The goals initially established to define successful therapy must be reconsidered as the time for discharge approaches. If the goals are recalibrated, this does not have to reflect a lack of success, but rather indicates realistic and functional expectations.

Considerations for Discharge

Discharge considerations can be both objective and subjective, but goals should also be functional and measurable. Within the context of potentially shifting definitions of success and dynamic goals for all the areas targeted, discharge questions should be consistent with traditional communication disorders therapy. These discharge questions may include:

- What does it mean when the client says I've met my goal?
- What is holding the client back if they continue to be unsure of success?
- Do therapy outcomes match the current statement of client need or hope for communication success?
- Has there been a desired and goal-appropriate change from baseline measures?

- Has the client reached or approximated their highest potential for communication and overall authenticity in everyday life outside of the therapy room?
- Is the client satisfied and comfortable with their current communication skills and techniques?
- If specific communication goals are not being met, is there indeed an opportunity for change?
- Is the client confident in using learned tools across unanticipated or uncomfortable contexts?
- Is the client able to maintain the new voice during "inner voice" tasks such as doing the dishes, changing their mind in mid-activity, searching for car keys, etc.?
- Is the client capable of flexibly using their voice and communications skills/techniques across a variety of situations and environments?
- Is the client capable of troubleshooting their voice and communication skills/techniques in the face of a challenging communication moment?
- If the client is not 100% where they want to be vocally, do they feel that they are on the right path? Do they know what their voice/communication goals are, and do they feel that they can address them independently?
- Does the client feel prepared to transition to less frequent training sessions or fully end training?
- Does the client have a plan for how they will continue to address their voice and communication goals in the absence of regularly scheduled training sessions?

Outcome Measures

When the time arrives to obtain outcome measures, clinicians may refer to the following recommendations. First, clients' experiences with and perception of their own voice are some of the most meaningful considerations for discharge. Hancock, Krissinger, and Owen (2011) showed that for trans women, quality of life was more strongly correlated with the speaker's self-ratings of voice compared with other listeners' perceptions, with regard to both likability and femininity. Thus, use of a voice-related quality-of-life scale such as those described in Chapter 7 on assessment and goal setting (e.g., TVQ) should be administered as a key outcome metric.

It is considered best practice to also quantify the final measure of success with the specific goals and objectives used during the assessment: pitch, intonation, semantics, resonance, non-verbal markers, and vocal hygiene. For example, the measurement of pitch and intonation, as outlined in Chapter 10, will obtain specific and meaningful "hard data" worth comparing across baseline and discharge time points. When measuring resonance and nonverbal criteria, even the implementation of a generic scale can provide some values for pre- and post-therapy measurement of these aspects of therapy (see Chapters 11 and 12). Parameters measured at the time of initial assessment can be re-measured, as these may be used as quantitative benchmarks for discharge. Assessment protocols have been thoroughly covered in Chapter 7.

It should be noted that a detailed survey of voice-specialized SLPs revealed a striking lack of agreement regarding the importance of improvement in acoustic and aerodynamic outcomes as a metric of readiness for discharge (Gillespie & Gartner-Schmidt, 2017). Some highly skilled voice-specialized SLPs find instrumental assessment to be of very high value, whereas others do not find it to be useful in their discharge considerations. At a minimum, clinicians—especially

those new to transgender voice and communication work—should be obtaining measures that help them gauge their clinical efficacy and develop reference points for how client satisfaction matches up with performance metrics. Toward this end, a high-value outcome measure is a comparison between the pre- and post-pitch and intonation measures during a standard reading protocol such as the Rainbow passage, and during a one-minute (at least) spontaneous speech sample. If other measures were taken at the time of initial assessment, then a comparison of these areas might also be useful. However, it is important to remember that from the client's perspective, it is most important to be able to show a perceptual change during spontaneous speech regardless of any objective acoustic changes that may have occurred. This can be achieved by comparing the client's perception of listener response (whether or not a client continues to be misgendered, for instance) in real-life settings (e.g., on the phone, playing online video games, at the store, waiting for a bus, managing the minutia of day-to-day activities, in business meetings).

If, as recommended, regular and frequent sessions are discontinued before clients have achieved their full vocal and communicative potential, all of the aforementioned measures might reasonably be adjusted down in terms of expected accuracy at the time of discharge. For instance, consider a transfeminine client who has been working on her voice for a couple of months but is not yet presenting regularly with gender congruence and thus has few opportunities to practice her target voice. In that situation, the clinician might focus on training until the client can maintain (a) the target pitch with 80% accuracy in conversation, (b) forward resonance with 80% accuracy in conversation, and (c) a specific variance in intonation with 80% accuracy in conversation. If the client is actually capable of aligning these three skills to culminate in the production of her desirable target voice, then she can hopefully understand that when she has the opportunity to use this voice more, the skills underpinning that target voice will have the opportunity to solidify. Thus, rather than seeking a high level of accuracy for maintaining that target voice, a clinician might choose to aim for a lower accuracy (e.g., 60%), while adding a set of goals pertaining to the client's demonstration of her ability to independently *find* her target voice across situations. Because the client's voice may improve, evolve, and "gel" over time, it may be more useful to ensure that the client can demonstrate skills in *adjusting* behaviors and *accessing* target behaviors readily, rather than *maintaining* them in the absence of a real-world opportunity to do so. This speaks specifically to the earlier mention in this chapter of ensuring that clients become their own clinician. The ability of a client to self-assess and adjust independently is critical.

Maintenance

Corollary to the closing statements in the preceding paragraph, consider this question: what is the difference between maintaining a target voice versus finding or accessing it repeatedly? Oftentimes clinical goals for skill maintenance focus on the former: that clients are expected to maintain their target voice for a period of time that is relevant to social communication. However, this perspective might lead to clients feeling as though every time they fall away from their target voice, they have failed at maintaining it. Indeed, clients are often disheartened and frustrated by their failure to maintain their target voice, and this can

have a negative impact on progress. An alternative framework is one in which clients are assessed on their ability to access and return to their target voice quickly and with ease. This framework involves the implicit expectation that clients *will* fall away from their target voice—indeed, it is a normal part of the process and not something to lament—and are measured on their ability to return to it independently as they deem necessary.

Clinicians are encouraged to shift their expectations and shape clients' expectations to align with this latter perspective on skill maintenance. It is a subtle but profound shift that can influence clients' sense of self-efficacy and ability to achieve their goals. This perspective can be valuable in the short term (e.g., within a conversation) as well as in the longer term (e.g., after discharge). That is, if clients have transitioned to less frequent sessions or are fully discharged and trying to maintain their target voice, they need to know that a failure to maintain their voice is simply an opportunity to call upon their skills. Too often, clients interpret a failure to maintain their target voice as evidence that they have no skills, or that their skills are inadequate. If clients are discharged from training with the perspective that a lapse away from the target voice is simply a cue to call upon their techniques, they will be more likely to report success in maintaining their target voice over time.

We are promoting a model wherein the clinical approach to the maintenance phase is that it overlaps with the training phase, both conceptually and practically. That is, as soon as clients are able to implement a target skill or technique, they are encouraged and expected to return to it as often as possible. As the individual skills and techniques converge to produce a more cohesive target voice or communication profile, clients have an evolving target that they are constantly trying to find, access, and maintain. This, then, becomes a cycle of behavior wherein clients' maintenance skills are developed early in training, strengthen throughout training, and seamlessly take precedence as direct training frequency decreases. This model may be in conflict with a more traditional approach to maintenance wherein the beginning of the maintenance phase is signified by discharge from training. In this paradigm, maintenance and readiness for discharge become essentially synonymous, and appear to best develop a client's overall confidence.

With regard to logistics, it can be useful to schedule maintenance sessions at the time of discharge from training. For instance, at the time of discharge, the client might estimate that they would benefit from checking back in with the clinician after three months have passed. Scheduling that session at discharge gives the client a clear mid-horizon expectation for maintenance rather than an open-ended period that might feel overwhelming or minimize a sense of accountability. Some clients might enter a note in their personal calendar to email the clinician one week prior to that scheduled session, letting the clinician know what they want to address in their maintenance session. This is, of course, something that reinforces a sense of accountability and ownership, so clinicians might consider requesting it of all clients at discharge.

Finally, the concept of maintenance as discussed herein is not just that clients are expected to maintain their target voice, but also that the clients are invited to maintain a relationship with the clinician. It is reasonable for clients and clinicians to anticipate having a long-term relationship wherein the bulk of their work is conducted in the early training phase, but then they return for refresher sessions as needed for months or even years after discharge from weekly sessions. Perhaps taking this approach will help some clinicians feel more comfortable with the idea of discharging clients before their communication goals are perfectly met. Clients also feel the need to wean from a strong support system developed throughout the therapy process. After all, as said earlier, the point of discharging early is so that clients function as their own clinician—this means less money out of their pocket, a greater sense of empowerment and self-efficacy, and a more rapid transition to their target communication behaviors. As such, clinicians should brainstorm ways to reinforce and support their clients even after discharge. For instance, clinicians might ask their clients to write reminders and goals on a postcard that they self-address; the clinician then files it away to mail to the client at a future point in time. Or, clinicians might ask clients to send a biweekly voicemail letting them know how their voice and communication is evolving. Regardless of the approach, a plan should be made for how the client will engage with the clinician after discharge from regularly scheduled training sessions.

All clinicians have a different set of tools and approaches for facilitating maintenance of therapy outcomes. A thoughtful and creative approach tailored for individual clients is likely to be most effective. Moreover, introducing the concepts and tasks of maintenance early on and throughout the therapy timeline, rather than just before discharge, will ideally promote more rapid independence and thus a shorter course of training.

Real-Life Tests

The ability to maintain skills across various situations is central to success in training.

Training environments often are poor replications of real-life environments. Even in excellent training environments, clients might feel that they are sitting beneath a spotlight and a microscope as they work to build their skills in the training situation. These environments also tend to be socially sterile, with low ambient noise, few distractions, and an unnaturally heightened degree of support provided by the clinician. These traits are desirable early in training before clients are ready to practice their communication in real-life situations. However, as their skills emerge and then solidify, real-life tests with the client and clinician together can be incredibly rich sources for identifying and troubleshooting challenges as well as for facilitating maintenance. Real-life tests may include:

- Genuine laughter
- Going out for coffee or to lunch
- Going for a walk in an environment with relatively high ambient noise to assess volume control and breath support, as well as ability to communicate in the presence of distractions
- Spending time with the client performing daily activities like driving, grocery shopping, or going to the post office
- If the client is presenting in their gender identity at work, observations in the setting will provide excellent information about whether old patterns of behavior and communication have changed
- Listen to the client making "chore" phone calls
- Recordings of speech samples derived from real-life interactions (e.g., phone calls, presentations)

When considering real-life tests, one of the areas difficult for transgender clients is "self-chat." Clients may revert to their "old" voice when they talk to themselves. One

powerful "real life" test is for the client to maintain (or not stray far from) a congruent voice for the entire day, even when alone in the quiet of the mind.

Maintenance/Generalization Tasks

Clients require differing levels of structure to maintain a variety of communication behaviors. It is the clinician's task to help clients strike a balance between needing a crutch versus having tools and techniques to which they can turn in times of communication breakdown. As with any client working toward communication change, it is necessary to ensure that "pull out" and re-set strategies have been practiced so that clients do not experience complete breakdown, a crisis of confidence, and in some instances a very real risk of danger. Clients need to know that they have the tools and techniques to troubleshoot through challenging and unpredictable situations. In order to be able do this, it is important that as part of therapy they learn how and why their communication will be altered. A firm understanding of vocal mechanics, vocal boundaries, and each of their techniques is essential for successful discharge.

Clients need to be able to identify when and how they will practice, as routine practice will assist with generalizing learned behaviors and techniques. A journal to document and monitor the client's progress could be beneficial for both the clinician and the client. Clients often benefit from seeing their own progress across time by listening to earlier recordings of their voice. Reminders about the use of the acoustic assumptions discussed in Chapter 11 are useful. For instance, clients might set a semi-regular alarm to remind them to bring acoustic awareness back into focus or do an occasional home-based "selfie" video-taping of an occupational or social activity. Following are additional approaches that a clinician might suggest to a client.

"Pull-Up List"

The "pull-up list" consists of a list of x words and fillers that can easily and seamlessly be interjected into most conversations (e.g., so, well, no, yeah, um, and, etc.). Clients practice the word at a pitch that will "pull" them toward their target pitch, and then practice subtly inserting this word—*in the calibrated and rehearsed pitch*— into running speech. This task initially feels awkward for a lot of clients, and thus they will benefit from hearing a good clinician model of the technique.

Vocal Warm-Up

The vocal warm-up is useful as a precursor to extended or important vocal/speech activity. The goal is not to warm up the voice *per se* (though this certainly might help), but rather to find and solidify the target voice before using it in important contexts. This warm-up might last only two minutes or extend toward 10 minutes, and involves clients engaging in a gentle vocal warm-up that consists of activities that take them through their accessible range of pitch, loudness, and resonance. Hopefully, clients can use the warm-up period to achieve their target voice, trouble-shooting any issues (e.g., sensations of strain or discomfort) along the way. The idea is for them to emerge with a firm command of their target voice, carrying it mindfully into speech.

"Best Voice Ever" File

For clients who are comfortable with making voice recordings (not all people are), encourage them to keep a sample of their self-identified "best voice yet" on a personal device (e.g., cell phone). The client's goal should be to replace that sample often. Some clients might not choose to listen to their samples after recording if they are not comfortable. Others might listen and actively try to improve on their most recent samples. If clients maintain even a semi-regular practice of recording their "best voice yet," then when they do choose to review the samples they will hopefully have a mechanism for helping them appreciate the evolution of their voice/communication over time. As a reminder, clinicians must be sensitive to the possibility of audio recordings triggering dysphoria, and thus not recommend audio recording and playback tasks universally.

Call-Around Task

Clients can get great benefit from calling businesses in order to practice their voice and communication techniques. Some clients might choose to call businesses whose representatives are more likely to use pronouns when speaking with customers (e.g., high-end retail stores), but that needn't be the goal. More and more businesses are being instructed not to use any pronoun-specific salutations. Clients can be provided a list of numbers, with the instruction to call *x* businesses using the target voice. Such calls will give them an opportunity to record their phone voice, prepare for a real-world communicative exchange with vocal warm-up tasks, and maybe even take care of some of their own errands. Recording business Skype sessions, or other webinar-based business meetings, is also an excellent approach, especially for checking and practicing complex cognitive tasks.

Voicemail Task

One outstanding way for clients to achieve some metric of accountability and real-world engagement is to leave x voicemails per week for their clinician. This task leads to a number of possible ways for the client and clinician to engage: if the voicemails are stored via VOIP, clinicians can forward them to clients with their feedback; clinicians can tally the number of weekly recordings delivered as a metric of practice; clinicians can download files to obtain a rough estimate of average f_o during speech; and so forth. At minimum, though, this task fosters a degree of accountability on the client's part, and can be an excellent task even without direct analysis of any recordings.

"10–30 Second Rule"

In this method, during the first 10–30 seconds of specific conversations, the client is directed to implement certain aspects of his or her new communication style. During this short time of the conversation, the client will focus on *how* to speak rather than *what* to say. It is important that the client not attempt to use the techniques throughout the entire conversation, as this puts too great a burden on the client to maintain skills that will come more effortlessly with continued practice. As clients become more comfortable and proficient with the elements of their new communication style, the 10–30 seconds become a minute and then 2 minutes and so on, until eventually the clients can think less about *how* they are speaking during an entire conversation.

Functional Phrases

Clients can be guided to identify 20-30 functional phrases they use on a daily basis (e.g., "See you tomorrow!" "How are things going?" "What are you up to this weekend?"). These phrases are useful to establish and practice early on in training. The more familiar and natural the phrases are for the client, the easier they will be to implement. These phrases should serve across different environments, including work, home, and social situations. Once the phrases are established, the client will aim to use specified communication skills as outlined in therapy, while calling upon these functional phrases each day. The client should alter the task demand on a regular basis, beginning with phrases that have a low cognitive load, and increasing to greater and greater complexity. This method will not only provide practice time, but will also serve to maintain vigilance during the vulnerable phase of generalization.

Selective Communication Partner or Situation

Clients might identify three to five people with whom they speak on a daily or near-daily basis (e.g., roommate, friend, colleague, family member) and three to five regular/daily speaking situations (e.g., speaking on the phone at work). The client can set a goal to use selected communication techniques particularly while speaking with these individuals or in these situations. The "10–30 second rule" may also be applied here. For example, each time clients speak with a sibling, they will use a targeted skill for the first 10–30 seconds of that particular conversation. Ideally, clients' groups of conversational partners comprise a mix of cis and gender diverse people and people who are associated with varying social contexts (e.g., a sibling, a work colleague, a neighbor).

Environment-Embedded Cues

If clients had an "angel on their shoulder" that reminded them throughout the day to modify their pitch, return to their target resonance when they strayed, minimize tension when it crept in, and so on, then it would obviously be easier for them to find and maintain their target voice. Indeed, this is why clients often develop a beautiful "therapy room voice" but struggle to maintain it outside of that training environment. Training environments are, of course, rich with built-in cues, not the least of which is the clinician sitting across from the client. Thus, a critical element of success is for clients to determine a variety of cues that they can build into their own life and that are salient enough to remind them of their various communication goals as they go through their day. This can take any number of forms. Several commonly implemented cues are listed below. Each is meant to get clients' attention in their natural environment, and serve as a cue for them to tune in to how they are speaking at that moment (if applicable), to speak in order to use their target voice or a target skill/technique (e.g., forward resonance), or simply to bring awareness to a certain behavior of interest (e.g., physical tension).

- If clients regularly wear a specific piece of jewelry or accessory (e.g., a watch, a pager), they can switch it to the opposite side of the body.
- Clients can add something to their attire or style that they don't typically wear (e.g., nail polish, longer earrings, different socks, a different belt).
- Clients might set random alerts on their phone.
- Clients can post notes throughout the house and/or office with written cues.
- Clients can add a note or a meaningful photo to key contacts in their cell phone, so that when they see who is calling, they are cued to access and prepare their target voice briefly before answering.
- Clients can identify a "Cue Person" in their lives that they will make a point of

having brief social exchanges with while using their target voice (e.g., a security guard, barista, specific person in their office).

The above list is, of course, far from exhaustive. Both clients and clinicians should be creative in identifying cues that will actually work for each individual. For instance, one previous client decided to hang colorful tassels from every ceiling-fan pull in her house, and found that this reminded her to access her target voice every time she walked into a new room. It should be noted that attention to most cues will fade over time as they become part of life's background noise. Thus, when a cue stops getting a person's attention, it is time for them to identify and implement new cues.

Setting the Stage for Independent Practice

Clients need to develop a clear sense of the definition of *practice* in terms of what will actually be effective for them. As with learning a language or musical instrument, there is a difference between "doing one's scales" or practicing a few rote phrases and playing the whole piece, or speaking fluently. Many clients need to engage in a simple daily warm-up routine in order to find and align their target voice before engaging in full conversations. This need might diminish over time, or it might be a lifelong practice. Regardless, clients should understand that their goal needn't necessarily be to move away from needing their foundation-building tasks, such as a warm-up or a lip trill or a flow phonation or semi-occluded vocal tract basic training gesture. Practicing those tasks individually is useful in developing basic skills, but is only truly valuable if clients provide a "thread to pull" that effectively and efficiently takes them toward their target voice. The mental capacity for self-monitoring and modifying communication has to be trained and requires conscious establishment of small patterns first.

The client, not the clinician, should decide on a specific plan for practicing learned therapy techniques and voice applications. Clients may select multiple, shorter practice times or one large block of time to best suit their personal schedule and learning style. Clinicians should try to encourage a relationship with practice that does *not* mimic a classic relationship with homework. That is, while focused practice time can be very useful, people often have a relationship with homework that results in them putting it off, not finding the time to do it, or only engaging with the material when they are actually engaged in their homework related to that material. Instead, every time a client opens their mouth to talk is an opportunity to practice their target voice. If they are not yet presenting in a manner congruent with their gender identity, they can still practice modifying their resonance, engaging ample airflow during speech, and minimizing physical tension that might be associated with speaking. The client who can come to view the daily collection of small communication moments as repeated opportunities to practice will often make faster and deeper gains than the client who simply practices techniques for 30 minutes a day. Ideally, both situations occur for any given client. One way or another, clients are all strengthening a habit.

At the outset of training it might be prudent to recommend that clients do not practice in the car. The basic training gesture for training pitch and resonance requires focus and aural acuity. Vocal health (and attention) can be comprised by trying to do this while driving, particularly for clients whose daily commute occurs on a

highway with the windows rolled down. Once a moderate level of vocal understanding has been established, the car is an excellent place to practice random utterances. Observations of life going by and street signs are an excellent set of endless stimuli!

Keeping in Touch

It is our opinion that the best practice in voice training might involve long-term engagement with the clinician, at least for a proportion of clients. Historically, clients might have engaged in regularly scheduled sessions for many months, and then been discharged with the expectation that their goals are now met and they should function independently. In such a model, a client's return to the speech-language pathologist is often viewed in the context of a "relapse" or failure to maintain their skills. Indeed, some clients might be reluctant to return to their voice therapist even in the face of voice difficulties, for fear that doing so would reflect some failure on their part.

As an alternative to this situation, we promote a model that reinforces and normalizes a long-term professional relationship between clinician and client. Some techniques, behaviors, and personal insights simply must be revisited multiple times before they "click" and "stick." This is true for many voice patients irrespective of their gender identity. Clinicians should consider ways to keep in touch with their clients after official discharge, both to track their progress over time and to remain a resource for the clients (as needed). Indeed, Gelfer and Tice (2013) showed that voice improvements observed immediately after a course of therapy were not maintained fully in the long term. Although Gelfer and Tice were reporting from a small sample, their findings are fully consistent with anecdotal report by experienced clinicians. At a minimum, clinicians should make it clear that returning for follow-up services as needed is normal, perfectly acceptable, and perhaps even preferred. Some ideas for achieving this long-term relationship are bulleted below.

- At the time of discharge, clients can schedule a follow-up session for one, three, or six months in the future.
- At the time of discharge, clinicians can ask clients to enter reminders in their personal calendar to contact the SLP with updates on how they are doing (in terms of their voice and communication), e.g., at 1, 3, 6, and 12 months post-discharge.
- Clinicians can offer small-group "refresher" sessions on a regular schedule (e.g., quarterly) to all clients who have been officially discharged. Topics might include vocal hygiene refreshers, troubleshooting bad voice days, et cetera.
- As is often done in dental practice, clients can self-address postcards that are then sent to them by the clinician at a specified time. Clinicians might design the postcard to convey generic information about vocal health and training, tailor the information to specific clients' needs, and/or simply use the postcard to remind the clients that they remain a resource.

Summary

The journey to successful gender diverse voice and communication training/therapy is neither swift nor simple. Communication change takes time and dedication on the part of both the client and the clinician. It is thought that 60–80,000 repetitions are needed for behavioral changes to become subconscious (Schiffren & Schneider,

1977). Although no one ever reaches that high number in direct training, the underlying message from the research is that a large number of repetitions is needed for clients to truly internalize and automate their target communication behaviors. As previously stated, the length of treatment is influenced by several variables, including the number of sessions available per week or month. However, a key determinant of training duration is the client's participation outside the clinic and his or her willingness to be challenged and to take risks. In some cases, a written practice contract helps to guarantee full commitment and participation. Successful discharge from therapy is only partially controlled by the clinician. It is our duty to guide the client to take personal responsibility for the enormous task at hand. The importance of such resolve must be made very clear to the client at the outset of therapy, so as to dispel any notions that the client may have of a "quick fix" or a "magic technique." Successful carryover should be, and is, the ultimate criterion for discharge. It also happens to be the true measure of therapeutic success across any behavioral change.

References

Gelfer, M. P., & Tice, R. M. (2013). Perceptual and acoustic outcomes of voice therapy for male-to-female transgender individuals immediately after therapy and 15 months later. *Journal of Voice: Official Journal of the Voice Foundation, 27*(3), 335–347. https://doi.org/10.1016/j.jvoice.2012.07.009

Gillespie, A. I., & Gartner-Schmidt, J. (2017). Voice-specialized speech-language pathologist's criteria for discharge from voice therapy. *Journal of Voice: Official Journal of the Voice Foundation.* https://doi.org/10.1016/j.jvoice.2017.05.022

Hancock, A. B., Krissinger, J., & Owen, K. (2011). Voice perceptions and quality of life of transgender people. *Journal of Voice: Official Journal of* the *Voice Foundation, 25*(5), 553–558. https://doi.org/10.1016/j.jvoice.2010.07.013

Helou, L. (2017). Crafting the dialogue: Metatherapy in transgender voice and communication training. *Perspectives of the ASHA Special Interest Groups, SIG 10, 2*(2), 83–91.

Safer, J. D., Coleman, E., Feldman, J., Garofalo, R., Hembree, W., Radix, A., & Sevelius, J. (2016). Barriers to healthcare for transgender individuals. *Current Opinion in Endocrinology, Diabetes, and Obesity, 23*(2), 168–171. https://doi.org/10.1097/MED.0000000000000227

Shiffrin, R. M., & Schneider, W. (1977). Controlled and automatic human information processing: II. Perceptual learning, automatic attending, and a general theory. *Psychological Review, 84,* 127–190.

Van Leer, E., & Connor, N. P. (2010). Patient perceptions of voice therapy adherence. *Journal of Voice: Official Journal of the Voice Foundation, 24*(4), 458–469. https://doi.org/10.1016/j.jvoice.2008.12.009

Ziegler, A., Dastolfo, C., Hersan, R., Rosen, C. A., & Gartner-Schmidt, J. (2014). Perceptions of voice therapy from patients diagnosed with primary muscle tension dysphonia and benign mid-membranous vocal fold lesions. *Journal of Voice: Official Journal of the Voice Foundation, 28*(6), 742–752. https://doi.org/10.1016/j.jvoice.2014.02.007

17

A Call to Action: Meeting the Unique Needs of Trans and Gender Diverse Young People

Sandy Hirsch, Richard K. Adler, and Jack Pickering

Of all the issues parents face when raising a transgender or gender variant child, the one they often struggle with most is how to work with their child's school. . . . A child's experience at school can significantly enhance or undermine their sense of self.
—Brill and Pepper, 2008, p. 153

Introduction

"Young people" is a term used by the World Health Organization (n.d.) to include adolescent youth and young adults, 10–24 years of age. As the age of gender dysphoria shifts farther and farther down, we are charged as clinicians, coaches, educators, and multidisciplinary teams to understand the unique characteristics of this young population in order to best serve them, and to prepare them for school and life success. The complexities of weaving together a strong tapestry of support are not insignificant. This chapter presents information on the unique needs of young people who identify as trans, gender diverse, or indeed cisgender. It will present some of the more commonly known

coexisting medical diagnoses with gender dysphoria, the creativity required to best serve a young population, the challenges inherent in school individual educational plan (IEP) inclusion, and the role that speech-language pathologists (SLPs) might play in moving the narrative forward to seamless multidisciplinary team approaches. With the exception of Hancock and Helenius (2012), there is to date a paucity of literature in our field to guide us in working on voice and communication with young trans people. The authors do not profess to provide any firm answers in this chapter, but rather hope to bring to light the next crucial discussion in moving the care of young trans and gender diverse people forward. SLPs do not shy away from being agents of change: here we may again be tasked to do just that.

We acknowledge that the thoughts and ideas presented below are largely from the perspective of the American public (state) school and medical systems. Wherever possible, an international perspective has been added with the help of the anecdotal input of a few colleagues.

Young People: They Are Not Simply Miniature, or Underdeveloped Adults

A 13-year-old trans girl comes into Hirsch's office for an evaluation, and when asked at the end of the intake about her own goals for therapy, she shrugs and says, "I don't know. I mean I do know, but I don't know. Do you know what I mean?" Hirsch laughs with her and says, "I do know what you mean, actually. It's very hard to explain, isn't it? How about we start with x,y,z to get you used to working on your voice and communication, and then we can settle on some goals together soon when you feel more comfortable. How does that sound?" Shrug. "Sure, OK. Yes. Sounds good."

A 14-year old trans girl, still presenting male and going by him/his pronouns lumbers into the office for his third session. He rolls his eyes, screws up his face, asks, "What did you want me to do again for my homework? I lost the book where I wrote it. Oh yeh, I did do that pitch thingy a couple times." He sits in the chair and starts spinning it around perseveratively, stops, and then stares out of the window with no apparent plan to turn and face Hirsch. "Hey, X, how about if you turn around now so we can talk to each other? We'll go over the homework again, and then do the session standing up and moving around so you can focus a bit better. How does that sound?." "Sounds about right. [smirk] I can see you've done this before . . ." "Yes, a few times, but you're the first YOU that I've met!" Laughter together.

A 17-year-old trans girl, brought in by her father, looks relieved once her dad has signed off on policy and procedure papers, HIPAA (Health Insurance Portability and Accountability Act) forms, and ROI (release of information) and has left the office. She turns to Hirsch and says, "My dad means well [her father seemed utterly charming, articulate, and supportive] but he can be pretty awkward and inappropriate sometimes. He has a lot to learn."

Young people from approximately age 11 to 24 are working feverishly to develop the skills that they need to negotiate life and relationships successfully. They are working overtime to "get it right" while fumbling around in the dark of their rapidly developing selves. The prefrontal cortex limbic systems of their brain are developing rapidly, shifting hormonal and cortical balances. It is a stressful, confusing period of life (Spear, 2000). These hormonal and cortical changes during a young person's life may also be involved in their cognitive and social function: young people tend to be more self-conscious, they question their identity (gender or otherwise), and they are cognitively un-cemented (Blakemore, 2008). We may all remember, or if we are parents, that life can be an emotional roller coaster for many young people; they may experience being "left out" and have to navigate the perceived treacherous landscape of multiple social contexts (Blakemore & Mills, 2014; Kilford, Garrett, & Blakemore, 2016). According to Beesdo, Pine, Lieb, and Wittchen (2010) and Stein (2006), rates of the diagnosis of social anxiety disorders increase at approximately age 10, with 50% of cases presenting at around age 13 and 90% of cases presenting by age 23. Young people are often highly motivated by what their peers think of them, but also desperately fear rejection or indeed humiliation (Caouette & Guyer, 2014; Lucock & Salkovskis, 1988). This may well be in part why there are frequent flare-ups in friendships, tears and laughter in one hour and "I love you/I hate you" in one breath.

Misinterpretation of a direction, a comment, or a facial expression is common in young people. Significant neurobiological changes that take place during adolescence may in part contribute to "a range in cognitive and affective behavior seen during adolescence" Yurgelun-Todd (2007, p. 1). Yurgelun-Todd conducted a telling brain mapping study that looked at the differences between adult and teenage brains. One of the most interesting findings was that adults interpreted a facial expression of fear with 100% consistency, whereas approximately half of teens saw fear, whereas the rest variously saw shock, confusion, or sadness, and in some cases anger. Yurgelun-Todd's findings have strong implications for how widely young people may misinterpret or misperceive the feelings of those with whom they are communicating. "Their own behavior is not going to match that of the adult. So you'll see miscommunication, both in terms of what they think the adult is feeling, but also what the response should then be to that" (Yurgelun-Todd, 2002). No wonder that young people sometimes look at adults sideways.

Fostering Successful Therapy and Training: Tailoring Clinical Approaches to the Young Mind

It is evident from the above summary of some of the research on adolescent brain development that it is incumbent on clinicians, trainers, and coaches to creatively tailor their approaches when working with young minds. The scope of this chapter does not allow for a comprehensive discussion on learning theory and strategies for school success, but a few bullet points on setting the stage for success may be worthwhile. Hirsch has found the approaches below to help teens succeed. They are a compilation of thoughts from her own clinical experience with working with this age group.

- Check in carefully but gently on the day's mood and energy level. A young person may just have come from doing a test, or an exam, or may have started with a very early class that day.
- Be positive, kind, but firm. Provide positive reinforcement where it is due. Young people smell "adult gushing over-praise" a mile away and grow weary of it quickly.
- Provide clear written directions for therapy/training instructions. Young people say "got it" enthusiastically, and then immediately demonstrate that they didn't "get" anything. They want to succeed.
- Be clear about the plan for the session and keep the plan moving. Young minds flag easily without a plan.
- Recognize the need for a "change up."
- Where allowable, have beverages and snacks on hand. There's nothing like a fed mind to make therapy go better.
- Be current, but don't profess to be "super hip." Bring a sense of humor to the table.
- Be prepared to have your session standing, moving, or both. Movement is excellent for breath support at all ages, but young minds may need a little oxygen jolt after a long day. Since they usually come after school, they are often burned out and need to move around, rather than sit.
- Vary the medium in directions given. Some young people need directions recorded on their phone, some need a dedicated composition or notebook, some need directions emailed. It is important to know the mind of each young client rather than assuming that one size fits all.

These suggestions are by no means exhaustive. They are ideas gleaned from working with middle and high schoolers in the schools, private practice, and rehabilitation programs. There are numerous excellent resources available to help adolescent students succeed. A few of these have been listed in the online resources as part of this publication. Readers are invited and encouraged to learn as much as possible through reading and continuing education about the unique needs of young minds. The greater discussion lies ahead of us now: specifically, how do we best serve the needs of young trans people?

Statement of the World Professional Association for Transgender Health: Differences to Consider When Working with Young People

The World Professional Association for Transgender Health (WPATH) published a Standards of Care version 7 (SOC-7) in 2012 (revisions toward a version 8 are in their nascent stages). The document emphasizes that "there are a number of differences in the phenomenology, developmental course, and treatment approaches for gender dysphoria in children, adolescents, and adults. In children and adolescents, a rapid and dramatic developmental process (physical, psychological, and sexual) is involved" (World Professional Association for Transgender Health, 2012, pp. 10–11). The SOC-7 offers specific and extensive guidelines for the assessment and treatment of gender dysphoric children and adolescents. An important difference between gender dysphoric children and adolescents is in the proportion for whom dysphoria persists into adulthood. Gender dysphoria during childhood does not inevitably continue into adulthood.

The Phenomenology of Trans Children

Children as young as age 2 may show features that could indicate gender dysphoria.

They may express a wish to be of the other gender and be unhappy about their physical sex characteristics and functions. In addition, they may prefer clothes, toys, and games that are commonly associated with the other gender and prefer playing with other-gender peers. There appears to be heterogeneity in these features: some children demonstrate extreme gender nonconforming behavior and wishes, accompanied by persistent and severe discomfort with their primary sex characteristics. In other children, these characteristics are less intense or only partially present (Cohen-Kettenis et al., 2006; Knudson, DeCuypere, & Bockting, 2010).

It is relatively common for gender dysphoric children to have coexisting internalizing diagnoses such as anxiety and depression (Bradley & Zucker, 2003; Cohen-Kettenis, Owen, Kaijser, Wallien, Swaab, & Cohen-Kettenis, 2007; Zucker, Owen, Bradley, & Ameeriar, 2002). In addition, the prevalence of autistic spectrum disorder (ASD) seems to be higher in clinically referred, gender dysphoric children than in the general population (de Vries, Noens, Cohen-Kettenis, van Berckelaer-Onnes, & Doreleijers, 2010; Strang et al., 2016). These comorbidities should be carefully considered when working with trans young people. The scope of this chapter does not allow for an in-depth discussion of the nuanced approaches necessary in working with people on the autism spectrum, but suffice to say that SLPs and trainers would do well to feather their clinical nests with current knowledge, especially in the area of video modeling (Franzone & Collet-Klingenberg, 2008; Merrill & Risch, 2014) and storyboarding (Pierson & Glaeser, 2007). The nonprofit organization Talk About Curing Autism (TACA) provides a succinct and thought-provoking summary of working with teens with ASD on their website at https://www.tacanow.org/family-resources

/teens-with-asd-social-skills/ (retrieved February 27, 2018).

As discussed earlier in the chapter, the young developing mind is already buckling under the stress of rapid change, while being full of potential. Trans teens, already navigating the social anxieties inherent in many teenagers, are more likely to be bullied than teens in the general population. In a 2015 School Climate Survey (Kosciw, Greytak, Giga, Villenas, & Danischewski, 2016), 43.3% of gender diverse students reported feeling unsafe at school. "Compared to LGBQ cisgender students, transgender, genderqueer, and other non-cisgender students faced more hostile school climates. Gender nonconforming cisgender students (students whose gender expression did not align to traditional gender norms) experienced worse school climates compared to gender conforming cisgender students" (https://www.glsen.org/article/2015-national -school-climate-survey retrieved February 25, 2018). While district policies and procedures are beginning to change in some areas regarding umbrella issues such as terminology and "trans 101" training for staff and administrators, we have yet to overcome the hurdles of communication challenges faced by trans young people in the schools and pediatric clinics. Conversations and emails with colleagues internationally (Georgia Dacakis and Jenni Oates [Australia] and Christella Antoni [United Kingdom] suggest that this is an area that begs attention globally. In a telephone conversation, Aidan Key, executive director of the nonprofit organization Gender Diversity, raised this glaring point: "This is the first time in my 10 years of doing my work that anyone has presented the thought of having a cogent plan in the schools for trans youth" (personal communication, March 6, 2018). He is serendipitously working on a book about trans teens in the schools, entitled *Transgender Children in Today's Schools*. He feels that the time is more than ripe for formally rising to these challenges.

The Role of the SLP with Pediatric and Adolescent Transgender Teams

It is often SLPs, fluently versed in the needs of gender diverse students, who initiate a discussion about their potential role on a pediatric or adolescent gender team. Adler has communicated with such gender teams on the U.S. West and East Coasts and in the Midwest. A short opinion questionnaire was sent to 20 random gender teams from a list of large Children's hospitals in the United States. To ensure anonymity, each letter asking for opinions was sent with a self-addressed stamped envelope asking the participant to not use identifying information when sending it back because this was just an opinion poll and not a formal qualitative or quantitative study. It was made clear in the letter that someone on the gender team should fill out the opinion poll.

Limitations of This Small Opinion Poll

One limitation of this poll is that the total number of gender teams contacted was very small. In addition, it was not clear which gender team member actually returned the opinion poll. And finally, the distribution of responses across states and teams was not clear. It was not possible to know what gender team from what hospital was returning the poll, since responses were anonymous. That said, the overall purpose of the poll was to find out if an SLP was part of the team as either a full-time member or an adjunct. Nine participants (45%) returned the opinion poll. Themes emerged that were common amongst these teams. An outline of the findings will be discussed here to help the SLP/speech-language therapist (SLT) learn the importance of being a member of such a care team, when appropriate.

Survey Questions (Table 17–1)

Most gender teams are aware that some of their transmasculine and transfeminine patients seek voice modification as part of

their transition journey. However, most adolescent/pediatric gender team members did not consider an SLP's role on the team in *any* capacity. Results of the poll follow here.

Question 1: Is there an SLP/SLT on your team in any capacity?
Response: 100% said No.
Question 2: Sometimes, children have a difficult time expressing their emotions, feelings, cares, and concerns regarding growing up in general, as well as their gender dysphoria. Do you think an SLP on your team could help?

Table 17–1. Opinion Survey Questions

1. Is there an SLP/SLT on your team in any capacity?
Yes: _____   No: _____
All of the following questions were answered using this modified Likert scale:

1	2	3	4
Yes	**No**	**Maybe**	**Never crossed my mind**

2. Sometimes, children have a difficult time expressing their emotions, feelings, cares, and concerns regarding growing up in general as well as their gender dysphoria. Do you think an SLP on your team could help?
3. Sometimes, a child is referred to the gender team and that child also has an additional/dual diagnosis on the Autism Spectrum, or ADD/ADHD/Learning Disability, Developmental Disability, Oppositional Defiant Disorder, General Language or Speech Delay, Fluency or Stuttering difficulty, etc. Do you see an SLP as having a role in helping the child express him/herself to make progress in transition as a transfeminine or transmasculine member (patient) of your team?
4. Think about how you deal with children or adolescents who have difficulty reading facial expressions, the nuances of voice differences, tones/intonation variations, misreading nonverbal signals, etc. Do you think an SLP could help with these matters?
5. Think about how you deal with parents or children who have difficulty with matters of social language, pragmatic language, and rules of language to be adequately prepared to discuss the gender dysphoria issues that come up during an intake interview. Do you think consulting an SLP from your team (or the child's school) could help the team get more complete and honest answers?
6. Think about your patient referrals. Before the social worker meets the parents/child for an initial intake interview, would the SLP report from the school (if there is one) or would the SLP on your team (if there is one) help the team to verify that the child has adequate articulation, language development, vocabulary, social language to be able to express him/herself in the interview?
7. Have you ever had a patient referral (child or parent) who was very concerned with "coming out" at school as transgender?
8. Did you ever have a situation where the IEP team at a child's school asked to get some help to address the privacy issues and needs of a transgender or gender diverse/non-binary student who is not out to his/her parents?
9. Do you think an SLP on your team could be valuable to address the concerns in question #8 above?

Response: Yes: 11%, No: 22%, Maybe: 11%, Never crossed my mind: 56%

Question 3: *Sometimes, a child is referred to the gender team and that child has an additional/dual diagnosis on the Autism Spectrum, or ADD/ADHD/Learning Disability, Developmental Disability, Oppositional Defiant Disorder, General Language or Speech Delay, Fluency or Stuttering difficulty, etc. Do you see an SLP as having a role in helping the child express him/herself to make progress in transition as a transfeminine or transmasculine member (patient) of your team?*

Response: Yes: 0%, No: 0%, Maybe: 56%, Never crossed my mind: 44%

Question 4: *Think about how you deal with children or adolescents who have difficulty reading facial expressions, the nuances of voice differences, tones/intonation variations, misreading nonverbal signals, etc. Do you think an SLP could help with these matters?*

Response: Yes: 0%, No: 0%, Maybe: 67%, Never crossed my mind: 33%

Question 5: *Think about how you deal with parents or children who have difficulty with matters of social language, pragmatic language, and rules of language to be adequately prepared to discuss the gender dysphoria issues that come up during an intake interview. Do you think consulting an SLP from your team (or the child's school) could help the team get more complete and honest answers?*

Response: Yes: 0%, No: 0%, Maybe: 0%, Never crossed my mind: 100%

Question 6: *Think about your patient referrals. Before the social worker meets the parents/child for an initial intake interview, would the SLP report from the school (if there is one) or would the SLP on your team (if there is one) help the team to verify that the child has adequate articulation, language development, vocabulary, social language to be able to express him/herself in the interview?*

Response: Yes: 0%, No: 0%, Maybe: 44%, Never crossed my mind: 56%

Question 7: *Have you ever had a patient referral (child or parent) who was very*

concerned with "coming out" at school as transgender?

Response: Yes: 44%, No: 56%, Maybe: 0%, Never crossed my mind: 0%

Question 8: *Did you ever have a situation where the IEP team at a child's school asked to get some help to address the privacy issues and needs of a transgender or gender diverse/non-binary student who is not out to his/her parents?*

Response: Yes: 0%, No: 100%, Maybe: 0%, Never crossed my mind: 0%

Question 9: *Do you think an SLP on your team could be valuable to address the concerns in question #8 above?*

Response: Yes: 0%, No: 0%, Maybe: 56%, Never crossed my mind: 44%

Summary of Results from the Poll

The results of the poll may not be entirely surprising to most SLPs/SLTs. The scope of practice in the field is still misunderstood by many who have not had personal need for the services of an SLP, or whose discipline is outside the realm of communication disorders and differences. It is evident from the responses given by people on the gender teams, that (a) SLPs are underrepresented on such teams for young people, (b) there is little to no understanding of the potential role that SLPs might play on gender teams serving to improve the care of young trans and gender diverse people, and (c) there is a paucity of knowledge within IEP teams of the resources available to trans youth and their parents. There should be no wonder that the final finding on the poll is that teens are still experiencing a high degree of fear in coming out at school. These findings have helped in guiding our thinking regarding overriding themes and issues of concern that beg further attention.

Important Themes Revealed by the Survey

The survey appears to reveal four themes that require attention. They are as follows:

1. The survey raises our consciousness to the needs of trans youth in schools.
2. The survey forces our attention to the major issues facing trans youth and their parents in the schools.
3. The survey heightens our awareness to actions that may be taken by SLPs in concert with state education agencies, school districts, and gender teams to help children and parents through transition.
4. The survey triggers an urgency to increase our efforts to reach out to communities, cities, states, and all parties involved in enhancing the experience of trans youth and their parents in the schools.

Any seasoned clinician, educator, coach, or trainer knows full well that greater clarity may lead to greater confusion before solutions may be revealed. As stated earlier in the chapter, the authors do not profess to have any concrete answers to these issues. The aforementioned themes reveal a number of concerns, and show us that the hurdles to improving care and support are not insignificant. Hurdles are of course designed to be overcome. In that spirit, possible solutions will be discussed later in the chapter.

Issues and Concerns Inherent in the Emerging Themes

There are a number of inherent issues that are raised when delving deeper into a discussion of how to increase and improve the support of young trans people.

1. While it is evident that gender teams need to be educated and become more familiar with the role that SLPs might play in helping their young patients, it needs to be said that a good majority of SLPs in the public schools do not know about transgender and gender nonconforming youth. To date, SLPs in the schools are generally not trained in the area of transgender issues. If there is *one* trans expert on a school SLP team, it is still a rare percentage within the SLP group. Referrals of trans students are often ignored or never brought up at an IEP meeting, not because the SLP doesn't want to help but because he/she is not sure who to speak with or how to begin an informed conversation. Anecdotally, the SLP first chooses the school psychologist or counselor for a discussion, but the issue soon becomes complicated and ignored for lack of clear guidance and limited research to which they might turn. SLPs therefore often turn to this text, the internet, scant research such as Hancock and Helenius (2012), ASHA Perspectives articles on the topic (see reference list) or flailingly reach out to colleagues far and wide in order to do the best research they can in the face of never before having encountered a gender diverse student.
2. In the United States, public schools are federally regulated by Public Law (P.L.) 94-142 and P.L. 99-457. We now refer to P.L. 94-142 as the Individuals with Disabilities Education Act (IDEA), which requires that public schools make "available to eligible children with disabilities a free appropriate public education in the least restrictive environment appropriate for their individual needs." This

law was designed to serve the needs of students age 3–21 years (National Education Association of the United States, 1978).

There are some inherent conceptual and semantic challenges to the interpretation of this law with respect to transgender and gender diverse students, and how they might access communication services in the school setting. Gender diverse students, like gender diverse adults, often experience severe communication dysphoria if there is a mismatch in voice and gender identity. Commonly this can lead to a decrease in participation in class, or a fear of coming to school. Grades quickly begin to drop and anxieties increase. To date, Gender Dysphoria is not one of the listed categories for qualification for special education services. In trying to find a reasonable work-around for this lack of category, SLPs with some knowledge of the issues have had solution-focused discussions with psychologists and special education teachers. Students who have coexisting diagnoses such as severe social anxiety might qualify under Emotional Behavioral Disorder (ESB), or indeed those who have already been diagnosed with an Autism Spectrum Disorder would qualify under *that* category. There is some question as to whether a student could qualify under Health Impaired (HI) with a diagnosis of Gender Dysphoria, since this is not a disorder in and of itself, though it IS a diagnosis. Speculating for a moment that the solution to a category has been found, proving eligibility for communication services is the next challenge. There are no standardized tests for a mismatch between voice and gender identity, and to qualify for services at the time of an initial evaluation, results need to fall at or below 1.5 standard deviations from the mean. Professional opinion is usually not considered

adequate at the initial phases of eligibility. In the Washington State school districts, voice therapy also requires an ear nose and throat (ENT) referral for voice therapy. An ENT could report a mismatch of pitch range and gender. ASHA's Practice Portal quotes the following: "A voice disorder occurs when voice quality, pitch, and loudness differ or are inappropriate for an individual's age, gender, cultural background, or geographic location" (ASHA, n.d.).

The arguments and discussions begin to circle around. There is a strong need for clarifications of definition and policy around inclusion criteria, diagnosis, and referral. Brill and Pepper (2008) state: "Each and every parent who has a significantly gender variant or transgender student will have to work with their child's schools to ensure physical and emotional safety for their child"(p. 154). As things stand, parents might spend an unreasonable amount of time, time that young people do not have, advocating for communication and support services in the public schools.

3. Many transgender/ non-binary children and their parents appear not to know how to express themselves using the vocabulary and language as needed to be self-advocates. This is especially true for transgender students who have coexisting diagnoses such as ASD, language/ learning disabilities, speech or cognitive developmental delays, articulation or stuttering diagnoses, or indeed ones who speak English as a second language. Brill and Pepper (2008) stated: "If your child has additional qualities that put them at greater risk for bias and therefore teasing or discrimination, their gender identity or expression can compound and confuse the situation" (p. 160). Parents become aware of this problem and often speak out about their frustrations. One

parent, quoted in Brill and Pepper (2008, p. 161) stated, "My transgender child has a speech impediment. Somehow this combination of less common characteristics positions him as the target of unending teasing.... [I]t seems that the teacher does not intervene as much as she would for other children."

Students with a diagnosis on the autism spectrum typically have difficulty interpreting facial expressions, vocal tone, perspective, or abstract language. As was mentioned earlier in the chapter, many gender diverse children are victims of bullying. These students and their parents may have a greater challenge finding the vocabulary and resources to best advocate for their needs. A student may be called into the principal's office as a result of disruption, a student might stay at home, and a student might then pretend to be sick to stay out of school; grades may begin to drop, the student might inevitably begin to feel isolated and, not uncommonly, suicidal. According to the Centers for Disease Control and Prevention, the suicide rate among LGBTQ youth is twice the rate of that of non-LGBTQ young people (Centers for Disease Control and Prevention, 2017).

The cruelty of teenagers toward each other is not confined to transgender students, but the pain can be compounded by a greater complex of issues, as noted above. Hirsch spoke with a young transmasculine neighbor, now in his early 20s, who attended an alternative public school, a school that was purportedly "safe." He shared the following: "I did not feel supported on the whole. With the exception of my counselor and one teacher, who both made a huge difference, teachers, the administration, and even friends kept using my old name and pronouns. I gave them 2nd, 3rd, 4th 5th, 50th, 60th, 70th chances to get it right—they

still didn't get it! Each time that cuts a little deeper" (F. F-B personal communication, March 4, 2018). Close friends undermined him, one of them saying, "You don't look male, act male *and*, I'm a straight, man, and I'm attracted to you, so you *can't* be a man!" It is time to discuss possible solutions to challenges that have heretofore felt intractable to students, their parents, and some well-minded team members.

In a More Perfect World

It requires time, focus, intention, and resources in the form of monetary funds to educate, change attitudes, and increase overall confidence in how to support gender diverse young people. As has been admitted many times already in this chapter, the authors do not claim to have any concrete answers, but we offer below some possible starting places on the path toward a service model with integrity.

1. Gender teams across the world need to be educated about the scope of practice of SLPs, and their strong advocacy potential for young patients and clients. This should be done by SLPs well versed in gender issues, as well as the full scope of the SLP and audiology practices. They might suggest that they become adjunct members of a pediatric gender team.

2. SLPs with familiarity and knowledge of transgender issues could be assigned to school districts in order to mentor SLP groups in the schools. Districts should be encouraged to include this in their hiring expectations and goals.

3. SLPs with expertise in gender issues could serve as committee members and consultants for gender diverse students, their parents, teachers, counselors, ad-

ministrators, etc. These SLPs need to have a strong knowledge of common coexisting diagnoses of gender diverse students. The SLP would serve as a networking or referral source for appropriate support staff.

4. The whole school district and school "family" can do a great deal to support gender diverse students. Brill and Pepper (2008) stated that "there are a number of relatively simple things each school can do to dramatically increase the comfort and safety of gender variant and transgender students" (p. 163). They emphasize the need for the school to be committed to implement change that involves the administration of the school as well as the school system overhaul of policies and procedures. The SLP in the school could easily be a part of this educational endeavor as a part of the IEP team and overall school culture.

The following bullet points emphasize what Brill and Pepper (2008, pp. 163–178) describe as essential steps in order for schools to become a safe place for transgender/non-binary/gender variant children. Each point is described in more detail in their book:

- Create a supportive organizational school culture
- Adopt zero tolerance for discrimination
- Update policies and forms including suggestions of vocabulary usage such as sex/gender identity: male, female, transgender/gender diverse, non-binary, queer, nonconforming, agender.
- Honor stated names and pronouns
- Develop guidelines for transgender students such as ID cards, use of locker rooms and bathroom, legal name changes, etc.
- Provide staff training on the use of pronouns, keeping the gender variant child

safe, and very importantly, provide "a review of what an emerging awareness of gender identity in children may look like and how families and schools can support a child through the process" (p. 169).

- Provide parent education that would include the school's policy on gender. Some schools use handouts to do this and some use a PTA meeting to address gender variance or gender identity to all parents. An ideal meeting would include a speaker who could dispel rumors or stereotypes surrounding transgender people in general. One could also invite a gender team or at least the director of a pediatric or adolescent gender team from a local hospital or children's hospital to address a PTA meeting to describe the process of referral and answer questions from the parent body.
- Provide student education: If there is a gender policy in the school, students must be made aware of this as well as educated in this area. If the school has a chapter of GLSEN (pronounced Glisten), or the Gay, Lesbian, Straight Education Network, this organization would be essential to provide students with education on transgender issues as well as other aspects of being safe in the schools. GLSEN also has a teaching/learning part of their programming called "GLSEN UP." The purpose of this program is to teach people to take action and create "change-makers" for social change.
- Ensure bathroom safety for all students
- Document harassment of gender/variant/non-binary or transgender students
- Provide resources and support for families with gender variant, non-binary, or transgender children
- Address parents' fears of the child in the classroom who identifies as gender variant, non-binary, or transgender
- Conduct a gender sensitivity inventory in the school

■ Be prepared to confront gender issues in the classroom

Collaborative Efforts

It is well known that if you want to get a job done, ask a busy person . . . or an SLP. SLPs/SLTs internationally are already making efforts to reach out to professional organizations such as ASHA and state organizations in order to collaborate with clinics, hospitals, schools, and organizations. Workshops on transgender voice and communication exist in the private sector; there is a Gender Spectrum Facebook page and there are more and more live chats and webinars available that address general and specific trans and gender diverse issues; however, organizational efforts need to be increased. Speech and hearing associations, like ASHA, could provide annual workshops at the annual school conferences in order to provide school SLPs with a "starter kit" of knowledge in order to be prepared for the ever-growing potential that they will serve a gender diverse student on their caseload. Conferences and meetings are marvelous breeding grounds for advocacy groups within schools, but also at the local state and national levels. Hirsch and Adler already receive frequent calls for advice from school SLPs who may have some knowledge of gender diversity but want more information on how to present information to their staff and administration.

Expert SLPs might collaborate to develop information booklets for students, parents, and staff. Gender Odyssey in Seattle and now Los Angeles is already an excellent resource for such information and has grown exponentially over the past five years. SLPs can attend such conferences and learn about how best to work with their schools and teams on these issues, as well as increase their own knowledge across all transgender areas. This information can then be organized to share with additional disparate teams and groups.

Begin at the Source: Preparation at the Graduate School Level

A very informal set of email conversations to colleagues across the world has revealed an omission of formal transgender programs in the majority of SLP graduate programs. Hancock and Haskin (2015) highlight the need for SLPs to gain greater knowledge of the needs of the transgender and gender-diverse population. To date, La Trobe University in Australia (Oates & Dacakis, 2017) and the Karolinska Institutet in Sweden appear to be unique SLP graduate programs that fully address information on how to work with transgender and gender diverse people. Both of these programs are comprehensive, and the Karolinska Institutet has a textbook on voice, which includes transgender voice and communication therapy, that is compulsory (M. Södersten personal email communication, March 7, 2018). There are otherwise many programs in the United States and internationally that provide a series of short lectures (personal communication Shelagh Davies, Teresa Hardy, Christella Antoni, Georgia Dacakis, and Jenni Oates, March 2018, as well as Kathe Perez on the Gender Diverse Facebook page, n.d.), occasional classes taught by a guest lecturer, last minute add-ons, or a cursory mention with a PowerPoint slide or two. Increasingly, university-based speech, language, and hearing centers are providing services for gender diverse people. However, it is evident that there is still a general lack of adequate preparatory transgender courses. Jordan Jakomin, a recent graduate now working as a clinician in Los Angeles, is particularly interested in the topic of providing comprehensive teaching on transgender issues in graduate programs. In an informal survey that he conducted and is in the process of formalizing, he found that many professors reported that it didn't occur to them to teach this material, or that they didn't have time. "Those professors aren't even touching on the topic of transgender voice and communication therapy. This is an opportunity missed for students who could be moving transgender history forward" (J. Jakomin, personal communication, February 26, 2018).

It is time for SLPs internationally to begin advocating to graduate program planners that there is a need and desire for regular and formal courses in the area of transgender voice and communication. Students particularly interested in voice should be strongly advocating for this information. It should also be said that this is recognized as a problem amongst colleagues working in academia. In the United States, for instance, it is certainly a challenge to include trans services in the curriculum, since ASHA's standards for program accreditation mandate that masters-level education be broad, covering numerous clinical areas of practice (American Speech-Language-Hearing Association, 2017). The response on the Gender Spectrum Facebook page (now topping a thousand members), ASHA convention presentations, and conversations with colleagues suggest an increase in clinical services in college and university clinics, as well as more content in an already packed curriculum. It is clearly not adequate, particularly as it relates to trans youth. Colleges and universities the world

over need to find creative ways of increasing information in classes and connecting the growing clinical services with the classroom. Doctoral programs can provide leadership in promoting research, and more faculty/student research can support our understanding of trans voice and communication services. Excellent efforts are being made; just not enough, or fast enough.

Conclusion

Since the second edition of this text, the supports for transgender people have continued to strengthen and gel. The creation of more multidisciplinary teams is a testament to this fact. There has been a rapid increase in pediatric gender teams across the United States, as well as other parts of the world. We should all be proud of these advancements and the contributions that so many have made to increase the integrity of care for the gender diverse population. However, voice and communication services for young gender diverse people still lag behind. It is time, indeed overdue, for an organized, comprehensive, and integral approach to serving young people while they are in school. So far, we have had to address these vulnerable students as best as we can with the resources of staff and time haphazardly available. The best among those staff take care to attend gently to each student on a case by case basis, without placing them in a box for inspection when it is convenient or shying away from gently prying to learn what they need. Aidan Key shared that "inaction is so detrimental to young people" and that "as soon as they feel heard, and that validation is happening, is when you see the curled up person turn back into a flower" (A. Key, personal communication,

March 7, 2018). When asked what made his gender diverse students appear more comfortable and less fearful, Scott Peacock, once principal of Centennial Middle School and now Assistant Superintendent for Leadership and Learning in the Snohomish, Washington, school district, reported that meetings with parents and teachers go best when there is a student intervention team (SIT) meeting "without borders." The students have reported that they get "a sense that there is an overwhelming relief when they sit down with an adult who says, 'How can we help you? Are there friends who can help you? With whom do you feel comfortable?'" "I've heard it over and over again" (S. Peacock, personal communication, March 2, 2018). This is a call to action that we simply cannot ignore.

References

Additional resources and references are available on the chapter web-based resource links.

American Speech-Language-Hearing Association (n.d.). *ASHA practice portal: Voice disorders, overview*. Retrieved March 8, 2018 from https://www.asha.org/Practice-Portal/Clinical-Topics/Voice-Disorders/

American Speech-Language-Hearing Association (2017). Standards for *accreditation of graduate education programs in audiology and speech-language pathology*. ASHA Council on Academic Accreditation. Retrieved from https://caa.asha.org/wp-content/uploads/Accreditation-Standards-for-Graduate-Programs.pdf

Beesdo, K., Pine, D. S., Lieb, R., & Wittchen, H. (2010). Incidence and risk patterns of anxiety and depressive disorders and categorization of generalized anxiety disorder. *Archives of General Psychiatry, 67*, 47–57.

Blakemore, S. J. (2008). Development of the social brain during adolescence. *Quarterly Journal of Experimental Psychology, 61*(1), 40–48.

Blakemore, S. J., & Mills, K. L. (2014). Is adolescence a sensitive period for sociocultural pro-

cessing? *Annual Review of Psychology, 65*(2), 187–207.

Bradley, S. J., & Zucker, K. J. (2003). Children with gender nonconformity. *Journal of the American Academy of Child and Adolescent Psychiatry, 42*(3), 266–268.

Brill, S., & Pepper, R. (2008). *The transgender child: A handbook for families and professionals*. San Francisco, CA: Cleis Press.

Bumiller, K. (2008). Quirky citizens: Autism, gender, and reimagining disability. *Signs: Journal of Women in Culture and Society, 33*(4), 967–991.

Caouette, J. D., & Guyer, A. E. (2014). Gaining insight into adolescent vulnerability for social anxiety from developmental cognitive neuroscience. *Developmental Cognitive Neuroscience., 8*, 65–76. 10.1016/j.dcn.2013.10.003

Centers for Disease Control and Prevention (2017). *Lesbian, gay, bisexual, and transgender health*. US Department of Health and Human Services. Retrieved March 8, 2018 from http://www.cdc.gov/lgbthealth/youth.htm

Cohen-Kettenis, P. T. , Owen, A., Kaijser, V. G., Bradley, S. J. Zucker, K. J., & Zucker, K. J. (2003). Demographic characteristics, social competence, and behavior problems in children with gender identity disorder: A cross-national, cross-clinic comparative analysis. *Journal of Abnormal Child Psychology, 31*(1), 41–53.

Cohen-Kettenis, P. T., Wallien, M., Johnson, L. L., Owen-Anderson, A. F. H., Bradley, S. J., & Zucker, K. J. (2006). A parent-report gender identity questionnaire for children: A cross national, cross-clinic comparative analysis. *Clinical Child Psychology and Psychiatry, 11*(3), 397–405. doi: 10.1177/1359104506059135

de Vries, A. L. C., Noens, I. L. J., Cohen-Kettenis, P. T., van Berckalaer-Onnes, A. & Dereleijers, T. A. (2010). Autism spectrum disorders in gender dysphoric children and adolescents. *Journal of Autism and Developmental Disorders, 40*, 930. doi:10.1007/s10803-101-0935-9.

Franzone, E., & Collet-Klingenberg, L. (2008). *Overview of video modeling*. Madison, WI: The National Professional Development Center on Autism Spectrum Disorders, Waisman Center, University of Wisconsin. Retrieved from http://autismpdc.fpg.unc.edu/sites/autismpdc.fpg.unc.edu/files/VideoModeling _Overview_1.pdf

Gender and autism: A preliminary survey post. one woman's thoughts about life on the spec-

trum. Retrieved January 2017 from https://musingsofanaspie.com/2013/12/05/gender-and-autism-a-preliminary-survey-post/

Glidden, D., Bouman, W. P., Jones, B. A., & Arcelus, J. Gender dysphoria and autism spectrum disorder: A systematic review of the literature. *Sexual Medicine Review, 4*(3), 3–14.

Hancock, A. B., & Haskin, G. (2015). Speech-language pathologists' knowledge and attitudes regarding lesbian, gay, bisexual, transgender & queer (LGBTQ) populations. *American Journal of Speech-Language Pathology, 24*(2), 206–221. doi: 10.1044/2015_AJSLP-14-0095

Hancock, A. B., & Helenius, L. (2012). Adolescent male-to-female transgender voice and communication therapy. *Journal of Communication Disorders, 45*(5), 313–324.

Kilford, E. J., Garrett, E., & Blakemore, S. J. (2016). The development of social cognition in adolescence: An integrated perspective. *Neuroscientific Biobehavioral Review, 70*, 106–120.

Knudson, G., De Cuypere, G., & Bockting, W. (2010). Process toward consensus on recommendations for revision of the DSM diagnoses of gender identity disorders by the World Professional Association for Transgender Health. *International Journal of Transgenderism, 12*(2), 54–59. doi:10.1080/15532739.2010.509213

Kosciw, J. G., Greytak, E. A., Giga, N. M., Villenas, C., & Danischewski, D. J. (2016). *The 2015 National School Climate Survey: The experiences of lesbian, gay, bisexual, transgender, and queer youth in our nation's schools*. New York, NY: GLSEN.

Lucock, M. P., & Salkovskis, P. M. (1988). *Cognitive factors in social anxiety and its treatment. Behaviour Research and Therapy, 26*, 297–302. 10.1016/0005-7967(88)90081-2

Merrill, A., & Risch, J. (2014). Implementation and effectiveness of using video self-modeling with students with ASD. *The Reporter, 19*(6), 1–5.

National Education Association of the United States. (1978). *P.L. 94-142: Related federal legislation for handicapped children and implications for coordination*. Washington, DC: National Education Association.

Oates, J., & Dacakis, G. (2017). Inclusion of transgender voice and communication training in a university clinic. *Perspectives of the ASHA Special Interest Groups, SIG 10, Vol. 2(Part 2)*, 108–114.

Parkinson, J. (2014). Gender dysphoria in Asperger's syndrome. *Australasian Psychiatry, 22*(1), 84–85.

Pasterski, V., Giligan, L., & Curtis, R. (2014). Traits of autism spectrum disorders in adults with gender dysphoria. *Archives of Sexual Behavior, 43*, 387. doi: 10.1997/s10508-013-0154-5.

Pierson, M. R., & Glaeser, B. C. (2007). Using comic strip conversations to increase social satisfaction and decrease loneliness in students with autism spectrum disorder. *Education and Training in Developmental Disabilities, 42*(4), 460–466.

Shumer, D. E., Reisner, S. L., Edwards-Leeper, L., & Tishelman, A. (2016). Evaluation of Asperger syndrome in youth presenting to a gender dysphoria clinic. *LGBT Health, 3*(5), 387–390.

Spear, L. P. (2000). The adolescent brain and age-related behavioral manifestations. *Neuroscience and Biobehavioral Reviews, 24*(4), 417–463.

Stein, M. B. (2006). An epidemiologic perspective on social anxiety disorder. *Journal of Clinical Psychiatry, 67*(Suppl 12), 3–8.

Strang, J. F., Meagher, H., Kenworthy, L., de Vries, A. L.C., & Menvielle, E., Leibowitz, S, . . . Mandel, F. (2016). Initial clinical guidelines for co-occurring autism spectrum disorder and gender dysphoria or incongruence in adolescents. *Journal of Clinical Child and Adolescent Psychology*, 47(1), 105–115.

Talk About Curing Autism (2015, November). Teens with ASD: Social skills. Retrieved March 8, 2018 from https://www.tacanow.org/family-resources/teens-with-asd-social-skills/

Wallien, M. S. C., Swaab, H., & Cohen-Kettenis, P. T. (2007). Psychiatric comorbidity among children with gender identity disorder. *Journal of the American Academy of Child & Adolescent Psychiatry, 46*(10), 1307–1314. doi:10.1097/chi.0b013e3181373848

World Health Organization (n.d.). *Health for the world's adolescents: A second chance in the second decade. adolescence: a period needing special attention*. Retrieved February 24, 2018 from http://apps.who.int/adolescent/second-decade/section2/page1/recognizing–adolescence.html

World Professional Association for Transgender Health (2012). Standards of Care, VII. Retrieved November 2017 from https://s3.amazonaws.com/amo_hub_content/Association140/files/Standards%20of%20Care%20V7%20-%202011%20WPATH%20(2)(1).pdf

Yurgelun-Todd, D. (2002). Interview. Inside the teenage brain. *Frontline*. PBS. January 31, 2002.

Retrieved February 26, 2018 from https://www.pbs.org/wgbh/frontline/film/inside-the-teenage-brain/

Yurgelun-Todd, D. (2007). Emotional and cognitive changes during adolescence. *Current Opinion in Neurobiology, 17*(2), 251–257.

Zucker, K. J., Owen, A., Bradley, S. J., & Ameeriar, L. (2002). Gender-dysphoric children and adolescents: A comparative analysis of demographic characteristics and behavioral problems. *Clinical Child Psychology and Psychiatry, 7*(3), 398–411.

Index

Note: Page numbers in **bold** reference non-text material

Fundamental frequency (*continued*)
  speaking. *See* Speaking fundamental
    frequency
  in transgender women
    description of, 8
    voice training for, 91–92, 96

G

Gait, 256, 265–266
Gatekeepers
  definition of, 24
  mental health professionals as, 26–27,
    33, 35
Gatekeeping, 26
Gender
  affirmed, 59–61
  arm movements and, 256
  articulation differences, 235
  biological differentiation of, 59–60
  blogging and, 274–275
  definition of, **58**
  dichotomous view of, 34, 37
  facial expression and, 257–258
  finger movements and, 256
  foot movements and, 256
  gait differences, 256
  gestural styles and, 256–257
  hand movements and, 256
  haptics and, 252, 258–259
  head movements and, 256
  hip movements and, 256
  instant messaging, 273–274
  leg movements and, 256
  movement differences based on, 255–256
  nonverbal communication and, 253–254
  oculesics and, 258
  proxemics and, 252, 259
  psychotherapy and, 30–31
  texting, 273–274
  trunk movements and, 256
  written communication differences,
    270–272
Gender and Discourse, 253
Gender binary
  clothing selections based on, 269
  definition of, 23
  identifying information regarding, 110

*Gender Differences in Language Use: An
  Analysis of 14,000 Text Samples*, 271
Gender diverse populations
  assessment in. *See* Voice assessments
  goal setting for, 105
  Lessac-Madsen resonant voice therapy
    for, 226–227
  loss of friends, 113
  preparing to work with, 105–106
  societal responses toward, 106
  terminology associated with, **58**
  voice and communication training in,
    105
  voice assessment of. *See* Voice
    assessments
  volume-related problems in, 244
Gender dysphoria
  in adolescents, 60–61
  autism spectrum disorder and, 4, 378
  awareness of, 60–61
  in children, 378
  clinical presentation of, 1
  definition of, 1, 24, 28, 59
  *Diagnostic and Statistical Manual for
    Mental Disorders, Fifth Edition*
    diagnosis for, 2, 28–29
  national quality registry for, 16
  psychiatric care for, 111
  as psychiatric diagnosis, 2
  psychosocial challenges coexisting with,
    25
  psychotherapy for, 24–25
  puberty blockers for, 61
  self-awareness of, 60–61
  socially adaptive measures for, 24–25
  statistics regarding, 3
  in transmasculine individuals, 167
  treatment for, 59, 61–62
  in young children, 60–61
Gender Dysphoria Program, 110
Gender expression
  definition of, **58**
  history-taking, 156
Gender Guesser, 276
Gender identification, vocal intensity in,
  240–244
Gender identity
  binary, 23

resonance in, 214, 219
self-perceptions of, 196–197
singing voice in. *See* Singing voice,
	transfeminine
stress in speech, 200–201, **202**
therapy in
	case study of, 209–210
	conversational pitch range, 207–210,
		208
	general considerations, 206–207
	speaking fundamental frequency, 207
vocal quality in, 196, 214
vocal tension in, 196
vowels in, 236–237
Transgender, defined, 2, 22–23
Transgender adolescents, 379
Transgender children, 378–379
Transgender Children in Today's Schools,
	379
Transgender congruence scale, 118
Transgender health
	clinicians in, 65
	collaborative care, 35
	continuing education for, 15, 107
	diagnosis in, 27–28
	speech-language pathologist's
		understanding of, 106
Transgender health care
	global variations in, 1
	growth of, 291
Transgender men. *See also* Transmasculine
	voice and communication
	audio recordings for, 8, **12–15**
	definition of, 2, 59
	gender-affirming voice therapy in
		audio recordings before, 8, **12–15**,
			13–14
		elements of, 15
		self-ratings of voice, 15
		testosterone effects, 13–14
	hormone treatments in, 63
	marriage by, 113
	prevalence of, 3
	self-acceptance by, 170
	self-ratings of voice by, 15
	surgical treatments for, 64–65
	transition of, psychological issues in,
		138
	treatment options for, **5**

voice assessments in
	description of, 7–8, **12–15**
	referrals for, 107
voice change in, 69
voice of, 131
Transgender persons. *See also*
		Transfeminine clients; Transgender
		men; Transgender women;
		Transmasculine voice and
		communication
	assessment in. *See* Voice assessments
	case study of experience as, 21–22
	clinician resources, 72
	collaborative care for, 35
	cultural competence in dealing with, 80,
		105
	definition of, 2, 22–23
	diagnosis of, 27–28
	goal setting for, 105
	guilt felt by, 46
	Lessac-Madsen resonant voice therapy
		for, 226–227
	loss of friends, 113
	in mainstream media, 57
	multidisciplinary approach to, 39
	preparing to work with, 105–106
	psychiatric disorders among, 5
	public awareness of, 21
	rejection by, 112–114
	societal responses toward, 106
	terminology associated with, **58**
	voice and communication. *See also* Voice
		and communication training
		counseling goals, 45
		training in, 105
	voice assessment of. *See* Voice assessments
	volume-related problems in, 244
Transgender Self Evaluation of Voice
		Questionnaire, 76, 116–117
Transgender teams. *See also* Gender
		teams
	adolescents, 379–384
	pediatric, 379–384
Transgender women. *See also* Transfeminine
		clients
	audio recordings for, 7, **8–9**
	case study of, 21–22
	cisgender women and, voice differences
		between, 91